T0259497

Advanced Imaging in Gastroenterology

Editor

SHARMILA ANANDASABAPATHY

GASTROINTESTINAL ENDOSCOPY CLINICS OF NORTH AMERICA

www.giendo.theclinics.com

Consulting Editor
CHARLES J. LIGHTDALE

July 2013 • Volume 23 • Number 3

ELSEVIER

1600 John F. Kennedy Boulevard • Suite 1800 • Philadelphia, Pennsylvania, 19103-2899

http://www.theclinics.com

GASTROINTESTINAL ENDOSCOPY CLINICS OF NORTH AMERICA Volume 23, Number 3
July 2013 ISSN 1052-5157, ISBN-13: 978-1-4557-7590-3

Editor: Kerry Holland
Developmental Editor: Donald Mumford

Gastrointestinal Endoscopy Clinics of North America (ISSN 1052-5157) is published quarterly by Elsevier Inc., 360 Park Avenue South, New York, NY 10010-1710. Months of issue are January, April, July, and October. Business and Editorial Offices: 1600 John F. Kennedy Blvd., Suite 1800, Philadelphia, PA, 19103-2899. Periodicals postage paid at New York, NY and additional mailing offices. Subscription prices are $319.00 per year for US individuals, $441.00 per year for US institutions, $169.00 per year for US students and residents, $351.00 per year for Canadian individuals, $538.00 per year for Canadian institutions, $445.00 per year for international individuals, $538.00 per year for international institutions, and $235.00 per year for Canadian and foreign students/residents. To receive student/resident rate, orders must be accompanied by name of affiliated institution, date of term, and the *signature* of program/residency coordinator on institution letterhead. Orders will be billed at individual rate until proof of status is received. Foreign air speed delivery is included in all *Clinics* subscription prices. All prices are subject to change without notice. **POSTMASTER:** Send address change to *Gastrointestinal Endoscopy Clinics of North America*, Elsevier Health Sciences Division, Subscription Customer Service, 3251 Riverport Lane, Maryland Heights, MO 63043. **Customer Service: 1-800-654-2452 (US). From outside the United States, call 1-314-447-8871. Fax: 1-314-447-8029. E-mail: JournalsCustomerService-usa@elsevier.com (for print support) or JournalsOnlineSupport-usa@elsevier.com (for online support).**

Reprints. For copies of 100 or more, of articles in this publication, please contact the Commercial Reprints Department, Elsevier Inc., 360 Park Avenue South, New York, NY 10010-1710. Tel. (212) 633-3812; Fax: (212) 482-1935; E-mail: reprints@elsevier.com.

Gastrointestinal Endoscopy Clinics of North America is covered in *Excerpta Medica, MEDLINE/PubMed (Index Medicus), and MEDLINE/MEDLARS.*

Printed and bound by CPI Group (UK) Ltd, Croydon, CR0 4YY

Transferred to digital print 2012

Contributors

CONSULTING EDITOR

CHARLES J. LIGHTDALE, MD
Professor of Clinical Medicine, Director of Clinical Research, Division of Digestive and Liver Diseases, Department of Medicine, New York-Presbyterian Hospital/Columbia University Medical Center, New York, New York

EDITOR

SHARMILA ANANDASABAPATHY, MD
Director of Endoscopy, Associate Professor of Medicine, Division of Gastroenterology, The Mount Sinai Medical Center, New York, New York

AUTHORS

SUNIL AMIN, MD, MPH
Division of Gastroenterology, Department of Medicine, Mount Sinai School of Medicine, New York, New York

SHARMILA ANANDASABAPATHY, MD
Director of Endoscopy, Associate Professor, Division of Gastroenterology, Mount Sinai Medical Center, New York, New York

MARCIA IRENE CANTO, MD, MHS
Professor of Medicine and Oncology, Division of Gastroenterology and Hepatology, Department of Medicine, The Johns Hopkins Medical Institutions, Baltimore, Maryland

JENNIFER CARNS, PhD
Research Scientist, Department of Bioengineering, Rice University; Richards-Kortum Laboratory, BioScience Research Collaborative, Houston, Texas

JENNIFER CHENNAT, MD
Associate Professor of Medicine, Director of Therapeutic Endoscopy, Director of Interventional Endoscopy Fellowship Program, Co-Director of EUS Program, Division of Gastroenterology, Hepatology, and Nutrition, Liver-Pancreas Institute, University of Pittsburgh Medical Center, Pittsburgh, Pennsylvania

CHRISTOPHER J. DIMAIO, MD
Director of Therapeutic Endoscopy, Division of Gastroenterology, Department of Medicine, Mount Sinai School of Medicine, New York, New York

KERRY B. DUNBAR, MD, PhD
Assistant Professor of Medicine, VA North Texas Healthcare System – Dallas VA Medical Center, University of Texas Southwestern Medical Center, Dallas, Texas

JEFFREY EASLER, MD
Division of Gastroenterology, Hepatology, and Nutrition, University of Pittsburgh Medical Center, Pittsburgh, Pennsylvania

CHARLES GABBERT, MD
Division of Gastroenterology, Hepatology, and Nutrition, University of Pittsburgh Medical Center, Pittsburgh, Pennsylvania

MARTIN GOETZ, MD, PhD
Professor, Department of Medicine I, Universitätsklinikum Tübingen, Tübingen, Germany

SUSANA GONZALEZ, MD
Assistant Professor of Medicine, Henry D. Janowitz Division of Gastroenterology, Mount Sinai School of Medicine, New York, New York

CESARE HASSAN, MD
Digestive Endoscopy Unit, IRCCS Istituto Clinico Humanitas, Rozzano, Milan, Italy

VIJAY KANAKADANDI, MD
Division of Gastroenterology and Hepatology, Veterans Affairs Medical Center, University of Kansas School of Medicine, Kansas City, Kansas

PELHAM KEAHEY, BS
Graduate Student, Department of Bioengineering, Rice University; Richards-Kortum Laboratory, BioScience Research Collaborative, Houston, Texas

RALF KIESSLICH, MD, PhD
Professor of Medicine, Director, Medical Clinic, St. Marienkrankenhaus, Katharina-Kasper gGmbH, Frankfurt am Main, Frankfurt, Germany

MICHELLE KANG KIM, MD, MSc
Director of Endoscopic Ultrasound, Division of Gastroenterology, Department of Medicine, Mount Sinai School of Medicine, New York, New York

CHARLES J. LIGHTDALE, MD
Professor of Clinical Medicine, Director of Clinical Research, Division of Digestive and Liver Diseases, Department of Medicine, New York-Presbyterian Hospital/Columbia University Medical Center, New York, New York

JAMES F. MARION, MD, AGAF
Associate Clinical Professor of Medicine and Gastroenterology, Henry D. Janowitz Division of Gastroenterology, Icahn School of Medicine at Mount Sinai, New York, New York

STEVEN NAYMAGON, MD
Henry D. Janowitz Division of Gastroenterology, Icahn School of Medicine at Mount Sinai, New York, New York

HELMUT NEUMANN, MD, PhD
Professor of Medicine, Interdisciplinary Endoscopy, Department of Medicine I, University of Erlangen-Nuremberg, Erlangen, Germany

TIMOTHY QUANG, BS
Graduate Student, Department of Bioengineering, Rice University; Richards-Kortum Laboratory, BioScience Research Collaborative, Houston, Texas

ALESSANDRO REPICI, MD
Digestive Endoscopy Unit, IRCCS Istituto Clinico Humanitas, Rozzano, Milan, Italy

REBECCA RICHARDS-KORTUM, PhD
Stanley C. Moore Professor, Department of Bioengineering, Rice University;
Richards-Kortum Laboratory, BioScience Research Collaborative, Houston, Texas

PAYAL SAXENA, MBBS (Hons), FRACP
Division of Gastroenterology and Hepatology, Department of Medicine, The Johns
Hopkins Medical Institutions, Baltimore, Maryland

PRATEEK SHARMA, MD
Division of Gastroenterology and Hepatology, Veterans Affairs Medical Center, University
of Kansas School of Medicine, Kansas City, Kansas

MATTHEW WARNDORF, MD
Division of Gastroenterology, Hepatology, and Nutrition, University of Pittsburgh Medical
Center, Pittsburgh, Pennsylvania

JEROME D. WAYE, MD
Clinical Professor of Medicine, Mount Sinai Medical Center, The Icahn School of Medicine
at Mount Sinai, New York, New York

ANGELO ZULLO, MD
Digestive Endoscopy Unit, IRCCS Istituto Clinico Humanitas, Rozzano, Milan, Italy

Contents

> The key to detection and treatment of early neoplasia in Barrett's esophagus (BE) is thorough and careful inspection of the Barrett's segment. The greatest role for red flag techniques is to help identify neoplastic lesions for targeted biopsy and therapy. High-definition white light endoscopy (HD-WLE) can potentially improve endoscopic imaging of BE compared with standard endoscopy, but little scientific evidence supports this. The addition of autofluorescence imaging to HD-WLE and narrow band imaging increases sensitivity and the false-positive rate without significantly improving overall detection of BE-related neoplasia.

> The incidence of Barrett's-related adenocarcinoma of the esophagus continues to increase at an alarming rate. Studies to date show great promise for optical coherence tomography (OCT) in screening, surveillance, and guiding management of Barrett's esophagus. With continued innovation in rapid, accurate scanning systems, such as volumetric laser endomicroscopy or optical frequency domain imaging, advanced OCT seems likely to have an important impact. The next few years are likely to see the initiation of large clinical studies that will define the extent and significance of this impact.

> Barrett's esophagus has been a focus of confocal laser endomicroscopy (CLE) research. There are two CLE systems available, one probe-based and the other with a microscope embedded in the tip of an endoscope. Several CLE image classification systems are available. Studies suggest that CLE has good sensitivity, negative predictive value, and accuracy for detecting neoplasia, with good interobserver agreement using the CLE image classification systems. Larger, multicenter studies have been completed evaluating the impact of CLE on treatment of patients with BE. Future developments may include more specific contrast agents and new types of endomicroscopes.

criteria, and study within the context of comparative, randomized trials are needed and will contribute greatly to expedient patient care.

 Video of the inferior lip of the ileocecal valve as seen by a Third Eye Retroscope accompanies this article

Many different techniques for colon cancer screening are available. The fecal immunochemical test is best for fecal-based screening, although the DNA investigation may be more specific when further developed. Computed tomographic colonography is as good as colonoscopy for detecting colon cancer and is almost as good as colonoscopy for detecting advanced adenomas, but has limitations. The flexible sigmoidoscopic examination markedly decreases the incidence of cancer in the visualized segments, but colonoscopy is currently the best procedure for evaluating the large bowel. Techniques for retroflexion or backward view of the colon have been investigated, with all showing increased polyp detection.

Colorectal cancer represents a major cause of mortality in Western countries, and population-based colonoscopy screening is supported by official guidelines. A significant determinant of the cost of colonoscopy screening/surveillance is driven by polypectomy of diminutive (≤ 5 mm) lesions. When considering the low prevalence of advanced neoplasia within diminutive polyps, the additional cost of pathologic examination is mainly justified by the need to differentiate between precancerous adenomatous versus hyperplastic polyps. The aim of this review is to summarize the data supporting the clinical application of a resect and discard strategy, also addressing the potential pitfalls associated with this approach.

Patients with long-standing inflammatory bowel disease (IBD) have an increased risk of developing colorectal cancer. Performing periodic dysplasia screening and surveillance may diminish this risk. To date, chromoendoscopy is the only technique that has consistently yielded positive results in large, well-designed dysplasia-detection trials. Most major society guidelines endorse chromoendoscopy as an adjunct, accepted, or preferred dysplasia-detection tool. This review outlines the available endoscopic technologies for the detection of dysplasia in IBD, considers the evidence supporting their use, and assesses which modalities are ready for use in clinical practice.

Two types of endomicroscopy systems exist. One is integrated into a standard, high-resolution endoscope and one is probe-based, capable of passage through the working channel of a standard endoscope. Endocytoscopy allows visualization of the superficial mucosal layer. Endoscope-integrated and probe-based devices allow magnification of the mucosa up to 1400-fold. Endomicroscopy can differentiate histologic changes of Crohn disease and ulcerative colitis in vivo in real time. Endocytoscopy can discriminate mucosal inflammatory cells, allowing determination of histopathologic activity of ulcerative colitis. Molecular imaging with fluorescence-labeled probes against disease-specific receptors will enable individualized management of inflammatory bowel diseases.

 Video of high-resolution microendoscopy for the early detection of esophageal neoplasia accompanies this article

Recent developments in optical molecular imaging allow for real-time identification of morphologic and biochemical changes in tissue associated with gastrointestinal neoplasia. This review summarizes widefield and high-resolution imaging modalities in preclinical and clinical evaluation for the detection of colorectal cancer and esophageal cancer. Widefield techniques discussed include high-definition white light endoscopy, narrow band imaging, autofluoresence imaging, and chromoendoscopy; high-resolution techniques discussed include probe-based confocal laser endomicroscopy, high-resolution microendoscopy, and optical coherence tomography. New approaches to enhance image contrast using vital dyes and molecular-specific targeted contrast agents are evaluated.

GASTROINTESTINAL ENDOSCOPY CLINICS OF NORTH AMERICA

FORTHCOMING ISSUES

October 2013
Pancreatic Diseases
Martin Freeman, MD, *Editor*

January 2014
EUS-guided Tissue Acquisition
Shyam Varadarajulu, MD
and Robert Hawes, MD, *Editors*

April 2014
Endoscopic Submucosal Dissection
Norio Fukamin, MD, *Editor*

RECENT ISSUES

April 2013
Endoscopic Approach to the Patient with Biliary Tract Disease
Jacques Van Dam, MD, PhD, *Editor*

January 2013
Endolumenal Therapy
Steven A. Edmundowicz, MD, *Editor*

October 2012
Celiac Disease
Peter H.R. Green, MD and
Benjamin Lebwohl, MD, *Editors*

RELATED INTEREST

Gastroenterology Clinics of North America, March 2013 (Vol. 42, No. 1)
Esophageal Diseases
Nicholas Shaheen, MD, *Editor*

NOW AVAILABLE FOR YOUR iPhone and iPad

Foreword
Advanced Imaging for GI Endoscopy

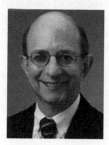

Charles J. Lightdale, MD
Consulting Editor

Seeing is believing. Most gastrointestinal endoscopists have a predisposition to appreciate the visual aspects of reality, and as endoscopes and cameras have changed from fiberoptic and analog to digital, the view has become even better. Most of us have strong visual memory and can picture aspects of the gut lumen and abnormalities long after completion of the examination. Now, in the digital age, pictures and videos are more easily obtained, stored, and retrieved for further analysis and interpretation. However, despite the availability of high-resolution endoscopes and high-definition video screens, there are still limitations.

The view we see is pretty much similar to the naked eye view. Many diseases are still best diagnosed when we remove tissue for pathology analysis, where the dead tissue is processed and sliced, mounted on a glass slide, stained, and looked at under a microscope by a highly trained specialist.

This system works quite well overall, but there are aspects that can be improved. The pathologist can only look at the tissue we provide, and if we can't see where the occult disease lurks because it is too small and scattered, our biopsies can miss the diagnosis. Then there is the issue of expense. If we take more random biopsies to get a better sample, the cost goes up, and the results may not be all that much better.

Enter the brave new world of endoscopic imaging. It started with magnification endoscopes and spraying dyes for contrast or surface staining and led to new digital contrast enhancements. This magnifying glass view allowed classification of surface patterns that had good correlation with biopsy results. Still, smaller and more subtle abnormalities could be missed. The really big leap came during the past decade as optical science and powerful computers led to the development of extraordinary new tools that can be utilized during endoscopic inspection.

These new tools, such as advanced optical coherence tomography and confocal laser endomicroscopy, let us see at the level of what the pathologist can see under

Gastrointest Endoscopy Clin N Am 23 (2013) xiii–xiv
http://dx.doi.org/10.1016/j.giec.2013.03.014
1052-5157/13/$ – see front matter © 2013 Published by Elsevier Inc.

giendo.theclinics.com

a microscope but in living tissue. Scanning views comparable to low-power microscopy at the 10-micron level and point views at less than the 1-micron level are possible that allow architectural and even cellular analysis in real time. Other spectroscopic techniques are being tested, and molecular imaging is in the development pipeline, using specific biochemical probes tagged with fluorescent markers that can be seen with specially designed endoscopes.

Other enhancements currently available include changing the direction of view with angled optics and reverse view to avoid missing visible lesions hidden by curves and folds. Endoscopic ultrasonography, increasingly used with fine-needle aspiration and biopsy, is being enhanced with elastography predicting tissue texture and echo signatures for needle guidance.

There are so many questions that will have to be answered. How much time will these new capabilities add to standard endoscopy? Will they be reliable, efficient, and accurate? How much will they cost, and will they be cost-effective? Will they be user-friendly or too complicated for routine use? Will the images be easy to interpret or will there be long learning curves? Can we send fewer but more accurate biopsies? Can we avoid sending biopsies at all in some cases? Can we use the results in real time to guide endoscopic therapy?

Getting a grasp on all this is the problem. Dr Sharmila Anandasabapathy, a leader in the field of endoscopic imaging, is the guest editor for this issue of the *Gastrointestinal Endoscopy Clinics of North America* on Advanced Imaging in Endoscopy. She picked all the key topics and rounded-up expert authors. Whether you just need an introduction to what is available or on the way, whether you are deciding to jump in now, or whether you are already using the new technologies and want an expert perspective, you must read this issue. The new imaging methods are upon us and will play a major role in defining the future of gastrointestinal endoscopy.

Charles J. Lightdale, MD
Department of Medicine
Columbia University Medical Center
161 Fort Washington Avenue, Room 812
New York, NY 10032, USA

E-mail address:
CJL18@columbia.edu

Preface
The Evolving Field of
Endoscopic Imaging

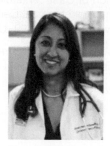

Sharmila Anandasabapathy, MD
Editor

Endoscopy is a visual field. Our ability to effectively manage patients is directly dependent on the image before us. From identifying neoplasia in patients with ulcerative colitis to delineating the border of a lesion prior to endoscopic resection in Barrett's esophagus, the success of our diagnostic or therapeutic intervention is only as good as *what we see*.

This edition of *Gastrointestinal Endoscopy Clinics of North America* is dedicated to the evolving field of endoscopic imaging. The world's leading experts in this area have written comprehensive articles spanning a variety of modalities from optical coherence tomography and confocal laser endomicroscopy to new digital software enhancement technologies. The role of these technologies in both enhancing screening and surveillance is discussed as well as the emerging role of imaging in endoscopic therapy.

Moving one step further into the realm of targeted imaging, part of the edition is dedicated to the role of optical molecular imaging. Indeed, the field of endoscopic imaging is being propelled by parallel advances in engineering, physics, and chemistry as novel, molecule-specific contrast agents are combined with fluorescent endoscopes to identify the particular molecular signature of a cancer and, potentially, predict a patient's risk of developing cancer. Equally exciting are advances in ultrasound and elastography, which give us textural information—a visual "touch" of a lesion without the surgeon's need for direct contact. While we move toward novel, targeted contrast agents, older technologies of nonspecific contrast dyes are becoming less frequently used as software-based enhancements seek to provide a "virtual" chromoendoscopic imaging with the push of a button. Last, even routine diagnostic colonoscopy is being viewed from new perspectives: forward, backward, *and* with an increased focus on reducing cost by predicting polyp histology in real-time.

Gastrointest Endoscopy Clin N Am 23 (2013) xv–xvi
http://dx.doi.org/10.1016/j.giec.2013.03.011
1052-5157/13/$ – see front matter © 2013 Published by Elsevier Inc.

I would like to thank my colleagues for their support, collaboration, and outstanding contributions to this edition. On behalf of all of the authors, I hope this collection broadens your perspective in this exciting, rapidly progressing area and raises new questions and challenges for the future.

Sharmila Anandasabapathy, MD
Division of Gastroenterology
The Mount Sinai Medical Center
New York, NY 10029, USA

E-mail address:
Sharmila.anandasabapathy@mountsinai.org

Red Flag Imaging Techniques in Barrett's Esophagus

Payal Saxena, MBBS, FRACP, Marcia Irene Canto, MD, MHS*

KEYWORDS

- Barrett's esophagus • Imaging • Red flag technique • White light endoscopy
- Chromoendoscopy

KEY POINTS

- The key to detection and treatment of early neoplasia in Barrett's esophagus (BE) is thorough and careful inspection of the Barrett's segment.
- The greatest role for red flag techniques is to help identify neoplastic lesions for targeted biopsy and therapy.
- High-definition white light endoscopy (HD-WLE) can potentially improve endoscopic imaging of BE compared with standard endoscopy, but little scientific evidence supports this.
- The addition of autofluorescence imaging to HD-WLE and narrow band imaging increases sensitivity and the false-positive rate without significantly improving overall detection of BE-related neoplasia.
- Evidence is insufficient to support the use of any single wide-field imaging technique over others in routine imaging of BE.

INTRODUCTION

Barrett's esophagus (BE) is defined by the presence of specialized intestinal metaplasia (SIM) of the esophagus and affects 1% to 2% of the general population.[1] BE is associated with increased cellular proliferation and turnover that may result in progression to dysplasia, and is therefore a precursor lesion of esophageal adenocarcinoma (EAC).[2] In a recent retrospective population-based cohort study, the presence of BE conferred a relative risk of EAC of 11.2 compared with that of the general population (95% confidence interval [CI], 8.8–14.4).[3] Early detection results in improved patient outcomes,[4] and therefore endoscopic surveillance of BE is recommended to detect

Conflicts of Interest: The authors have no relevant conflicts of interest to disclose.
Division of Gastroenterology and Hepatology, Department of Medicine, The Johns Hopkins Medical Institutions, 1830 East Monument Street, Baltimore, MD 21287, USA
* Corresponding author. Johns Hopkins Hospital, 1830 East Monument Street, Suite 427, Baltimore, MD 21287.
E-mail address: Mcanto1@jhmi.edu

Gastrointest Endoscopy Clin N Am 23 (2013) 535–547
http://dx.doi.org/10.1016/j.giec.2013.03.002
1052-5157/13/$ – see front matter © 2013 Elsevier Inc. All rights reserved.

giendo.theclinics.com

dysplasia or cancer at an early stage and instigate therapy.[2] Over the past decade, remarkable progress has been made in the endoscopic treatment of BE-related neoplasia, including endoscopic resection of focal lesions and ablative therapies.[5]

Endoscopy is a key approach for detection and treatment of BE-related neoplasia. Random biopsies are susceptible to sampling variability and have been shown to miss up to 57% of neoplastic lesions,[6] particularly flat neoplasias. Gastroenterology society guidelines and expert consensus statements recommend endoscopic surveillance using white-light endoscopy (WLE), with targeted biopsies of any endoscopically visible lesions, and random 4-quadrant biopsies of every 1 to 2 cm of the BE segment (Seattle protocol).[7,8] Endoscopic techniques that might improve visualization of endoscopic features associated with neoplastic change would greatly enhance the diagnostic yield, efficacy, cost, and efficiency of current surveillance practices.[9] This article describes a variety of "red flag" diagnostic techniques that have been developed with the goal of increasing the sensitivity for detecting lesions during a wide-field endoscopic examination.

CHARACTERISTICS OF IDEAL ENDOSCOPIC ENHANCEMENTS FOR WIDE-FIELD DETECTION OF BE-RELATED NEOPLASIA

In clinical practice, most patients with BE do not harbor dysplasia. These patients have a very low incidence of high-grade dysplasia (HGD) and EAC development, and thus most patients undergoing surveillance have multiple biopsy specimens showing no evidence of HGD/EAC. For populations with a low prevalence of disease, the most important metrics for a diagnostic test are the sensitivity and negative predictive value (NPV).[10]

The American Society for Gastrointestinal Endoscopy (ASGE) convened a PIVI (Preservation and Incorporation of Valuable Endoscopic Innovations) initiative to develop a priori diagnostic and/or therapeutic thresholds for endoscopic technologies designed to resolve relevant clinical questions.[10] The PIVI for BE provided thresholds for diagnosis of BE and associated neoplasia. The current 4-quadrant, 1- to 2-cm biopsy protocol has a reported sensitivity ranging from 28% to 85% for detecting HGD/EAC.[11-15] In studies in which cost-effectiveness of a surveillance program has been demonstrated, sensitivity of 85% to 90% has been assumed.[16,17] To eliminate the need for random mucosal biopsies during the endoscopic surveillance of patients with nondysplastic BE, an imaging technology with targeted biopsies should have a per-patient sensitivity of 90% or greater and an NPV of 98% or greater for detecting HGD or early EAC compared with the current standard protocol (WLE and targeted and random 4-quadrant biopsies every 2 cm).[10] The specificity of biopsy protocols in patients with BE has ranged from 56% to 100%. Hence, the new imaging technology should have a specificity that is sufficiently high (80%) to allow a reduction in the number of biopsies (compared with random biopsies). Because abnormal imaging requires biopsies for confirmation, new imaging methods should not result in more biopsy specimens being obtained than would a random biopsy protocol.

The various "red flag" endoscopic imaging techniques are summarized in **Table 1**.

HIGH-DEFINITION WLE

Standard WLEs are the most commonly used method of endoscopic imaging, generating 300,000-pixel images.[18] In contrast, modern high-definition endoscopes offer high pixel densities (600,000–1,000,000 pixels) and, when combined with high-definition monitors, provide marked improvement in image resolution (**Fig. 1**).[7] In a study by Kara and colleagues,[15] high-definition WLE (HD-WLE) alone had a 79%

Table 1
Characteristics of "red flag" endoscopic imaging techniques

Technique	Description	Device	Red Flag
HD-WLE	High-definition white light endoscope and monitor	>800,000 pixels Olympus, Pentax, Fujinon endoscopes	Improved resolution of white light image; highlights columnar (SIM = reticular or nonround pit pattern, gastric = round)
NBI	Narrows band width of blue and green light	Olympus endoscope GIF-H180, H190	Highlights from columnar from squamous and irregular mucosal and vascular patterns (neoplasia)
AFI	Natural fluorescence generated from endogenous tissue fluorophores	Olympus light source XCLV-260HP	Dysplastic tissues appear magenta
Chromoendoscopy			
Acetic acid	Topical spray of 1%–3% solution	All endoscopes	Accentuation of villi and pit pattern
Methylene blue	Topical spray	All endoscopes	Highlights IM and dysplasia, but not squamous epithelium
Digital chromoendoscopy			
I-Scan	Digital enhancement of WLE using postprocessing techniques	Pentax	Improves visualization of mucosal and vascular patterns
FICE	Digital enhancement of WLE using postprocessing techniques	Fujinon	Improves visualization of mucosal and vascular patterns

Abbreviations: AFI, autofluorescence imaging; HD-WLE, high-definition white light endoscopy; IM, intestinal metaplasia; NBI, narrow band imaging; WLE, white-light endoscopy.

sensitivity for detecting lesions with HGD. Gupta and colleagues[19] performed HD-WLE in 112 patients, and 34% had HGD or EAC detected across 130 locations. Most importantly, longer inspection time was associated with a significant increase in the number of lesions detected; an average inspection time of greater than 1 minute per centimeter of BE enabled a higher lesion detection rate (54.2% vs 13.3%; $P = .04$), with a trend toward a higher detection rate of HGD/EAC (40.2% vs 6.7%; $P = .06$). Hence, most experts would recommend high-definition (>850,000 pixels) endoscopy over standard endoscopy in evaluating patients with BE.[8] Standard-resolution endoscopes are not recommended, although scant scientific evidence exists for this recommendation.[8]

NARROW BAND IMAGING

Narrow band imaging (NBI) was first described in 2004 (Olympus Corporation, Tokyo, Japan).[20] Endoscopes equipped with NBI contain an additional filter that can be

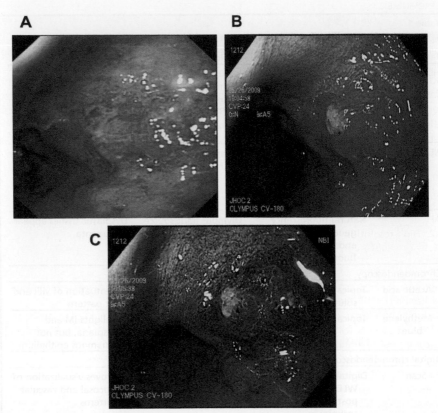

Fig. 1. Endoscopic endoscopy images of BE with a macroscopic Paris 2A neoplastic lesion seen with (*A*) standard-resolution WLE, (*B*) high-resolution WLE, and (*C*) high-resolution endoscopy with narrow band imaging.

activated by the endoscopist. The filter narrows the bandwidths of the emitted blue (440–460 nm) and green light (540–560 nm), and the relative intensity of blue light is increased. The narrow band blue light displays superficial capillary networks, whereas green light displays the subepithelial vessels. A combination of the 2 images produces a high-definition image of the mucosal surface, allowing visualization of subtle mucosal irregularities and alterations in vascular patterns (see **Fig. 1**; **Figs. 2** and **3**).[4,21]

In a small prospective study of 28 patients, NBI did not increase the number of cases diagnosed with HGD/EAC compared with high-resolution WLE.[15] More areas of HGD were detected with NBI than with WLE (4 additional lesions in 3 patients); however, given the small size of the study, statistical significance was not reached. A prospective, blinded study by Sharma and colleagues[22] in 2006 using a standardized classification of mucosal (ridge/villous, circular, and irregular/distorted) and vascular pattern (normal and abnormal) suggested that NBI had a high sensitivity and specificity for detecting HGD (100% and 99%). In a tandem crossover study, Wolfsen and colleagues[17] showed that high-resolution NBI was superior to standard-resolution WLE in detecting dysplasia (57% vs 43%), with a sensitivity and specificity of 89% and 95%, respectively. Additionally, in the NBI group, fewer numbers of biopsies were required (mean, 4.7 vs 8.5; *P*<.001). However, the higher-resolution endoscopes used in the NBI group may have accounted for the higher detection rate.

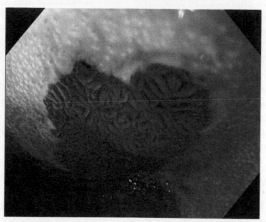

Fig. 2. High-resolution NBI of flat nondysplastic BE showing the contrast between squamous mucosa (*greenish*) and columnar Barrett's mucosa (*brown-blue*) and regular mucosal pit pattern.

Classification of mucosal and vascular patterns by NBI is key for the correct prediction of BE histology. Studies by Curvers and colleagues[23] and by Herrero and colleagues[24] have shown that NBI does not improve inter-observer agreement or accuracy over HD-WLE. In a study involving ex vivo examination of pedigreed NBI and WLE BE images, the interobserver agreement for NBI diagnosis ranged from 0.40 to 0.56 (moderate) and did not significantly differ between expert and nonexpert endoscopists.[23] The overall yield for correctly identifying images of early neoplasia was 81% for high-resolution WLE, 72% for NBI, and 83% for high-resolution WLE with NBI, with no significant difference between experts and nonexperts. These kappa scores and accuracy rates are slightly lower than those reported for NBI in the colon ($\kappa = 0.63$; substantial agreement for prediction of polyp histology; accuracy rates 80%–85%).[25] Widespread training will be needed for recognition of irregular NBI patterns in BE and a study of interobserver variability when used by community gastroenterologists to determine the incremental benefit of NBI over careful HD-WLE examination for routine imaging in BE.

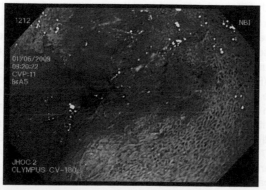

Fig. 3. Irregular mucosal pattern and highlighted subtle nodularity in neoplastic BE (3–5 o'clock position) by high-resolution NBI.

Sharma and colleagues[26] recently reported results of an international randomized controlled trial involving experts comparing NBI with HD-WLE, which showed that both techniques detected 92% of patients with intestinal metaplasia, but NBI required fewer biopsies per patient (3.6 vs 7.6; $P<.0001$). NBI also detected a higher proportion of areas with dysplasia (30% vs 21%; $P = .01$). All areas of HGD and cancer had an irregular mucosal or vascular pattern when examined with NBI and, importantly, no area of regular mucosal/vascular pattern harbored HGD or cancer, suggesting biopsies of these areas can be avoided. Not surprisingly, the accuracy of NBI for detecting low-grade dysplasia was limited. This trial showed that NBI-targeted biopsies are more efficient than random 4-quadrant biopsies.

AUTOFLUORESCENCE

Autofluorescence imaging (AFI) produces real-time pseudocolor images based on the detection of natural tissue fluorescence generated from endogenous tissue fluorophores, such as elastin, collagen, porphyrins, flavins, aromatic amino acids, and NADH. When exposed to short-wavelength light, fluorophores are excited and emit fluorescent light of longer wavelength (ie, autofluorescence). Normal and neoplastic tissue have different autofluorescence characteristics, enabling their differentiation.[4,18,27]

During AFI, normal tissue is pseudo-colored as green, blood vessels as dark green, and dysplastic/neoplastic areas appear as magenta. Suspected neoplasia (AFI-positive lesion) is defined as any area that is different in color from the surrounding mucosa and that has a defined circumferential margin.[27] The following characteristics of neoplastic tissue enable abnormal AFI: (1) increase in the nuclear-cytoplasmic ratio, (2) loss of collagen, and (3) neovascularization, inducing increased hemoglobin concentration, which absorbs autofluorescence light.[27] Autofluorescence in BE is believed to result primarily from collagen in the stroma that is reabsorbed by hemoglobin.[28]

Autofluorescent intensity can be low and earlier AFI systems failed to produce sufficient image quality for clinical use. However, the integration of AFI with high-resolution video endoscopes and a second, more sensitive, charge-coupled device that converts light into a digital image has significantly improved image quality.[18,21]

In a feasibility study, Kara and colleagues[29] examined 22 patients with HGD using both WLE and AFI. HGD was detected in 6 of these subjects with AFI alone. The sensitivity for detecting HGD was 91%; however, a high rate of false-positives as seen, yielding a specificity of only 43%. To overcome this inadequacy, subsequent studies combined NBI with AFI, hoping to improve the specificity of the technique. In a study of 20 patients with suspected HGD, Kara and colleagues[30] showed that the addition of NBI to AFI reduced the false-positive rate from 40% to 10%. However, NBI also resulted in the misclassification of 8% to 17% of true-positive areas as nonneoplastic.

The combined use of WLE, NBI, and AFI resulted in the development of endoscopic trimodal imaging (ETMI), which incorporates the 3 platforms into 1 endoscope and is currently available in the United Kingdom and Asia.[16] WLE and ETMI were compared in 87 patients with suspected HGD/EAC. Targeted detection of HGD/EAC was higher with ETMI than with WLE (65% vs 45%), but the overall detection rate for neoplasia was not statistically significant (84% vs 72%). Higher false-positive rates were also still noted with ETMI (71% vs 53%). Random 4-quadrant biopsies identified more areas of HGD/EAC than targeted biopsies (84% vs 64%).[31] A subsequent randomized crossover study of 99 patients with low-grade intraepithelial neoplasia compared the use of ETMI versus WLE and found an improved targeted detection with ETMI (54% vs 34%), but no statistically significant increase in overall detection.[16]

In summary, the major limitation of AFI seems to be the high false-positive rate, and data in the current literature have not yet supported its widespread use.

CHROMOENDOSCOPY

Chromoendoscopy is a diagnostic method in which a chemical substance is sprayed onto the esophageal mucosa in an attempt to highlight and improve detection of abnormalities. The dyes most commonly used for chromoendoscopy in BE are acetic acid and methylene blue.

Acetic Acid Chromoendoscopy

When sprayed on Barrett's epithelium at a low concentration (1%–3%), acetic acid (AA) eliminates the superficial mucus layer by breaking down glycoprotein disulfide bonds. The unbuffered acid on the mucosal cell surface then causes a reversible deacetylation of cellular proteins and a change in the spatial properties of nuclear and cytoplasmic proteins. The transient disruption of the single-layered columnar mucosal barrier occurs in a few minutes, leading to whitening of the tissue with vascular congestion, and marked accentuation of the villi and mucosal pit pattern when the AA reaches the capillaries in the stroma (**Fig. 4**). The whitening effect is lost in dysplastic areas earlier than in the surrounding mucosa, helping the endoscopist differentiate between the 2 tissues. The effect is transient, lasting 2 to 3 minutes; therefore, repeated applications of AA may be required.[32–35]

Guelrud and colleagues[36] first described 4-pit patterns identifiable in Barrett's epithelium after AA spray (round, reticular, villous, and ridged) and using high-magnification WLE. Ridged and villous patterns were associated with intestinal metaplasia. Subsequently, studies have shown that AA-assisted chromoendoscopy increases the diagnostic yield of dysplasia over standard WLE.[37–39] In one of the larger studies,[38] 190 procedures were performed in 119 patients. Excellent correlation was seen between the lesions predicted to be neoplastic by AA and those diagnosed by histologic analysis (r = 0.99). A 2.5-fold increase in detection of visible abnormalities during endoscopy was seen with AA spray compared with WLE alone. Dysplasia or cancer was identified with AA with a sensitivity of 95.5% and a specificity of 80%. In a United Kingdom–based cost-effective study,[39] 263 procedures were performed in 197 patients over a 5-year period. AA chromoendoscopy correctly identified dysplasia in 96% of cases, although the false-positive rate was significant at 25%. No adverse

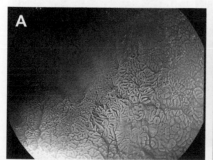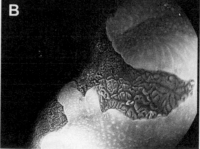

Fig. 4. High-resolution white light (*A*) and I-Scan digital chromoendoscopy (*B*) images of nondysplastic BE after application of AA. Note that visible mucosal pit pattern in both unmagnified images.

events were seen in the 14-day follow-up period. AA spray enabled a 2-fold increase in the detection rate of neoplasia when compared with WLE (96% vs 48%; $P = .001$). Most remarkably, the authors concluded that if AA-guided targeted biopsies were performed rather than 4-quadrant random biopsies, a cost reduction of 91% to 97% could be achieved.

In summary, AA chromoendoscopy requires an additional spray catheter and adds minimal time (few minutes) to the surveillance procedure; however, it seems to be a promising red flag technique and cost-effective in reducing the number of random biopsies required for detecting neoplastic lesions.[8]

Methylene Blue Chromoendoscopy

Methylene blue (MB) is a vital dye that is taken up by absorbent intestinal-type epithelium in BE and dysplastic cells but not by squamous or gastric mucosa or gastric-type metaplasia within the distal esophagus.[40] During MB chromoendoscopy, specialized intestinal metaplasia typically stains blue (**Fig. 5**), whereas a lighter intensity and increased heterogeneity in the staining pattern predict HGD and/or EAC.[41] The heterogeneous appearance of dysplastic or malignant tissue aids in its endoscopic identification resulting in a "red flag" (see **Fig. 5**B).

MB chromendoscopy in BE was first introduced more than a decade ago,[42] with many subsequent studies[11–13,41,43–47] showing variable results, with sensitivities 53% to 98% and specificities of 32% to 97%. However, there is great heterogeneity in study design, MB staining techniques, and interpretation of staining patterns. A meta-analysis comparing detection rates of neoplasia in BE with MB staining versus random 4-quadrant biopsies showed no significant increased yield for the detection of HGD and early cancer.[48] MB staining is considered safe. However, one small study by Olliver and colleagues[49] suggested that MB may cause DNA changes, but no proof showed that these are permanent or clinically significant.

Currently, chromoendoscopy is not widely used in clinically practice to assess patients with BE. Contributing factors include the inconsistent evidence and practical limitations in preparing for and performing the procedure. Furthermore, the outcomes can be dependent on the experience and expertise of the individual endoscopist, which can also limit its usefulness outside of academic referral centers.

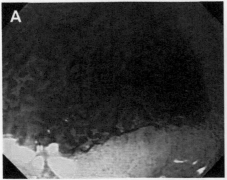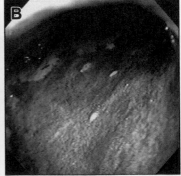

Fig. 5. High-resolution white light image of Barrett's mucosa after MB chromoendoscopy showing the blue stain in nondysplastic intestinal-type epithelium (*A*) and dysplastic flat Barrett's mucosa (note heterogeneous staining, with unstained areas corresponding to decreased MB uptake) (*B*).

DIGITAL ELECTRONIC ENHANCEMENTS (CHROMOENDOSCOPY)

As opposed to conventional chromoendoscopy, which involves the application of stains or substances to the gastrointestinal mucosa, digital chromoendoscopy uses arithmetic processing techniques instead of filters to manipulate red, green, and blue components of a white light digital image. The major advantage of digital chromoendoscopy is the ease of use, involving just the press of a button on the endoscope. No additional catheters or messy dyes are required.

FICE (Fujinon Corporation, Saitama, Japan) and I-Scan (Pentax Medical, subsidiary of Hoya Corporation, Tokyo, Japan) use postprocessing techniques combined with high-definition imaging to increase the relative intensity of narrowed blue light to maximum and decrease narrowed green and red lights to a minimum. This technique improves visualization of the microvasculature and mucosal pit patterns because of the differential absorption of light by hemoglobin.[18,21]

Very limited data exist on the role of FICE in BE. A randomized crossover study by Pohl and colleagues[50] found that FICE had comparable sensitivity (87%) to AA chromoendoscopy. In a recent pilot study, Camus and colleagues[51] showed that FICE in combination with AA chromoendoscopy was superior to HD-WLE in detecting HGD (100% vs 14%), with 100% specificity.

Various combinations of enhanced contrast and sharpness can be used with I-Scan. It consists of 3 types of algorithms: surface enhancement (SE), contrast enhancement (CE), and tone enhancement (TE).[52] SE enhances light-dark contrast through obtaining luminance intensity data for each pixel and applying an algorithm that allows detailed observation of a mucosal surface structure. CE digitally adds blue color in relatively dark areas through obtaining luminance intensity data for each pixel and applying an algorithm that allows detailed observation of subtle irregularities around the surface. Both enhancement functions work in real time without impairing the original color of the organ; therefore, SE and CE are suitable for screening endoscopy to detect gastrointestinal tumors at an early stage. TE dissects and analyzes the individual red, green, blue components of a normal image. The algorithm then alters the color frequencies of each component and recombines the components to a single new color image. This image is designed to enhance minute mucosal structures and subtle changes in color (see **Fig. 4**B; **Fig. 6**).

The advantages of I-Scan include enhanced customization during in vivo endoscopic imaging (similar to Photoshop but "live"), whereas the disadvantages include

Fig. 6. High-resolution WLE with I-Scan digital enhancement of BE. Note the near-field enhancement of contrast and sharpness and relative darkness or blurring of areas distally.

variability in settings and lack of consistency across different processors. A paucity of literature exists on the assessment of BE with I-Scan technology. However, in patients with gastroesophageal reflux disease, I-Scan may significantly improve detection of small esophageal reflux lesions when used with WLE.[53–55] Several studies have reported the use of I-Scan during colonoscopy, suggesting that it is equivalent to NBI for predicting histology in diminutive colon polyps,[56] good interobserver agreement exists,[57] and it shows improvement over HD-WLE for predicting neoplastic versus nonneoplastic polyps.[58] Prospective, randomized, controlled studies are yet to be conducted to determine the true added value of digital chromoendoscopy in routine clinical practice.

SUMMARY

The key to the detection and treatment of early neoplasia in BE is thorough and careful inspection of the Barrett's segment. If Barrett's inspection time was considered a surrogate marker for vigilant assessment, longer inspection time is associated with higher lesion detection rates in the hands of experienced endoscopists.[19] The greatest role for red flag techniques is to help identify neoplastic lesions for targeted biopsy and therapy. The ideal endoscopic red flag technique should be simple, highly sensitive, sufficiently specific, consistent (result in minimal interobserver variability), and be readily available.

HD-WLE can potentially improve endoscopic imaging of BE compared with standard endoscopy, but little scientific evidence supports this. NBI is readily available and can improve the efficiency of detecting dysplasia (comparable detection of neoplasia with fewer biopsies); however, this has been shown in expert centers only. The addition of AFI to HD-WLE and NBI increases sensitivity and the false-positive rate without significantly improving overall detection of BE neoplasia. AA chromoendoscopy is the only proven red flag technique that is cost-effective and improves overall detection of BE neoplasia. Overall, evidence is insufficient to support the use of any one wide-field imaging technique over others in routine imaging of BE.

REFERENCES

1. Ronkainen J, Aro P, Storskrubb T, et al. Prevalence of Barrett's esophagus in the general population: an endoscopic study. Gastroenterology 2005;129:1825–31.
2. Evans JA, Early DS, Fukami N, et al. The role of endoscopy in Barrett's esophagus and other premalignant conditions of the esophagus. Gastrointest Endosc 2012;76:1087–94.
3. Hvid-Jensen F, Pedersen L, Drewes AM, et al. Incidence of adenocarcinoma among patients with Barrett's esophagus. N Engl J Med 2011;365:1375–83.
4. Almond LM, Barr H. Advanced endoscopic imaging in Barrett's oesophagus. Int J Surg 2012;10:236–41.
5. Pouw RE, Wirths K, Eisendrath P, et al. Efficacy of radiofrequency ablation combined with endoscopic resection for Barrett's esophagus with early neoplasia. Clin Gastroenterol Hepatol 2010;8:23–9.
6. Vieth M, Ell C, Gossner L, et al. Histological analysis of endoscopic resection specimens from 326 patients with Barrett's esophagus and early neoplasia. Endoscopy 2004;36:776–81.
7. Spechler SJ, Sharma P, Souza RF, et al. American Gastroenterological Association medical position statement on the management of Barrett's esophagus. Gastroenterology 2011;140:1084–91.

8. Bennett C, Vakil N, Bergman J, et al. Consensus statements for management of Barrett's dysplasia and early-stage esophageal adenocarcinoma, based on a Delphi process. Gastroenterology 2012;143:336–46.
9. Thekkek N, Anandasabapathy S, Richards-Kortum R. Optical molecular imaging for detection of Barrett's-associated neoplasia. World J Gastroenterol 2011;17:53–62.
10. Sharma P, Savides TJ, Canto MI, et al. The American Society for Gastrointestinal Endoscopy PIVI (Preservation and Incorporation of Valuable Endoscopic Innovations) on imaging in Barrett's esophagus. Gastrointest Endosc 2012;76: 252–4.
11. Canto MI, Setrakian S, Willis J, et al. Methylene blue-directed biopsies improve detection of intestinal metaplasia and dysplasia in Barrett's esophagus. Gastrointest Endosc 2000;51:560–8.
12. Wo JM, Ray MB, Mayfield-Stokes S, et al. Comparison of methylene blue-directed biopsies and conventional biopsies in the detection of intestinal metaplasia and dysplasia in Barrett's esophagus: a preliminary study. Gastrointest Endosc 2001;54:294–301.
13. Ragunath K, Krasner N, Raman VS, et al. A randomized, prospective cross-over trial comparing methylene blue-directed biopsy and conventional random biopsy for detecting intestinal metaplasia and dysplasia in Barrett's esophagus. Endoscopy 2003;35:998–1003.
14. Kara MA, Smits ME, Rosmolen WD, et al. A randomized crossover study comparing light-induced fluorescence endoscopy with standard videoendoscopy for the detection of early neoplasia in Barrett's esophagus. Gastrointest Endosc 2005;61:671–8.
15. Kara MA, Peters FP, Rosmolen WD, et al. High-resolution endoscopy plus chromoendoscopy or narrow-band imaging in Barrett's esophagus: a prospective randomized crossover study. Endoscopy 2005;37:929–36.
16. Curvers WL, van Vilsteren FG, Baak LC, et al. Endoscopic trimodal imaging versus standard video endoscopy for detection of early Barrett's neoplasia: a multicenter, randomized, crossover study in general practice. Gastrointest Endosc 2011;73:195–203.
17. Wolfsen HC, Crook JE, Krishna M, et al. Prospective, controlled tandem endoscopy study of narrow band imaging for dysplasia detection in Barrett's Esophagus. Gastroenterology 2008;135:24–31.
18. Lee MH, Buterbaugh K, Richards-Kortum R, et al. Advanced endoscopic imaging for Barrett's Esophagus: current options and future directions. Curr Gastroenterol Rep 2012;14:216–25.
19. Gupta N, Gaddam S, Wani SB, et al. Longer inspection time is associated with increased detection of high-grade dysplasia and esophageal adenocarcinoma in Barrett's esophagus. Gastrointest Endosc 2012;76:531–8.
20. Gono K, Obi T, Yamaguchi M, et al. Appearance of enhanced tissue features in narrow-band endoscopic imaging. J Biomed Opt 2004;9:568–77.
21. Mannath J, Ragunath K. Era of Barrett's surveillance: does equipment matter? World J Gastroenterol 2010;16:4640–5.
22. Sharma P, Bansal A, Mathur S, et al. The utility of a novel narrow band imaging endoscopy system in patients with Barrett's esophagus. Gastrointest Endosc 2006;64:167–75.
23. Curvers WL, Bohmer CJ, Mallant-Hent RC, et al. Mucosal morphology in Barrett's esophagus: interobserver agreement and role of narrow band imaging. Endoscopy 2008;40:799–805.

24. Herrero LA, Curvers WL, Bansal A, et al. Zooming in on Barrett oesophagus using narrow-band imaging: an international observer agreement study. Eur J Gastroenterol Hepatol 2009;21:1068–75.
25. Rastogi A, Pondugula K, Bansal A, et al. Recognition of surface mucosal and vascular patterns of colon polyps by using narrow-band imaging: interobserver and intraobserver agreement and prediction of polyp histology. Gastrointest Endosc 2009;69:716–22.
26. Sharma P, Hawes RH, Bansal A, et al. Standard endoscopy with random biopsies versus narrow band imaging targeted biopsies in Barrett's oesophagus: a prospective, international, randomised controlled trial. Gut 2013;62:15–21.
27. Filip M, Iordache S, Saftoiu A, et al. Autofluorescence imaging and magnification endoscopy. World J Gastroenterol 2011;17:9–14.
28. Herrero LA, Weusten BL, Bergman JJ. Autofluorescence and narrow band imaging in Barrett's esophagus. Gastroenterol Clin North Am 2010;39:747–58.
29. Kara MA, Peters FP, Ten Kate FJ, et al. Endoscopic video autofluorescence imaging may improve the detection of early neoplasia in patients with Barrett's esophagus. Gastrointest Endosc 2005;61:679–85.
30. Kara MA, Peters FP, Fockens P, et al. Endoscopic video-autofluorescence imaging followed by narrow band imaging for detecting early neoplasia in Barrett's esophagus. Gastrointest Endosc 2006;64:176–85.
31. Curvers WL, Herrero LA, Wallace MB, et al. Endoscopic tri-modal imaging is more effective than standard endoscopy in identifying early-stage neoplasia in Barrett's esophagus. Gastroenterology 2010;139:1106–14.
32. Canto MI. Acetic-acid chromoendoscopy for Barrett's esophagus: the "pros". Gastrointest Endosc 2006;64:13–6.
33. Lambert R, Rey JF, Sankaranarayanan R. Magnification and chromoscopy with the acetic acid test. Endoscopy 2003;35:437–45.
34. Rey JF, Inoue H, Guelrud M. Magnification endoscopy with acetic acid for Barrett's esophagus. Endoscopy 2005;37:583–6.
35. Costello S, Singh R. Endoscopic imaging in Barrett's oesophagus: applications in routine clinical practice and future outlook. Clin Endosc 2011;44:87–92.
36. Guelrud M, Herrera I, Essenfeld H, et al. Enhanced magnification endoscopy: a new technique to identify specialized intestinal metaplasia in Barrett's esophagus. Gastrointest Endosc 2001;53:559–65.
37. Fortun PJ, Anagnostopoulos GK, Kaye P, et al. Acetic acid-enhanced magnification endoscopy in the diagnosis of specialized intestinal metaplasia, dysplasia and early cancer in Barrett's oesophagus. Aliment Pharmacol Ther 2006;23:735–42.
38. Longcroft-Wheaton G, Duku M, Mead R, et al. Acetic acid spray is an effective tool for the endoscopic detection of neoplasia in patients with Barrett's esophagus. Clin Gastroenterol Hepatol 2010;8:843–7.
39. Bhandari P, Kandaswamy P, Cowlishaw D, et al. Acetic acid-enhanced chromoendoscopy is more cost-effective than protocol-guided biopsies in a high-risk Barrett's population. Dis Esophagus 2012;25:386–92.
40. Trivedi PJ, Braden B. Indications, stains and techniques in chromoendoscopy. QJM 2013;106(2):117–31.
41. Canto MI, Setrakian S, Willis JE, et al. Methylene blue staining of dysplastic and nondysplastic Barrett's esophagus: an in vivo and ex vivo study. Endoscopy 2001;33:391–400.
42. Canto MI, Setrakian S, Petras RE, et al. Methylene blue selectively stains intestinal metaplasia in Barrett's esophagus. Gastrointest Endosc 1996;44:1–7.

43. Kiesslich R, Hahn M, Herrmann G, et al. Screening for specialized columnar epithelium with methylene blue: chromoendoscopy in patients with Barrett's esophagus and a normal control group. Gastrointest Endosc 2001;53:47–52.
44. Kouklakis GS, Kountouras J, Dokas SM, et al. Methylene blue chromoendoscopy for the detection of Barrett's esophagus in a Greek cohort. Endoscopy 2003;35:383–7.
45. Sharma P, Topalovski M, Mayo MS, et al. Methylene blue chromoendoscopy for detection of short-segment Barrett's esophagus. Gastrointest Endosc 2001;54:289–93.
46. Dave U, Shousha S, Westaby D. Methylene blue staining: is it really useful in Barrett's esophagus? Gastrointest Endosc 2001;53:333–5.
47. Gangarosa LM, Halter S, Mertz H. Methylene blue staining and endoscopic ultrasound evaluation of Barrett's esophagus with low-grade dysplasia. Dig Dis Sci 2000;45:225–9.
48. Ngamruengphong S, Sharma VK, Das A. Diagnostic yield of methylene blue chromoendoscopy for detecting specialized intestinal metaplasia and dysplasia in Barrett's esophagus: a meta-analysis. Gastrointest Endosc 2009;69:1021–8.
49. Olliver JR, Wild CP, Sahay P, et al. Chromoendoscopy with methylene blue and associated DNA damage in Barrett's oesophagus. Lancet 2003;362:373–4.
50. Pohl J, May A, Rabenstein T, et al. Comparison of computed virtual chromoendoscopy and conventional chromoendoscopy with acetic acid for detection of neoplasia in Barrett's esophagus. Endoscopy 2007;39:594–8.
51. Camus M, Coriat R, Leblanc S, et al. Helpfulness of the combination of acetic acid and FICE in the detection of Barrett's epithelium and Barrett's associated neoplasias. World J Gastroenterol 2012;18:1921–5.
52. Kodashima S, Fujishiro M. Novel image-enhanced endoscopy with i-scan technology. World J Gastroenterol 2010;16:1043–9.
53. Hoffman A, Basting N, Goetz M, et al. High-definition endoscopy with i-Scan and Lugol's solution for more precise detection of mucosal breaks in patients with reflux symptoms. Endoscopy 2009;41:107–12.
54. Kang HS, Hong SN, Ko SY, et al. The efficacy of i-SCAN for detecting reflux esophagitis: a prospective randomized controlled trial. Dis Esophagus 2013;26(2):204–11.
55. Kim MS, Choi SR, Roh MH, et al. Efficacy of I-scan endoscopy in the diagnosis of gastroesophageal reflux disease with minimal change. Clin Endosc 2011;44:27–32.
56. Lee CK, Lee SH, Hwangbo Y. Narrow-band imaging versus I-Scan for the real-time histological prediction of diminutive colonic polyps: a prospective comparative study by using the simple unified endoscopic classification. Gastrointest Endosc 2011;74:603–9.
57. Masci E, Mangiavillano B, Crosta C, et al. Interobserver agreement among endoscopists on evaluation of polypoid colorectal lesions visualized with the Pentax i-Scan technique. Dig Liver Dis 2013;45(3):207–10.
58. Hong SN, Choe WH, Lee JH, et al. Prospective, randomized, back-to-back trial evaluating the usefulness of i-SCAN in screening colonoscopy. Gastrointest Endosc 2012;75:1011–1021.e2.

Optical Coherence Tomography in Barrett's Esophagus

Charles J. Lightdale, MD

KEYWORDS

- Barrett's esophagus • Optical coherence tomography
- Optical frequency domain imaging • Volumetric laser endomicroscopy

KEY POINTS

- The incidence of Barrett's-related cancer of the esophagus continues to increase at an alarming rate.
- Ablative therapies for Barrett's esophagus and for early neoplasia in Barrett's esophagus are increasingly being applied for cancer prevention.
- Studies to date show great promise for optical coherence tomography (OCT) in screening, surveillance, and guiding management of Barrett's esophagus.
- With continued innovation in rapid, accurate scanning systems, such as volumetric laser endomicroscopy or optical frequency-domain imaging, advanced OCT seems likely to have an important impact.
- The next few years are likely to see the initiation of larger clinical studies that will define the extent and significance of this impact.

INTRODUCTION

Optical coherence tomography (OCT) is emerging as perhaps the most important advance in imaging Barrett's esophagus in the modern era. High-resolution white-light endoscopy and digital chromoendoscopy with magnification provide superb imaging of the mucosal surface, but nothing below the surface.[1] Endoscopic ultrasonography (EUS) can image the entire esophageal wall thickness, but at insufficient resolution to satisfactorily detect dysplasia or early cancer.[2] Confocal laser endomicroscopy (CLE), both endoscope-based and probe-based, can obtain dramatic cellular level imaging of the esophageal mucosa, but of small areas and at specific limited depths.[1,3]

IMAGING OF BARRETT'S ESOPHAGUS

Barrett's esophagus presents a difficult problem for endoscopic imaging. The presence and extent of short-segment Barrett's esophagus may be difficult to detect at

Division of Digestive and Liver Diseases, Department of Medicine, New York-Presbyterian Hospital/Columbia University Medical Center, 161 Fort Washington Avenue, Room 812, New York, NY 10032, USA
E-mail address: CJL18@columbia.edu

Gastrointest Endoscopy Clin N Am 23 (2013) 549–563
http://dx.doi.org/10.1016/j.giec.2013.03.007
1052-5157/13/$ – see front matter © 2013 Elsevier Inc. All rights reserved.

giendo.theclinics.com

the esophagogastric junction.[4] The top of the gastric folds, used as a landmark for the esophagogastric junction, change with insufflation of air, and there is often a hiatal hernia causing bends and angles at the distal esophagus, making a complete view difficult.[5] These factors are further compounded by movement associated with swallowing, belching, coughing, peristalsis, respiration, and pulsation.

ENDOSCOPIC SURVEILLANCE OF BARRETT'S ESOPHAGUS

In patients with known Barrett's esophagus, endoscopic surveillance is performed to detect dysplasia as a risk factor for progression to cancer.[6–8] Low-grade dysplasia (LGD) involves primarily cytologic abnormalities. Though comparable with those in adenoma, in Barrett's esophagus the changes of LGD are usually flat and changes in mucosal appearance are usually not detectable by endoscopy.[9–11]

High-grade dysplasia (HGD) involves changes in both cytology and tissue architecture, and may be detected in some cases using high-resolution white-light endoscopy, digital chromoendoscopy with magnification, and CLE, but unless present in visible nodules or ulcers, detection of HGD can be subtle and difficult.[1] In addition, dysplastic changes usually occur in a mosaic-type unpredictable distribution within the Barrett's metaplasia.[11]

Endoscopic Biopsies

Four-quadrant random biopsies every 1 to 2 cm of Barrett's length are recommended as the standard approach to dysplasia detection, but are notoriously underperformed, and even when correctly done sampling error is common.[12–14]

Need for Red-Flag Technology

Using targeted biopsies based on abnormalities seen with high-resolution white-light endoscopy and narrow-band imaging increase the accuracy of dysplasia detection, and CLE further adds to the diagnostic yield, but sampling error persists.[1] The requirement is for a "red-flag" or scanning technology that can accurately locate all the dysplastic areas within the Barrett's segment for targeted biopsies or endoscopic therapy. Autofluorescence imaging combined with high-resolution white-light endoscopy and narrow-band imaging (trimodal imaging) was tested for this purpose, but false-positive rates were prohibitively high.[15] The use of fluorescent-tagged lectins and peptide probes with specialized endoscopic systems (molecular imaging) are the subject of ongoing research projects, which are designed to localize areas of dysplasia for targeted biopsy or therapy.[16,17]

ADVANCED OCT IN BARRETT'S ESOPHAGUS

It would seem that advanced OCT may have the ability to meet most of the challenges of imaging in Barrett's esophagus. The method has the potential to achieve wide-field scanning at a resolution comparable with that of low-power microscopy, detecting changes in tissue architecture that occur in Barrett's metaplasia, dysplasia, and cancer.

The technology has the potential to:

1. Identify Barrett's metaplasia
2. Detect HGD and early cancer
3. Locate subsquamous (buried) Barrett's glands
4. Guide endoscopic therapies.

ANALOGY OF EUS AND OCT

Gastrointestinal endoscopists have become increasingly familiar with EUS, which is now widely available in modern endoscopy units. There are some parallels between OCT and EUS imaging. In ultrasonographic imaging, tissue structures are imaged in depth by measuring the time delay between the interrogating sound wave (emitted by a piezoelectric crystal) and the time taken by reflected sound waves to return to the crystal detector. The total depth and resolution of the image depend on the sound frequency. The sound waves require a liquid medium between the ultrasound transducer and tissue, and the best high-frequency EUS axial resolution is in the range of 100 μm.[18]

OCT can be thought of as a technique analogous to ultrasonography; however, instead of producing an image from the scattering of sound waves, it uses infrared light from a laser and optical scattering, based on differences in tissue composition, to form a 2-dimensional image.[19] With OCT, depth intensity can be measured by time-domain measurements, allowing for image construction in all 3 dimensions.[20-22] OCT is a noncontact method. Air does not produce artifacts as in ultrasonography, and a liquid conducting medium is not required. The great benefit of OCT over ultrasonography is that it is capable of generating cross-sectional images of tissues with an axial resolution in the range of 10 μm or less, which is comparable with that of low-power (4×) bright-field microscopy. This resolution is sufficient to detect microscopic tissue architecture.

INTERFEROMETRY

The speed of light is so much faster than the speed of sound that no detector is capable of directly determining the time difference between incident and reflected light. OCT uses a method called interferometry to perform this task. OCT measurements are made using low-coherence interferometry typically configured as a Michelson-type interferometer, as illustrated in **Fig. 1**. The interferometer functions by splitting the beam into 2 independent paths and then recombining the 2 paths to

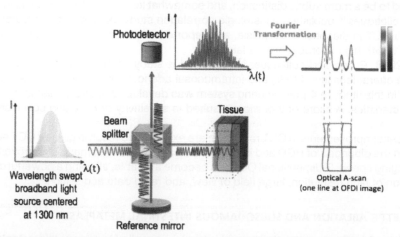

Fig. 1. The essential elements of advanced second-generation optical coherence tomography (OCT), known as optical frequency domain imaging (OFDI) or volumetric laser endomicroscopy (VLE). (*Courtesy of* Michalina J. Gora, Research Fellow, Massachusetts General Hospital, Boston, MA.)

generate interference. The depth-dependent tissue microstructure information is derived from the interference patterns. Signal-processing algorithms transform interference patterns into images than can be displayed in real time.[20–22]

INITIAL MEDICAL USES OF OCT

The first report of OCT imaging of human tissue was published in 1991 by a research group at the Massachusetts Institute of Technology, who used OCT in the laboratory for in vitro studies of the human retina and atherosclerotic plaques.[20] The first clinical applications were in ophthalmology, where OCT has found a solid role in diagnosing and monitoring diseases such as glaucoma and macular degeneration.[22,23]

In 1997, a catheter-based OCT probe was used to study the gastrointestinal tract in live animals,[19] and a pilot study in humans was reported using a different OCT catheter-based endoscope system.[24] In 2000, 3 different groups reported OCT imaging of the esophagus and stomach. Imaging depth in the esophagus was achieved to approximately 2 mm, allowing imaging of the submucosa. These studies showed that the normal squamous mucosa was routinely imaged as a layered structure, with layers corresponding to the epithelium, lamina propria, and muscularis mucosae.[25–27]

OCT IN BARRETT'S ESOPHAGUS

Barrett's metaplasia has a specific appearance on OCT imaging, easily distinguished from the appearance of the gastric cardia and normal squamous mucosa.[26–29] In 2001, Poneros and colleagues[30] published the first study examining the accuracy of in vivo OCT in diagnosing Barrett's metaplasia. Studies have found sensitivities ranging from 81% to 97% and specificities from 57% to 92% in comparison with histopathologic evaluation of endoscopic biopsies.[31]

OCT IN IMAGING OF DYSPLASIA

Initial studies differentiating nondysplastic Barrett's mucosa from Barrett's dysplasia proved to be a more subtle distinction, and somewhat less accurate. In 2005, Isenberg and colleagues[32] published a histologic correlation study examining the accuracy of in vivo OCT in diagnosing dysplasia, and reported sensitivity of 68% and specificity of 82% with high interobserver variability.

In 2006, Evans and colleagues[33] published a study further examining the OCT-image characteristics of HGD and intramucosal adenocarcinoma in Barrett's esophagus. In this study, a 4-point scoring system was developed based on histopathology characteristics. A score of 2 or more resulted in sensitivity of 83% and specificity of 75%.

Recent improvements in OCT resolution are expected to result in greater OCT accuracy in the diagnosis of HGD and intramucosal carcinoma. With marked improvement in imaging speed, 3-dimensional OCT has become available, allowing a powerful combination of high resolution, large field of view, and rapid data acquisition.[34]

BARRETT'S ABLATION AND SUBSQUAMOUS INTESTINAL METAPLASIA

A variety of endoscopic ablation therapies has been applied to remove the metaplastic mucosal lining that characterizes Barrett's esophagus. Most ablation procedures have been reported in patients in whom dysplasia has been detected within the Barrett's segment.

Photodynamic Therapy

Photodynamic therapy (PDT), in which a photosensitive chemical is usually given systemically followed by photoactivation in the Barrett's segment with a directed laser at a specific wavelength, was effective but was associated with many adverse reactions.[35,36] PDT using porfimer sodium as the chemical sensitizer resulted in deep injury in some cases, with a resulting high stricture rate. Despite this, on follow-up endoscopic biopsies Barrett's glands were detected in some patients underneath the neosquamous epithelium.

Buried Barrett's Glands Before Ablation Therapy

Further analysis has confirmed that such "buried" glands occur even before ablation therapy, at the Z-line (squamocolumnar junction), and are related to squamous islands within the Barrett's segment.[37] Buried glands that present after ablation are of unclear clinical significance; however, particularly in patients who have been treated for HGD, buried glands after therapy may contain or develop dysplasia or adenocarcinoma.

Argon Plasma Coagulation

Argon plasma coagulation (APC), widely available in modern endoscopy units, has been used for the ablation of Barrett's mucosa. However, the depth of ablation is variable, and an even ablation depth is difficult to achieve, particularly in larger segments. Buried glands and recurrent dysplasia and cancer have been reported following APC ablation of Barrett's esophagus.[38]

RADIOFREQUENCY ABLATION IN BARRETT'S ESOPHAGUS

The current standard for ablation of Barrett's esophagus is radiofrequency ablation (RFA).[7,8] RFA for Barrett's esophagus consists of a radiofrequency energy waveform delivered on contact with the targeted epithelium resulting in water vaporization, coagulation of proteins, and cell necrosis. The depth of injury is controlled by the electrode pattern and field geometry, as well as standardization of power density and energy density. Devices are available for circumferential and focal RFA.

RFA Results

Shaheen and colleagues[39] reported on a multicenter randomized, sham-controlled trial in the United States of RFA versus surveillance for dysplastic Barrett's esophagus including separate patient cohorts having HGD or LGD. In the per-protocol analyses complete eradication of HGD was 89.5%, compared with 20% in the control group, and eradication of LGD was reported as 95.0% in the ablation group compared with 26.3% in the control group ($P<.001$). The incidence of any neoplastic progression during the first year of the study was 3.6% in the ablation group, compared with 16.3% in the controls ($P<.05$).

RFA treatment was designed to remove Barrett's mucosa (with an emphasis on safety) just to the top of the submucosa. Transient chest pain and odynophagia are common after RFA, but in the 84 patients with dysplasia in this randomized controlled trial there was only 1 case of significant gastrointestinal bleeding and 3 cases of easily dilated esophageal strictures.[39]

Surveillance After RFA for Barrett's Esophagus

In an ongoing follow-up of the same cohorts including patients in the control group crossed over to treatment after 1 year, more than 85% of patients remained free of dysplasia, and more than 75% were free of intestinal metaplasia at 3 years. More than 90% of patients were free of dysplasia and intestinal metaplasia after a single additional treatment.[40]

In another study, Pouw and colleagues[41] showed a reversion of abnormal molecular markers in dysplastic Barrett's esophagus to normal in the neosquamous mucosa after RFA. With all this benefit, however, on further surveillance 7% to 32% of patients successfully ablated with RFA will over time be found to have intestinal metaplasia on endoscopic biopsies.[41–46] The great majority of these will be at the new squamocolumnar junction or within a few centimeters of the junction. Long-segment Barrett's esophagus and ablation performed in patients with HGD and intramucosal carcinoma have been identified as having a higher risk for recurrence of intestinal metaplasia.[45,46] Recurrent dysplasia and adenocarcinoma have also been reported, almost all in patients who had dysplasia or intramucosal cancer before ablation.[46,47] This phenomenon has once again raised the question of the significance of buried Barrett's glands.[47]

Buried Glands Before and After RFA

In a controlled study of RFA for Barrett's dysplasia, a systematic review of all biopsy specimens before and after RFA was performed by the central pathology laboratory.[39] Before ablation, buried glands were found to be common, and were a nearly identical (25% and 26%, respectively) in the treatment and control groups. Following the 1-year RFA protocol, the buried glands in the treatment group decreased to 5%, whereas the rate in the control group increased to 40% with the additional biopsies. In this rigorous analysis, clearly RFA was reducing, but not completely eliminating, buried Barrett's glands.

OCT for Detection of Buried Glands After RFA

In 2009, Adler and colleagues[48] published a case report detailing the use of 3-dimensional OCT in a patient with Barrett's esophagus following RFA. Buried Barrett's glands were identified on OCT beneath neosquamous mucosa. Challenged by a Letter to the Editor that histologic confirmation was inconclusive and that OCT might not be relevant in postablation patients, the investigators pointed out the much larger area sampled by OCT compared with the 4-mm^2 area sampled by a biopsy; they pointed out that buried biopsy glands usually occur in a sparse distribution, likely to be missed by biopsy sampling error.[49]

An ex vivo study by Cobb and colleagues[50] in 2009 supported the potential for OCT to detect buried Barrett's glands after ablation. The investigators conducted 2-dimensional OCT on esophagectomy specimens from 14 patients who underwent surgery for HGD or adenocarcinoma in Barrett's esophagus. Buried Barrett's glands in these ablation-naïve patients on OCT corresponded to histology. OCT showed buried glands in 10 of 14 patients, which were not detected by prior endoscopic biopsy.

In 2012, Zhou and colleagues[51] studied patients with 3-dimensional OCT at various stages of RFA treatment, evaluating the presence of buried glands in the area of the esophagogastric junction. A total of 18 patients were examined before they had complete response of intestinal metaplasia (CR-IM), and 16 patients were examined after CR-IM on endoscopy. OCT showed buried glands in 13 of 18 patients in the pre–CE-IM group and 10 of 16 patients in the post–CR-IM group. The number (mean [standard deviation]) of buried glands per patient in the post–CE-IM group (7.1 [9.3]) was significantly lower than that in the pre–CE-IM group (34.4 [44.6]; $P = .02$). The investigators concluded that while buried glands were markedly reduced by RFA, their continued presence at the esophagogastric junction could be localized with OCT for possible additional therapy.

OCT for Predicting Incomplete RFA

In a second article from this group in 2012, Tsai and colleagues[52] published a report evaluating 33 patients with 3-dimensional OCT. The patients had short-segment Barrett's esophagus (<3 cm in length). OCT was performed at the esophagogastric junction immediately before and after RFA treatment using the focal RFA device. Using OCT, the investigators measured the thickness of the Barrett's mucosa before treatment and looked for evidence of residual Barrett's glands immediately after completion of the ablation. After 6 to 8 weeks the patients were examined again with standard endoscopy, and biopsies were performed if there was no endoscopic evidence of residual Barrett's esophagus.

Results showed that the Barrett's mucosa was significantly thinner in patients who achieved complete eradication of intestinal metaplasia (257 ± 60 μm) than in patients who did not achieve complete eradication of intestinal metaplasia (403 ± 86 μm) on biopsy 6 to 8 weeks after an initial focal RFA ($P<.0001$).[52] A threshold thickness of 333 μm (derived from receiver-operating characteristic curves) corresponded to sensitivity of 93.3%, specificity of 85%, and accuracy of 87.9% in predicting the presence of Barrett's glands on follow-up biopsy. The presence of Barrett's glands on OCT imaging immediately after ablation also correlated with the finding of Barrett's glands on follow-up (sensitivity 83.3%, specificity 95%, accuracy 90.6%). The investigators postulated that OCT might be able to guide RFA by suggesting more aggressive treatment in selected patients based on the pretreatment thickness of the Barrett's mucosa or the detection of residual Barrett's glands immediately after treatment.[52]

GOALS FOR OCT IN BARRETT'S ESOPHAGUS

In an editorial on the use of OCT in Barrett's esophagus, Peery and Shaheen[53] emphasized that OCT has great potential. To meet this potential, they noted that OCT must be shown to be:

1. Accurate
2. Efficient
3. Reliable
4. User-friendly
5. Cost-effective

Peery and Shaheen suggested that image interpretation may be problematic in wide-scale use, and that studies must demonstrate high interobserver agreement concordant with histopathology. As an alternative they suggested a computer algorithm to assist in image analysis.[53]

VOLUMETRIC LASER ENDOMICROSCOPY

An advanced OCT method called volumetric laser endomicroscopy (VLE) seems to have achieved the critical postulate of Peery and Shaheen that OCT must be capable of rapid imaging of wide swatches of Barrett's tissue without compromising image resolution or quality.[54–58] Also known as Fourier-domain OCT or optical frequency-domain imaging (OFDI, see **Fig. 1**), VLE devices are being designed for commercial use in gastroenterology, with Barrett's esophagus the primary target.

VLE acquires cross-sectional images by using a focused, narrow-diameter beam to repeatedly measure the delay of reflections from within the sampled tissue.[57] Interferometry is used to measure the delay intervals, while Fourier transformation is used to compute traditional A-lines, or depth scans, which comprise the tissue reflectivity as a function of depth along the beam. Unlike previous time-domain OCT, VLE uses a fixed-wavelength or swept-source technology, whereby the wavelength of a monochromatic light source is rapidly scanned to measure the interference signal as a function of wavelength.[57]

The use of a balloon-based VLE system with helically scanning optics for esophageal imaging is particularly suited to the imaging of Barrett's esophagus.[59] With this system, the optical components of the catheter are positioned within the esophageal lumen via a balloon-centered probe placed over a guide wire under endoscopic control. After the balloon is inflated to 25 mm diameter, the optics become centered in the lumen. The optics are then slowly pulled back during the imaging procedure while the imaging optics are simultaneously rotated by a probe scanner. The entire portion of the esophageal mucosa in contact with the balloon is thus scanned in a circumferential and helical manner. Real-time volumetric images are obtained by scanning the imaging beam over the tissue surface in 2 dimensions.[60]

Preliminary data for the VLE system have shown its ability to image the distal esophagus at a higher speed, to obtain better-quality images than with previous OCT time-domain technology. VLE provides an axial resolution of less than 10 μm with a penetration depth of up to 3 mm.[61]

In the first clinical experience with this technique, VLE successfully imaged the microscopic architecture of the distal esophagus in 10 of 12 patients undergoing routine upper endoscopy for Barrett's esophagus screening, with surveillance with volumetric images being obtained in a 6-cm length of esophagus in less than 2 minutes.[61] The investigators proposed criteria for interpretation of the images based on prior experience,[30–33] which are outlined in **Table 1**.

Recent experience has shown that the distinction of Barrett's mucosa from the mucosa of the gastric cardia and from squamous mucosa has been readily performed (**Fig. 2**). The ability of this method to delineate layers of the normal squamous lining has

Table 1
Criteria for the interpretation of OCT images using VLE/OFDI of gastroesophageal tissue in patients with Barrett's esophagus

Diagnosis	Imaging Criteria on OCT
Squamous	1. Layered architecture
Cardia	1. Vertical pit and crypt architecture 2. Highly reflective surface 3. Broad, regular glandular architecture 4. Poor image penetration
SIM	1. Lack of layered or vertical pit and crypt architecture 2. Heterogeneous scattering 3. Irregular surface 4. Glands in epithelium with layered architecture
HGD/IMC	1. Increased surface/subsurface reflectivity (score 0–2) 2. Irregular gland/duct architecture (score 0–2)

The diagnosis of SIM requires any 2 of the first 3 criteria for SIM or criterion 4 alone. The diagnosis of HGD/IMC requires scoring the severity of both criteria on a scale of 0 (absence) to 1 (mild) or 2 (severe) abnormality. A total score of ≥2 indicates HGD/IMC.

Abbreviations: Cardia, gastric cardia; HGD, high-grade dysplasia; IMC, intramucosal carcinoma; OCT, optical coherence tomography; OFDI, optical frequency domain imaging; SIM, specialized intestinal metaplasia; VLE, volumetric laser endomicroscopy.

Adapted from Suter MJ, Vakoc BJ, Yachimski PS, et al. Comprehensive microscopy of the esophagus in human patients with optical frequency domain imaging. Gastrointest Endosc 2008;68:745–53; with permission.

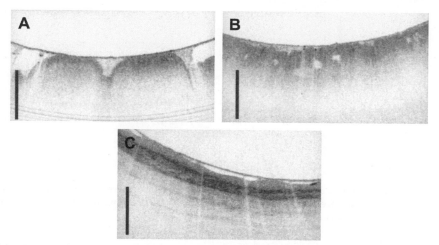

Fig. 2. Zoomed images (scale bars = 2 mm) obtained by VLE. (*A*) Normal gastric cardia, showing vertical pit and crypt architecture, highly reflective surface, broad regular glandular architecture, and poor image penetration. (*B*) Specialized intestinal metaplasia of Barrett's esophagus, showing neither a layered or pit and crypt architecture, but rather an appearance of heterogeneous scattering, with an irregular surface, and glandular epithelium. (*C*) Normal esophageal squamous epithelium, showing a layered architecture.

been demonstrated along with proposed histologic correlation (**Fig. 3**). The diagnosis of abnormal findings denoting dysplasia and early cancer in Barrett's mucosa has been also described (**Fig. 4**).

While pilot results with VLE continue to be encouraging, new larger clinical studies will be critical in determining the utility and significance of this new technology in improving the management of patients with Barrett's esophagus.

OCT-GUIDED LASER MARKING FOR TARGETED BIOPSY

Once potentially abnormal areas are identified on OCT, a frequently needed next step is to confirm the abnormality with biopsy. The key problem is to localize the area for

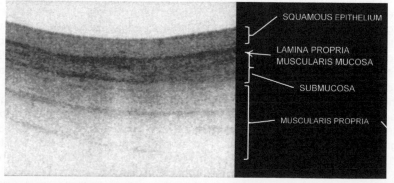

Fig. 3. Zoomed normal esophageal wall image obtained by VLE, showing proposed histologic correlates to the layered image.

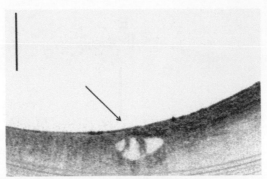

Fig. 4. Zoomed image (scale bar = 2 mm) obtained by VLE from the esophagus, showing an area of increased surface and subsurface reflectivity with enlarged and highly irregular epithelial glands (*arrow*).

endoscopy-directed biopsy. Although estimates can be made from the OCT images alone, a more precise method would likely be very helpful. Suter and colleagues[62] tested a system for image-guided biopsy using advanced OCT and laser marking of artificially placed targets in the esophagus in 5 living swine.

The researchers tested a system of OFDI or VLE deployed through a balloon-centering catheter, which allowed a scan length of 6.0 cm of the distal esophagus in approximately 2 minutes. Using this system, a laser was used to mark the esophagus where the artificial targets were placed.[62]

All of the laser-induced marks were visible at endoscopy. Target locations were correctly marked with a success rate of 97% (95% confidence interval, 89.8%–99.7%). Thermal damage was limited to the superficial mucosa and was observed to partially heal within 2 days. The investigators concluded that laser marking of the esophagus at sites found to be abnormal on their high-speed 3-dimensional OCT system was feasible, safe, and accurate, and provided sufficient visibility in their experimental model to guide endoscopic biopsy.[62] Testing this type of system in human subjects is anticipated.

TETHERED-CAPSULE ENDOMICROSCOPY

Tethered capsules designed to be swallowed for evaluation of Barrett's esophagus are a recent concept. A video-camera capsule has been developed for the acquisition of images, and also a sponge has been used that is compressed inside a dissolvable capsule for the acquisition of cytology and biomarkers.[63,64] A new approach to advanced OCT evaluation of the upper gastrointestinal tract using a capsule design was introduced in 2013 by Gora and colleagues,[65] using technology similar to that of balloon-based OFDI or VLE.

Rather than a balloon catheter passed over a guide wire with endoscopic control, engineers developed a tethered capsule-sized device, designed to be swallowed. The clear, transparent plastic capsule measures 12.8 mm in diameter and 24.8 mm in length, the size of a large vitamin pill. The tether measures just 0.96 mm. The tether sheath encloses a driveshaft and an optical fiber; the fiber transmits light to and receives light from the miniature optics inside the capsule.[65]

The driveshaft conveys rotational torque from the system's optical rotary junction to the capsule's optics. Circumferential cross-sectional images are acquired as the rotary junction, and thus the optical beam in the capsule, continuously spins. Tissue in the stomach and esophagus can be scanned, and the capsule can be retrieved by pulling it back out of the mouth via the tether. The capsule can be reused after standard chemical-soak disinfection.[65]

Initial Human Tests of Tethered-Capsule Endomicroscopy

The researchers at the Wellman Center for Photomedicine, Massachusetts General Hospital, Boston, tested the tethered-capsule device in 13 subjects, 7 healthy volunteers, and 6 persons with known Barrett's esophagus. All subjects successfully swallowed the device with a sip of water. The capsule was then propelled down the esophagus into the stomach by peristalsis. The esophageal lumen contracted around the capsule, allowing circumferential images. During transit multiple optical frequency domain, cross-sectional images are acquired at 30 μm (lateral) × 7 μm axial resolution, enabling the differential visualization of normal esophageal squamous mucosa, normal stomach mucosa, and Barrett's mucosa.[65]

Sequential cross sections may be compiled to reconstruct a 3-dimensional microscopic representation of the entire luminal organ. In the 13 subjects initially tested in the reported study, the esophagus remained in close apposition to the outer surface of the capsule, resulting in the production of high-quality images in an average of 94.5% of all frames acquired.[65]

The mean transit time for imaging an approximately 15-cm length of esophagus was 58 seconds. For 4 imaging passes (2 up and 2 down), resulting in 4 complete data sets, the entire procedure lasted an average of approximately 6 minutes (6 minutes 18 seconds) from capsule insertion to extraction. There were no complications in the 13 subjects who had the tethered-capsule endomicroscopy procedure. After the procedure, all but 1 of the subjects (12 of 13) reported that they would prefer the tethered-capsule procedure to conventional endoscopy.[65]

Comparison of Capsule and Balloon Endomicroscopy

Both the capsule-based and balloon-based methods use the same OFDI or VLE technology, and will likely share a compatible imaging console in the future. The capsule is a rigid device, whereas the balloon is a more conformable plastic material. In addition, the probe inside the capsule rotates at a single level, and axial images are created as the capsule is manually pulled upward by the tether or pushed down by peristalsis. In the balloon method, the placement is over a guide wire directed by endoscopy, and once inflated the balloon stays in a relatively fixed position while the probe is retracted axially inside the balloon via a drive mechanism.

The great advantage of an ingestible capsule scanner is that endoscopy and sedation are unnecessary, with associated potentially increased ease of use on a wide scale and significantly lower cost. Because the capsule can be reused, it has the potential to be sufficiently inexpensive for population-based screening for Barrett's esophagus. The device might also be useful for dysplasia and cancer surveillance in patients with known Barrett's esophagus. Larger studies to determine the efficacy of tethered-capsule endomicroscopy for these indications, and comparative studies with the balloon-based method, are clearly needed.

SUMMARY

The incidence of Barrett's-related cancer of the esophagus continues to increase at an alarming rate. Ablative therapies for Barrett's esophagus and for early neoplasia in Barrett's esophagus are increasingly being applied for cancer prevention. Studies to date show great promise for OCT in diagnosing and directing the management of Barrett's esophagus. With continued innovation in rapid, accurate scanning systems, such as VLE and OFDI, advanced OCT seems likely to have an important impact. The next few years are likely to see the initiation of larger clinical studies that will define the extent and significance of this impact.

REFERENCES

1. Sharma P, Meining AR, Coron E, et al. Real-time increased detection of neoplastic tissue in Barrett's esophagus with probe-based confocal laser endomicroscopy: final results of a multi-center prospective international randomized controlled trial. Gastrointest Endosc 2011;74:465–72.
2. Larghi A, Lightdale CJ, Memeo L, et al. EUS followed by EMR for staging of high-grade dysplasia and early cancer in Barrett's esophagus. Gastrointest Endosc 2005;62:16–23.
3. Kiesslich R, Tajiri H. Advanced imaging in endoscopy. In: Classen M, Tytgat GN, Lightdale CJ, editors. Gastroenterological endoscopy. 2nd edition. Stuttgart (NY): Thieme; 2010. p. 21–35.
4. Sharma P, Dent J, Armstrong D, et al. The development and validation of an endoscopic grading system for Barrett's esophagus: the Prague C & M criteria. Gastroenterology 2006;131:1392–9.
5. Amano Y, Ishimura N, Furuta K, et al. Which landmark results in a more consistent diagnosis of Barrett's esophagus, the gastric folds or the palisade vessels? Gastrointest Endosc 2006;64:206–11.
6. Wang KK, Sampliner RE. Updated Guidelines 2008 for the diagnosis, surveillance and therapy of Barrett's esophagus. Am J Gastroenterol 2008;103:788–97.
7. Spechler SJ, Sharma P, Souza RF, et al. American Gastroenterological Association medical position statement on the management of Barrett's esophagus. Gastroenterology 2011;140:1084–91.
8. Evans JA, Early DS, Fukami N, et al. ASGE Guidelines: the role of endoscopy in Barrett's esophagus and other premalignant conditions of the esophagus. Gastrointest Endosc 2012;76:1087–94.
9. Montgomery E, Bronner MP, Goldblum JR, et al. Reproducibility of the diagnosis of dysplasia in Barrett's esophagus: a reaffirmation. Hum Pathol 2001;32: 368–78.
10. Curvers WL, Ten-Kate FJ, Krishnadath KK, et al. Low-grade dysplasia in Barrett's esophagus: overdiagnosed and underestimated. Am J Gastroenterol 2010;105:1523–30.
11. Odze RD. Diagnosis and grading of dysplasia in Barrett's oesophagus. J Clin Pathol 2006;59:1029–38.
12. Abrams JA, Kapel RC, Lindberg GM, et al. Adherence to biopsy guidelines for Barrett's esophagus surveillance in the community setting in the United States. Clin Gastroenterol Hepatol 2009;7:736–42.
13. Cameron AJ, Carpenter HA. Barrett's esophagus, high-grade dysplasia, and early adenocarcinoma: a pathological study. Am J Gastroenterol 1997;92:586–91.
14. Kariv R, Plesec TP, Goldblum JR, et al. The Seattle protocol does not more reliably detect the detection of cancer at the time of esophagectomy than a less intensive surveillance protocol. Clin Gastroenterol Hepatol 2009;7:653–8.
15. Curvers WL, van Vilsteren FG, Baak LC, et al. Endoscopic trimodal imaging versus standard video endoscopy for detection of early Barrett's neoplasia: a

multicenter, randomized, crossover study in general practice. Gastrointest Endosc 2011;73:195–203.

16. Bird-Lieberman EL, Neves AA, Lao-Sirieix P, et al. Molecular imaging using fluorescent lectins permits rapid endoscopic identification of dysplasia in Barrett's esophagus. Nat Med 2012;18:315–21.

17. Joshi BP, Miller SJ, Lee CM, et al. Multispectral endoscopic imaging of colorectal dysplasia in vivo. Gastroenterology 2012;143:1435–7.

18. Botet JF, Lightdale CJ. Endoscopic ultrasonography of the upper gastrointestinal tract. Radiol Clin North Am 1992;30:1067–85.

19. Van Dam J, Fujimoto JG. Imaging beyond the endoscope. Gastrointest Endosc 2005;51:12–6.

20. Huang D, Swanson LA, Lin CR, et al. Optical coherence tomography. Science 1991;254:1178–81.

21. Tearney GJ, Brezinski ME, Bouma BE, et al. In vivo endoscopic optical biopsy with optical coherence tomography. Science 1997;276:2037–9.

22. Testoni PA. Optical coherence tomography. Scientific World Journal 2007;7: 87–108.

23. Hee MR, Puliafito CA, Wong C, et al. Quantitative assessment of macular edema with optical coherence tomography. Arch Ophthalmol 1995;113:1019–29.

24. Sergeev AM, Gelikonov VM, Gelikonov GV, et al. In vivo endoscopic OCT imaging of precancer and cancer states of human mucosa. Opt Express 1997;1:432–40.

25. Bouma BE, Tearney GJ, Compton CC, et al. High resolution imaging of the human esophagus and stomach in vivo using optical coherence tomography. Gastrointest Endosc 2000;51:467–74.

26. Sivak MV, Kobayashi K, Izatt JA, et al. High resolution endoscopic imaging of the GI tract using optical coherence tomography. Gastrointest Endosc 2000; 51:474–9.

27. Jäckle S, Gladkova N, Feldchtein F, et al. In vivo endoscopic optical coherence tomography of the human gastrointestinal tract–toward optical biopsy. Endoscopy 2000;32:743–9.

28. Jäckle S, Gladkova N, Feldchtein F, et al. In vivo endoscopic optical coherence tomography of esophagitis, Barrett's esophagus, and adenocarcinoma of the esophagus. Endoscopy 2000;32:750–5.

29. Chen Y, Aguirre AD, Hsiung P-L, et al. Ultrahigh resolution optical coherence tomography of Barrett's esophagus: preliminary descriptive clinical study correlating images with histology. Endoscopy 2007;39:599–605.

30. Poneros JM, Brand S, Bouma BE, et al. Diagnosis of specialized intestinal metaplasia by optical coherence tomography. Gastroenterology 2001;120:7–12.

31. Evans JA, Poneros JM, Bouma BE, et al. Identifying intestinal metaplasia at the squamocolumnar junction using optical coherence tomography. Gastrointest Endosc 2007;65:50–6.

32. Isenberg G, Sivak MV, Chak A, et al. Accuracy of endoscopic optical coherence tomography in the detection of dysplasia in Barrett's esophagus: a prospective, double-blinded study. Gastrointest Endosc 2005;62:825–31.

33. Evans JA, Poneros JM, Bouma BE, et al. Optical coherence tomography to identify intramucosal carcinoma and high-grade dysplasia in Barrett's esophagus. Clin Gastroenterol Hepatol 2006;4:38–43.

34. Yun SH, Tearney GJ, de Boer JF, et al. High-speed optical frequency-domain imaging. Opt Express 2003;11:2953–63.

35. Overholt BF, Lightdale CJ, Wang KK, et al. Photodynamic therapy with porfimer sodium for ablation of high-grade dysplasia in Barrett's esophagus:

international, partially blinded, randomized phase III trial. Gastrointest Endosc 2005;62:488–98.

36. Prasad GA, Wang KK, Buttar NS, et al. Long-term survival following endoscopic and surgical treatment of high-grade dysplasia in Barrett's esophagus. Gastroenterology 2007;132:1226–33.

37. Bronner MP, Overholt BF, Taylor SL, et al. Squamous overgrowth is not a safety concern for photodynamic therapy for Barrett's esophagus with high-grade dysplasia. Gastroenterology 2009;136:56–64.

38. Attwood SE, Lewis CJ, Caplin S, et al. Argon beam plasma coagulation as therapy for high-grade dysplasia in Barrett's esophagus. Clin Gastroenterol Hepatol 2003;1:258–63.

39. Shaheen NJ, Sharma P, Overholt BF, et al. Radiofrequency ablation in Barrett's esophagus with dysplasia. N Engl J Med 2009;360:2277–88.

40. Shaheen NJ, Sharma P, Overholt BF, et al. Durability of radiofrequency ablation in Barrett's esophagus with dysplasia. Gastroenterology 2011;142: 460–8.

41. Pouw RE, Gondrie JJ, Rygiel AM, et al. Properties of the neosquamous epithelium after radiofrequency ablation of Barrett's esophagus containing neoplasia. Am J Gastroenterol 2009;104(6):1366–73.

42. Fleischer DE, Overholt BF, Sharma VK, et al. Endoscopic radiofrequency ablation for Barrett's esophagus: 5-year outcomes from a prospective multicenter trial. Endoscopy 2010;42:781–9.

43. Pouw RE, Gondrie JJ, Sondermeijer CM, et al. Eradication of Barrett's esophagus with early neoplasia by radiofrequency ablation with or without endoscopic resection. J Gastrointest Surg 2008;12:1627–36.

44. Herrero LA, van Vilsteren FG, Pouw RE, et al. Endoscopic radiofrequency ablation combined with endoscopic resection for Barrett's esophagus with early neoplasia. Gastrointest Endosc 2011;73:682–90.

45. Vaccaro BJ, Gonzalez S, Poneros J, et al. Detection of intestinal metaplasia after successful eradication of Barrett's esophagus with radiofrequency ablation. Dig Dis Sci 2011;56:1996–2000.

46. Orman ES, Kim HP, Bulsiewicz WJ, et al. Intestinal metaplasia recurs infrequently in patients successfully treated for Barrett's esophagus with radiofrequency ablation. Am J Gastroenterol 2013;108:187–95.

47. Titi M, Overhiser A, Ulusarac O, et al. Development of subsquamous high-grade dysplasia and adenocarcinoma after successful radiofrequency ablation of Barrett's esophagus. Gastroenterology 2012;143:564–6.

48. Adler DC, Zhou C, Tsai TH, et al. Three-dimensional optical coherence tomography of Barrett's esophagus and buried glands beneath neosquamous epithelium following radiofrequency ablation. Endoscopy 2009;41:773–6.

49. Pouw RE, Bergman JJ. Biased assessment of 3D optical coherence tomography in a single post-radiofrequency ablation patient without histological correlation. Endoscopy 2010;42:179–80.

50. Cobb MJ, Hwang JH, Upton MP, et al. Imaging of subsquamous Barrett's epithelium with ultrahigh-resolution optical coherence tomography: a histologic correlation study. Gastrointest Endosc 2010;71:223–30.

51. Zhou C, Tsai TH, Lee HC, et al. Characterization of buried glands before and after radiofrequency ablation by using 3-dimensional optical coherence tomography (with videos). Gastrointest Endosc 2012;76:32–40.

52. Tsai TH, Zhou C, Tao YK, et al. Structural markers observed with endoscopic 3-dimensional optical coherence tomography correlating with Barrett's

esophagus radiofrequency ablation treatment response (with videos). Gastroint-est Endosc 2012;76:104–12.

53. Peery AF, Shaheen NJ. Optical coherence tomography in Barrett's esophagus: the road to clinical utility. Gastrointest Endosc 2010;71:231–4.
54. de Boer JF, Cense B, Park BH, et al. Improved signal to noise ratio in spectral domain compared with time-domain optical coherence tomography. Opt Lett 2003;28:2067–9.
55. Choma M, Sarunic M, Yang C, et al. Sensitivity advantage of swept source and Fourier domain optical coherence tomography. Opt Express 2003;11:2183–9.
56. Yun S, Tearney G, Bouma B, et al. High-speed spectral domain optical coher-ence tomography at 1.3 mum wavelength. Opt Express 2003;11:3598–604.
57. Vakoc BJ, Shishko M, Yun SH, et al. Comprehensive esophageal microscopy by using optical frequency-domain imaging (with video). Gastrointest Endosc 2007;65:898–905.
58. Bouma BE, Yun SJ, Vakoc BJ, et al. Fourier-domain optical coherence tomogra-phy: recent advances toward clinical utility. Curr Opin Biotechnol 2009;20: 111–8.
59. Yun SH, Tearney GJ, Vakoc BJ, et al. Comprehensive volumetric optical micro-scopy in vivo. Nat Med 2006;12:1429–33.
60. Carignan CS, Yagi Y. Optical endomicroscopy and the road to real-time, in vivo pathology: present and future. Diagn Pathol 2012;7:98.
61. Suter MJ, Vakoc BJ, Yachimski PS, et al. Comprehensive microscopy of the esophagus in human patients with optical frequency domain imaging. Gastroint-est Endosc 2008;68:745–53.
62. Suter MJ, Jillella PA, Vakoc BJ, et al. Image-guided biopsy in the esophagus through comprehensive optical frequency domain imaging and laser marking: a study in living swine. Gastrointest Endosc 2010;71:346–53.
63. Ramirez FC, Shaukat MS, Young MA, et al. Feasibility and safety of string, wire-less capsule endoscopy in the diagnosis of Barrett's esophagus. Gastrointest Endosc 2005;61:741–6.
64. Kadri SR, Lao-Sirieix P, O'Donovan M, et al. Acceptability and accuracy of a non-endoscopic screening test for Barrett's oesophagus in primary care: cohort study. BMJ 2010;341:4372.
65. Gora MJ, Sauk JS, Caarruth RW, et al. Tethered capsule endomicroscopy enables less invasive imaging of gastrointestinal tract microstructure. Nat Med 2013;19(2):238–40.

Endomicroscopy in Barrett's Esophagus

Kerry B. Dunbar, MD, PhD

KEYWORDS

- Confocal laser endomicroscopy • Confocal endomicroscopy
- Confocal microendoscopy • Barrett's esophagus • Esophageal imaging
- Barrett's neoplasia • Esophageal adenocarcinoma

KEY POINTS

- Confocal laser endomicroscopy (CLE) allows in vivo imaging of the epithelium during endoscopic procedures, providing 1000-fold magnification of the gastrointestinal mucosa.
- Two CLE platforms are currently available, endoscope-based CLE and probe-based CLE, which have both been used in multiple studies of Barrett's esophagus.
- CLE has good sensitivity, specificity, and accuracy for identifying neoplasia in patients with Barrett's esophagus.

INTRODUCTION

Confocal laser endomicroscopy (CLE) can provide live histology during the endoscopic examination, and thus has been the focus of numerous studies of mucosal gastrointestinal (GI) diseases. Barrett's esophagus (BE), the predominant risk factor for esophageal adenocarcinoma, has been a major focus of endoscopic imaging research. Surveillance of BE for development of neoplasia is recommended by all GI societies, with upper endoscopy with biopsy using a high-definition (HD) or a high-resolution endoscope (HRE) as the current standard of care.[1-3] However, the current standard of dysplasia surveillance has a low yield related to the focal nature of dysplasia and sampling error. Small areas of dysplasia are often difficult to identify, generating interest in new endoscopic imaging techniques.[4-6] CLE provides a magnification of 1000-fold allowing visualization of cells, capillaries, and the glandular architecture of BE, and has been evaluated in multiple studies of patients with BE.[7,8]

EQUIPMENT

There are two CLE platforms available: endoscope-based endomicroscopy (eCLE) and probe-based endomicroscopy (pCLE). Both systems provide 1000-fold

No disclosures.
VA North Texas Healthcare System – Dallas VA Medical Center, University of Texas Southwestern Medical Center, 4500 South Lancaster Road, Dallas, TX 75216, USA
E-mail address: Kerry.Dunbar@utsouthwestern.edu

Gastrointest Endoscopy Clin N Am 23 (2013) 565–579
http://dx.doi.org/10.1016/j.giec.2013.03.003
1052-5157/13/$ – see front matter Published by Elsevier Inc.

giendo.theclinics.com

magnification and use a laser with a wavelength of 488 nm (blue light). Images are acquired by placing the probe or endoscope tip on the mucosal surface and both systems use a separate screen to view the microscopic images, which can be saved and later exported as needed.

The pCLE system (Cellvizio; Mauna Kea Technologies, Paris, France) involves a flexible fiber-bundle probe, which can be inserted through the biopsy channel of most endoscopes. The Gastroflex UHD, the higher-resolution probe used in most recent studies of BE, has field of view of 240 μm, a resolution of 1 μm, and an imaging depth of 55 to 65 μm from the surface. The standard Gastroflex probe has a field of view of 600 μm and a resolution of 3.5 μm, with an imaging depth of 70 to 130 μm. pCLE images are acquired at a rate of 12 images per second, and images can be painted together using the mosaic function, giving a larger field of view.

The eCLE system (Pentax Medical Corporation, Tokyo, Japan) includes a microscope built into the end of a standard-resolution white-light endoscope. The field of view is 475 × 475 μm, with a lateral resolution of 0.7 μm and axial resolution of 1 μm. Pushing a button on the handle of the endoscope can change the depth of imaging, ranging from the mucosal surface to a depth of 250 μm. The imaging rate can be set to either 0.8 or 1.6 images per second.

CONTRAST AGENTS

Images are generated during confocal endomicroscopy when the laser reflects off the tissue of interest. Because of limited natural tissue fluorescence at the laser wavelength used for CLE, a fluorescent contrast agent is required for endomicroscopic imaging. Several contrast agents have been used, including intravenous fluorescein sodium, topical acriflavine hydrochloride, and topical cresyl violet.

Most CLE studies of BE have used intravenous fluorescein sodium for contrast, which is approved by the Food and Drug Administration for retinal angiography, and thus use in endomicroscopy is off-label. Fluorescein dosing varies by the CLE platform being used, but most published eCLE studies use 5 mL of 10% fluorescein sodium and the pCLE studies published have used either 2.5 mL of 10% fluorescein sodium or 0.1 mL/kg of 1% fluorescein sodium.[7-11] Fluorescein highlights the lamina propria, intercellular spaces, and fills the capillaries, but does not stain nuclei. A review of the safety of fluorescein in endomicroscopy has been published, which cataloged the adverse events from 16 academic medical centers where 2272 CLE procedures had been performed.[12] The most common side effects were nausea, transient hypotension, injection site erythema, self-limited diffuse rash, and mild epigastric pain, for an overall adverse event rate of 1.4%. No cases of anaphylaxis were reported, which has occurred rarely with fluorescein use in ophthalmologic procedures.[13] Most patients have temporary yellowing of the skin, eyes, and urine, which resolves in several hours.

Acriflavine hydrochloride 0.05% is a topical contrast agent applied with a spray catheter. It stains the nuclei of cells and provides imaging on the surface, but not of the deeper mucosa, and has predominantly been used in CLE studies of the colon.[14,15] Cresyl violet (0.13%–0.25%) is another topical contrast agent, which can be used for white-light chromoendoscopy and endomicroscopy.[16,17] Cresyl violet highlights the cytoplasm, causing the nuclei to appear dark.

TECHNIQUE

CLE has been used in numerous studies of BE and other GI disorders. Informed consent involves the usual risks and benefits of an endoscopic procedure, with additional discussion of the use of intravenous fluorescein sodium as a contrast agent. The risks of fluorescein were previously detailed, and most published research studies have excluded patients with a known fluorescein allergy and pregnant or lactating women.[7,8] During the endomicroscopy procedure, a standard white-light endoscopic (WLE) examination is performed, using either the eCLE endoscope or the endoscope to be used with the pCLE probe. Areas of interest are located, and then the contrast agent is applied (most often intravenous fluorescein sodium). The tip of the eCLE scope or pCLE probe is placed gently on the mucosa of interest, and images are acquired. A stable position is important for image acquisition, which can be obtained during eCLE by using suction and during pCLE by use of a translucent cap on the end of the endoscope. CLE and white-light images can be saved for later review.

CLE IMAGE CLASSIFICATION SYSTEMS FOR BE

The first study of CLE in BE was published in 2006 by Kiesslich and colleagues.[7] In this study, 63 patients with BE underwent eCLE and the images were used to create the Confocal Barrett's Classification system for distinguishing among BE, neoplastic BE, and gastric mucosa. A detailed description of the endomicroscopy procedure was included, which formed the basis for subsequent studies using CLE. The Mainz Confocal Barrett's Classification uses cellular and vessel architecture to distinguish between types of epithelium found in the esophagus, for surface and deep mucosal imaging (**Fig. 1**). Gastric epithelium has a cobblestone appearance, round glandular openings, a regular pattern, and regular-shaped capillaries seen in the deep mucosa. Nondysplastic BE shows columnar mucosa with goblet cells, a villiform pattern, and regular-shaped capillaries in the upper and deep mucosa. Neoplastic BE shows irregularly shaped cells, black cells, much darker than surrounding tissue with irregular, leaking, capillaries in the upper and deep mucosal layer. Testing the new classification system using masked evaluation of eCLE images, the classification system predicted histology findings of BE with sensitivity of 98%, specificity of 94%, positive predictive value (PPV) of 97%, negative predictive value (NPV) of 96%, and accuracy of 97%. Neoplastic BE was predicted with a sensitivity of 93%, specificity of 98%, PPV of 93%, NPV of 98%, and accuracy of 97% (**Table 1**). Interobserver and intraobserver agreement were almost perfect using Landis and Koch kappa interpretation,[18] with kappa of 0.84 and 0.89, respectively (**Table 2**).

Since the introduction of pCLE, several studies have been performed to develop a classification system for pCLE images of BE and BE neoplasia. Technical differences between eCLE and pCLE imaging, such as differences in field of view size, resolution, and differences in depth of imaging, led to development of separate pCLE image criteria for BE. The first pCLE study of BE and BE-associated neoplasia was published in 2008.[19] Two academic centers enrolled patients with BE and BE neoplasia and performed pCLE. Mucosal biopsies were taken at pCLE imaging sites for histopathologic confirmation. Data from the first 15 patients enrolled were used to develop pCLE-specific interpretation criteria for BE and neoplasia by participating gastroenterologists and pathologists. They identified five features suggestive of BE neoplasia and determined that if at least two of the five features were present, neoplasia was likely. Criteria they developed to identify neoplasia included irregular epithelial lining, variable width of the epithelial lining, irregular vascular pattern, fusion of glands, and dark areas of the image, thought to be suggestive of decreased fluorescein uptake (**Table 3**). The criteria that were developed were then applied to evaluate the esophageal mucosa of the next 23 patients referred for BE evaluation. Performance

Confocal diagnosis	Vessel architecture	Image Examples Upper and deeper parts of the mucosal layer
Gastric type epithelium	Capillaries of regular shape only visible in deeper parts of the mucosal layer.	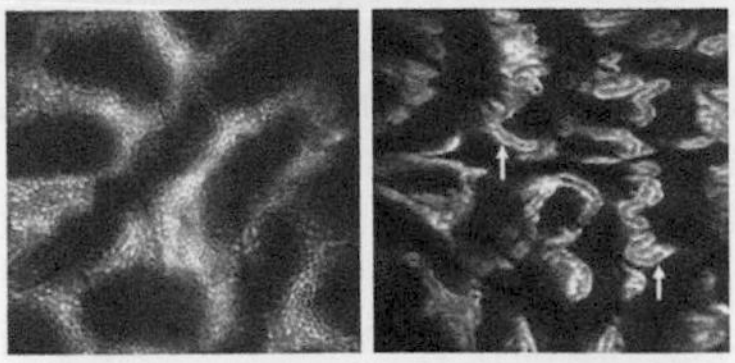
Barrett's epithelium	Subepithelial capillaries of regular shape beneath columnar lined epithelium visible in upper and deeper parts of the mucosal layer	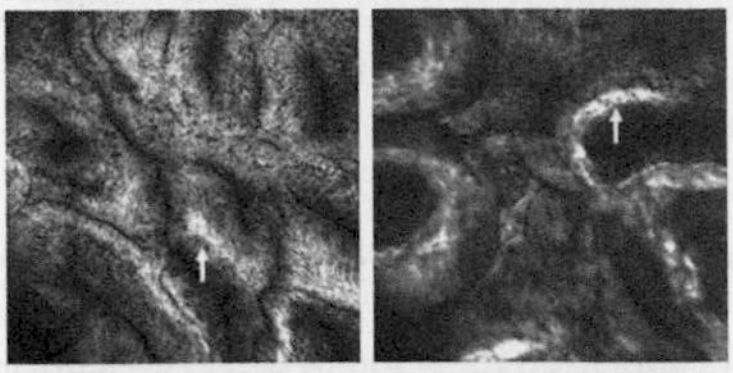
Neoplasia	Irregular capillaries visible in upper and deeper parts of the mucosal layer. Leakage of vessels leads to a heterogeneous and brighter signal intensity within the lamina propria.	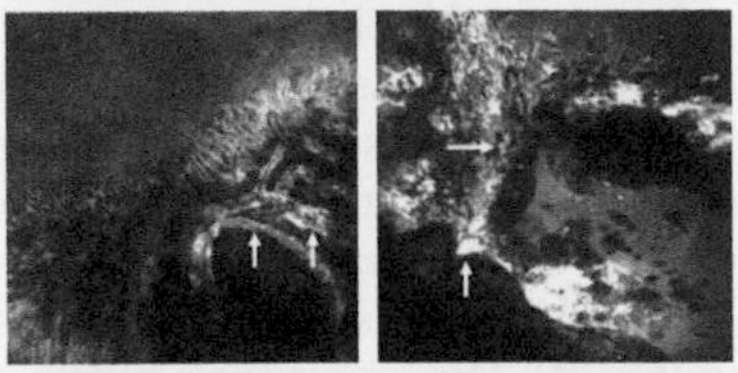
	Cell architecture	Image examples
Gastric type epithelium	Regular columnar lined epithelium with round glandular openings and typical cobble stone appearance	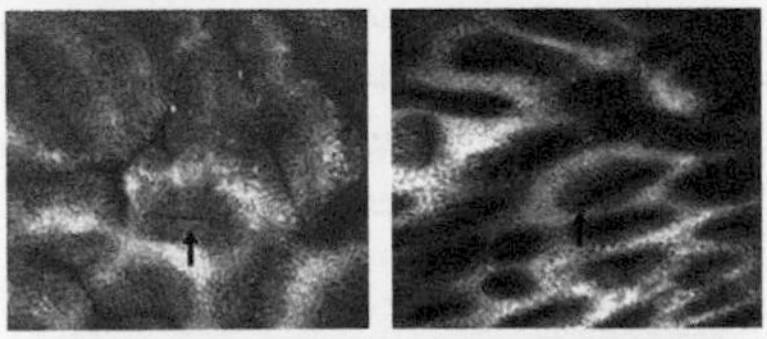
Barrett's epithelium	Columnar lined epithelium with in between dark mucin in goblet cells in upper parts of the mucosal layer. In deeper parts, villous like, dark shaped regular cylindrical Barrett's epithelial cells are present.	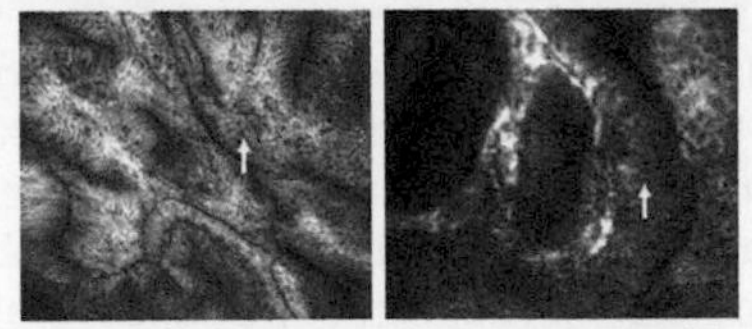
Neoplasia	Black cells with irregular apical and distal borders and shapes with high dark contrast to surrounded tissue	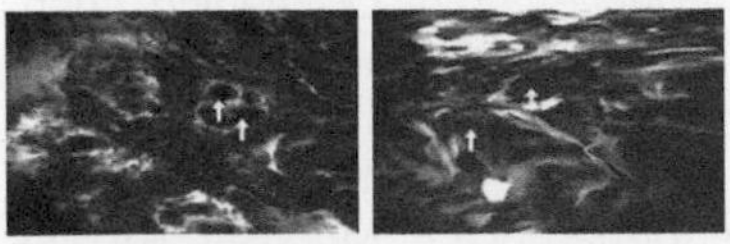

Fig. 1. Mainz confocal Barrett's classification system. (*From* Kiesslich R, Gossner L, Goetz M, et al. In vivo histology of Barrett's esophagus and associated neoplasia by confocal laser endomicroscopy. Clin Gastroenterol Hepatol 2006;4(8):984; with permission from Elsevier.)

characteristics for the two gastroenterologists using the pCLE classification for diagnosing high-grade intraepithelial neoplasia or early cancer included a sensitivity of 75%, specificity of 89% to 91%, PPV of 30% to 35%, NPV of 98%, and accuracy of 88% to 90% (see **Table 1**). The interobserver agreement was good, with a kappa

Table 1
Performance characteristics of CLE in studies of Barrett's esophagus

Modality	Year Published	Sensitivity	Specificity	Positive Predictive Value	Negative Predictive Value	Accuracy
eCLE: postprocedure interpretation[7] Per-image analysis	2006					
Nondysplastic BE		98%	94%	97%	96%	97%
Neoplastic BE		93%	98%	93%	98%	97%
pCLE: postprocedure interpretation[19] Per-image analysis	2008	75%	89%–91%	30%–35%	98%	88%–90%
pCLE: postprocedure interpretation[11] Per-image analysis	2010					
Endoscopists with pCLE experience		91%	100%			95%
Endoscopists inexperienced in pCLE		87%	94%			90%
pCLE: on-site (real-time) interpretation vs postprocedure interpretation[21]	2010					
Per-biopsy analysis						
On-site		12%	95%	18%	92%	NR
Masked		28%	97%	46%	93%	NR
Per-patient analysis						
On-site		60%	95%	67%	93%	NR
Masked		90%	59%	28%	97%	NR
pCLE: pCLE, NBI, HD-WLE, alone and in combination[8] Real-time interpretation	2011					
Per-location analysis						
HD-WLE		34%	93%	43%	90%	NR
HD-WLE + NBI		45%	88%	38%	91%	NR
HD-WLE + NBI + pCLE		76%	84%	43%	96%	NR
Per-patient analysis						
HD-WLE		87%	71%	57%	93%	NR
HD-WLE + NBI		97%	56%	49%	98%	NR
HD-WLE + NBI + pCLE		100%	56%	50%	100%	NR
pCLE: postprocedure review[10]	2011					
pCLE experts		75%	90%	82%	85%	84%
pCLE nonexperts		76%	81%	71%	85%	79%
pCLE: pCLE + HD-WLE[22] Real-time interpretation, per-patient analysis	2012	100%	83%	67%	100%	NR

(continued on next page)

Table 1
(continued)

Modality	Year Published	Sensitivity	Specificity	Positive Predictive Value	Negative Predictive Value	Accuracy
eCLE: sequential HD-WLE, NBI, eCLE[27] Real-time interpretation, per-location analysis	2012					
HD-WLE		79%	83%	28%	98%	83%
NBI		89%	81%	28%	99%	81%
eCLE		76%	80%	19%	98%	80%
eCLE: eCLE + HRE vs HRE alone[28] Real-time interpretation, per-biopsy analysis	2012					
HRE alone		36%	96%	38%	96%	93%
eCLE + HRE		75%	94%	73%	95%	91%

Studies using either eCLE or pCLE to detect BE-associated neoplasia.
Abbreviations: eCLE, endoscope-based endomicroscopy; HD-WLE, high-definition white-light endoscopy; NBI, narrow-band imaging; NR, not reported; pCLE, probe-based endomicroscopy.

of 0.6 (see **Table 2**). This initial study showed promise that neoplasia in BE could be detected with reasonable sensitivity and accuracy.

The pCLE criteria for diagnosis of BE neoplasia were further refined into the Miami classification of pCLE BE findings and tested in a subsequent study.[20] The interobserver agreement and accuracy of pCLE criteria was tested by a set of investigators, some with pCLE experience and the rest without specific pCLE experience.[11] They underwent structured training with pCLE images of dysplastic and nondysplastic BE, then applied the pCLE criteria to a test set of images. The criteria included irregular vessels; villi and crypt fusion; and three features associated with the epithelium (irregular epithelial thickness, epithelial inhomogeneity, and a dark epithelial border) (**Fig. 2**, see **Table 3**). Sensitivity for detection of neoplasia for the individual pCLE features ranged from 50% to 75%, with specificity of 93% to 97%. Applying the pCLE criteria to a test set of images, the investigators then compared image reviewers with pCLE experience with those without prior pCLE experience, which showed small differences

Table 2
Interobserver and intraobserver agreement for CLE image interpretation systems

Classification System	Interobserver Agreement	Intraobserver Agreement
eCLE: Mainz Confocal Barrett's Classification[7]	0.84	0.89
pCLE: initial pCLE BE paper[19]	0.6	NR
pCLE: Miami pCLE criteria[11]	0.83 (prior pCLE experience) 0.64 (inexperienced with pCLE)	NR
pCLE: KC Confocal criteria[10]	0.66 (pCLE experts) 0.56 (pCLE nonexperts)	NR

Abbreviations: eCLE, endoscope-based CLE; NR, not reported; pCLE, probe-based CLE.

Table 3
pCLE Barrett's esophagus image classification systems

Category of pCLE Finding	Original pCLE Criteria[19]	Miami pCLE Criteria[11]	KC pCLE Confocal Criteria[10]
Epithelial changes	Irregular epithelial lining Variable width epithelial lining	Epithelial inhomogeneity Irregular epithelial thickness Dark epithelial border	Saw-toothed epithelial surface
Vessel pattern	Irregular vascular pattern	Irregular vessels	
Glands	Fusion of glands	Fusion of villi and crypts	Unequal size and shape of glands Nonequidistant glands
Cells	Dark areas		Hard-to-identify goblet cells Pleomorphic cells Enlarged cells

Several image interpretation systems for pCLE images in Barrett's esophagus have been proposed. This table shows similarities and differences in the features addressed by each image classification system.

in performance characteristics. The sensitivity and specificity for investigators with pCLE experience was 91% and 100% compared with 87% and 94% for those less-experienced. The accuracy of the pCLE experts for diagnosis of neoplasia was 95%, compared with 90% for the inexperienced endomicroscopists (see **Table 1**). Interobserver agreement was also tested and found to be almost perfect (k = 0.83) for the experts and substantial (k = 0.64) for the less-experienced endomicroscopists (see **Table 2**).

A subsequent study was performed to determine criteria for pCLE image interpretation using a logistic regression model to identify image features that were most predictive of dysplasia, known as the KC Confocal Criteria.[10] This multipart study included development of criteria by an endomicroscopist and pathologist, based on 50 pCLE videos, followed by application to a test set of videos. Based on structured testing of the pCLE image features, the investigators selected criteria most sensitive for predicting of neoplasia, including unequal size and shape of glands, nonequidistant glands, hard-to-identify goblet cells, pleomorphic cells, enlarged cells, and a saw-toothed epithelial surface (see **Table 3**). Two or more of the criteria are needed to determine a diagnosis of dysplasia. The investigators then tested the criteria using expert and nonexpert endomicroscopists. For experts using the pCLE criteria, sensitivity for detection of neoplasia was 75%, specificity 90%, PPV 82%, NPV 85%, and accuracy 84%. For nonexperts, sensitivity for neoplasia was 76%, specificity 81%, PPV 71%, NPV 85%, with accuracy of 79% (see **Table 1**). Interobserver agreement using the criteria was substantial (k = 0.66) for experts and moderate (k = 0.56) for nonexperts (see **Table 2**).

With the Mainz Confocal Barrett's Classification System, the Miami pCLE, and the KC Confocal Criteria, BE with neoplasia can be readily identified. Expert and nonexpert users can apply the criteria to interpret endomicroscopic images of the esophagus. These image classification systems have been applied for clinical use and research studies of endomicroscopy in BE.

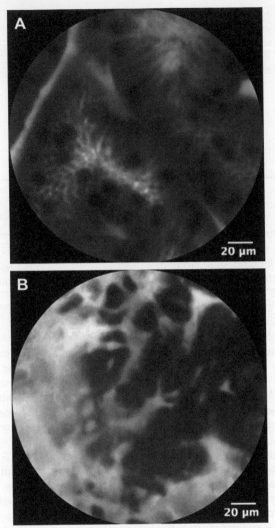

Fig. 2. pCLE images of Barrett's esophagus and Barrett's esophagus with neoplasia. (*A*) Shows Barrett's esophagus and (*B*) shows Barrett's esophagus with early adenocarcinoma. (*From* Sharma P, Meining AR, Coron E, et al. Real-time increased detection of neoplastic tissue in Barrett's esophagus with probe-based confocal laser endomicroscopy: final results of an international multicenter, prospective, randomized, controlled trial. Gastrointest Endosc 2011;74(3):469; with permission from Elsevier.)

STUDIES IN BE: ACCURACY FOR THE IDENTIFICATION OF DYSPLASIA

Since the original studies of eCLE and pCLE in BE, several studies have examined the ability of CLE to identify dysplasia in BE. One study of eCLE in BE addressed the issue of diagnostic yield, whether using eCLE would increase the yield for neoplasia compared with a standard endoscopic biopsy protocol.[9] In this crossover study, 23 patients referred for BE surveillance and 16 with suspected unlocalized neoplasia (biopsy suggestive of neoplasia, but no lesions or masses present) were enrolled. Each patient underwent standard endoscopy with four-quadrant biopsy protocol and eCLE with targeted biopsies, in randomized order. In the group of patients with suspected unlocalized neoplasia, the yield for neoplasia was 17% using standard endoscopy and 34% using eCLE to target biopsies, with 59% reduction in the number of mucosal biopsies needed for diagnosis. In the group referred for BE surveillance, there was an 87% reduction in the number of mucosal biopsies taken during eCLE compared with standard endoscopy, and two-thirds of the surveillance group had no mucosal biopsies taken during eCLE, because all their eCLE images showed non-dysplastic BE. This study suggested that compared with a standard endoscopic biopsy protocol, eCLE could be used to take targeted biopsies of BE and reduce the number of biopsies needed for a diagnosis of neoplasia.

In one study of pCLE, 68 patients with BE underwent endoscopy with pCLE and images were interpreted twice, first during the endoscopic procedure at the time of acquisition and then later were reviewed in a masked fashion.[21] The sites to be examined were marked with argon plasma coagulation (APC), pCLE image videos were acquired, and then biopsies were taken at the site to confirm the diagnosis. Performance characteristics were calculated for per-biopsy analysis and on a per-patient basis for pCLE image interpretation during the procedure and with later masked review. On-site review gave a per-biopsy sensitivity of 12%, specificity of 95%, PPV of 18%, and NPV of 92%. Post-procedure masked review improved the performance characteristics with sensitivity for neoplasia of 28%, specificity of 97%, PPV of 46%, and NPV of 93%. On a per-patient basis, on-site review had a sensitivity of 60%, specificity of 95%, PPV of 67%, and NPV of 93%. Masked review had sensitivity of 90%, specificity of 59%, PPV of 28%, and NPV of 97% (see **Table 1**). The authors concluded the NPV and specificity of pCLE for BE neoplasia were very good for both on-site and masked review, but further work was needed because the per-biopsy sensitivity and PPV were less than expected.

One recent study of detection of dysplasia using high-definition (HD) WLE and pCLE looked at patients with BE scheduled for surveillance endoscopy.[22] Participants were randomized to HD-WLE targeted biopsies or HD-WLE with pCLE. All patients then had four-quadrant random biopsies every 1 cm. Fifty patients were randomized to HD-WLE alone and 50 to HD-WLE with pCLE. Using pCLE, 42% of patients had imaging findings suggestive of neoplasia, with final pathology showing that 4% of patients in this group had high-grade dysplasia (HGD) and 24% had low-grade dysplasia (LGD). The authors report the detection rate for neoplasia using pCLE of 28% (2 with HGD, 12 with LGD) and HD-WLE of 10% (one case HGD, nine cases LGD) ($P = .04$), with a similar mean number of mucosal biopsies acquired in each group. Additionally, they calculated per-patient performance characteristics for pCLE detection of dysplasia of 100% sensitivity, 83% specificity, 67% PPV, and 100% NPV (see **Table 1**). No performance characteristics were reported for the HD-WLE alone group. This study had a high rate of suspected neoplasia (42%) using pCLE, whereas the actual rate of neoplasia found on mucosal biopsy was lower, but overall had good sensitivity and NPV for neoplasia detection. This study supports the role that CLE may play in patients with BE.

CLE provides excellent accuracy for identification of neoplasia in BE. There is some variability in performance characteristics between studies, which may be affected by the variable prevalence of neoplasia in these studies, but overall the outcomes have been good. Other studies have addressed the next step in new technology evaluation: what is the clinical impact of CLE in patients with BE?

ASSESSING THE POTENTIAL IMPACT OF CLE IN BE

Ideally, a novel imaging technique, such as CLE, would provide additional detection of neoplasia; reduce the number of biopsies taken of normal mucosa or nondysplastic

BE; and could be used to guide therapy, such as determining where an endoscopic mucosal resection (EMR) should be performed. Several case series and research studies have attempted to address the additional benefit of adding CLE to an endoscopic procedure for BE.

Several case reports and case series have used CLE to guide endoscopic therapy. One report discusses the use of eCLE to identify an area of flat HGD, for which an immediate EMR was performed, confirming the diagnosis.[23] Another case report used eCLE to examine an area of the esophagus previously treated with radiofrequency ablation (RFA), identifying the neosquamous mucosa and the untreated area of residual BE.[24] In one series of patients with BE neoplasia, pCLE was performed before endoscopic therapy (EMR or RFA).[25] Of seven patients with BE neoplasia who underwent pCLE, pCLE confirmed the diagnosis of HGD suspected on narrow-band imaging (NBI) in three patients, and influenced the management of one patient by leading to additional EMRs for neoplasia. Another case series reported four patients with neoplastic BE who underwent pCLE-guided endoscopic therapy.[26] In this series, the authors successfully used pCLE to examine EMR margins and the margins of areas treated with RFA. This led to additional EMR of residual neoplasia at the margin of an EMR in one case, and confirmation of negative margins in other cases.

One recently published research study assessed the added benefit of eCLE to HD-WLE and NBI, and enrolled 50 patients referred for evaluation and treatment of BE with dysplasia.[27] The patients were examined sequentially with HD-WLE, NBI, and then with eCLE, with the endoscopist predicting the histology at each stage of the examination. Imaging sites in the esophagus were marked for examination using APC and mucosal biopsies were acquired at each of the sites. Performance characteristics were calculated using mucosal histopathology as the reference standard. Sensitivity for detection of neoplasia using HD-WLE was 79%, with NBI it was 89%, and using eCLE it was 76% (see **Table 1**). Specificity for detection of neoplasia using HD-WLE, NBI, and eCLE was 83%, 81%, and 80%, respectively. No cases of intramucosal cancer were missed using any of the three imaging modalities. The authors also addressed the additional clinical benefit of adding NBI and CLE to HD-WLE and found that the most locations containing HGD or intramucosal cancer were detected when all three modalities were used. The addition of eCLE to HD-WLE and NBI detected one additional site of HGD, but this patient had HGD in another area of the esophagus seen by NBI, thus the authors concluded that the incremental benefit of adding endomicroscopy was not significant.

Two large multicenter studies have addressed the potential effect of CLE on management of patients with BE, but with more positive results. The interim results of a large multicenter international study of eCLE in BE have been reported, which addressed the real-time clinical impact of adding eCLE to HRE.[28] Patients with BE (N = 134) and suspected BE neoplasia (N = 44) were randomized to either HRE alone or HRE with eCLE and targeted mucosal biopsies. All patients had HRE and the endoscopist predicted the histology based on HRE examination and documented what the plan would be for each site examined, including the option to take a biopsy or perform an EMR. Patients randomized to the CLE group then had eCLE and the endoscopist's prediction of histology at each site was made using the Mainz Confocal Barrett's Classification. Mucosal biopsies were only acquired in areas where the eCLE imaging was abnormal. The overall diagnostic yield for neoplasia was 46% using HRE + eCLE compared with 8.8% for HRE alone (P<.001). Fewer biopsies were needed to make a diagnosis of neoplasia using eCLE. The per-biopsy sensitivity for neoplasia was 36% using HRE alone and 75% using HRE + eCLE. Specificity was 96% for HRE and 94% for HRE + eCLE. Examining small lesions found during the study, adding eCLE to HRE changed the diagnosis in 54% of cases and altered the treatment plan (biopsy vs EMR vs no intervention) in 35% of patients, suggesting that eCLE may have a role in impacting the management of patients with BE. Final results of the study are expected this year.

A large multicenter study of pCLE in BE examined the added benefit of pCLE to HD-WLE compared with HD-WLE and NBI.[8] The study enrolled 101 patients with BE or BE neoplasia who underwent HD-WLE, followed by NBI, and then pCLE. During the procedure, the endoscopist predicted the histology based on each imaging modality. Mucosal biopsies were acquired at each imaging location, which was marked with APC for accuracy. The per-location sensitivity for detection of neoplasia with HD-WLE alone was 34% with specificity of 93%. The addition of NBI to HD-WLE improved the sensitivity for detection of neoplasia to 45% and specificity decreased slightly to 88%. Adding pCLE to the other two modalities, the sensitivity for neoplasia was 76% with specificity of 84%, which generated a PPV of 43% and NPV of 96%. Per-patient analysis showed a sensitivity of 87% and specificity of 71% for HD-WLE alone. Adding NBI increased the sensitivity to 97% and decreased the specificity to 67%. Adding pCLE to HD-WLE and NBI increased the per-patient sensitivity for neoplasia to 100%, with a specificity of 56%. CLE also detected neoplasia in two patients that was missed using high-definition endoscopy alone. Overall, adding pCLE to HD-WLE and NBI increased the sensitivity of neoplasia detection.

Another potential role for CLE is assessing areas treated with ablative therapies in BE to look for residual dysplasia. An elegantly designed, multicenter randomized controlled trial was recently published that addressed this issue, whether pCLE could guide treatment of BE in patients undergoing ablative therapies.[29] In particular, the authors wanted to compare whether HD-WLE or HD-WLE with pCLE could guide therapy, reducing overtreatment or undertreatment of patients. They defined their outcome as the proportion of optimally treated patients, who were patients who had residual BE after ablation and were appropriately treated leading to complete ablation, or who had no BE, were not treated, and had no residual BE or dysplasia on follow-up endoscopy. The study enrolled patients with BE with or without dysplasia who were undergoing ablative therapy with RFA, photodynamic therapy, EMR, cryotherapy, or combination therapy. When patients returned for follow-up endoscopy after ablation, they were randomized to HD-WLE or HD-WLE with pCLE and underwent EGD to assess for residual BE or neoplasia. The endoscopist made a presumptive diagnosis of tissue type (ie, BE, dysplasia, and so forth) based on the HD-WLE findings. For patients in the pCLE group, the endoscopist also made a pCLE diagnosis for the sites examined. Mucosal biopsies were taken for histopathology confirmation. Patients with possible residual BE or neoplasia then underwent ablative therapy. Follow-up endoscopy with additional biopsies was performed 3 months later to assess completeness of treatment. The pathology results from the mucosal biopsies were used to see if overtreatment (ablation performed when no residual BE or neoplasia present) or undertreatment (no ablation performed but residual BE/neoplasia present) had occurred. Unfortunately, the study was halted after a planned interim analysis because of low conditional power, a result of finding no difference in optimal treatment rates between HD-WLE and HD-WLE with pCLE, a low rate of optimal treatment, and a higher-than-expected dropout rate. Another factors that the authors suggest contributed to the study outcome included the challenge of distinguishing nondysplastic BE from gastric metaplasia in the presence of postablation inflammation. With increased identification of early BE neoplasia through surveillance programs and successful BE ablation programs, assessment of treatment effect would be an ideal role for the instant histopathology that CLE can provide. However, further development of the technology and better understanding of the changes in postablation mucosa are needed for CLE to be of benefit in this role.

Several multicenter studies of CLE have started to address the impact of CLE on the care of patients with BE. Based on these studies, CLE may have a role in identifying flat neoplasia not identified by other endoscopic modalities. Imaging findings on CLE may also be used to guide therapy, such as performing an immediate EMR for flat neoplasia. Potential improvements in CLE technology could lead better identification of neoplasia and ease of use.

FUTURE DEVELOPMENTS IN CLE

New developments in CLE include development of new contrast agents and improved endomicroscopes. One new potential endomicroscopy contrast agent is fluorescent deoxyglucose, also known as 2-NBDG. In one preclinical study, biopsies from 26 patients with BE and BE neoplasia were treated with 2-NBDG and imaged with a fluorescent confocal microscope.[30] Neoplastic BE showed more fluorescence than nonneoplastic BE, which was measured quantitatively. Using the mean fluorescence intensity of the biopsy, neoplasia could be identified with a sensitivity of 96% and specificity of 90%.

2-NBDG has also been investigated in a study of patients undergoing EMR for BE neoplasia.[31] In this study, EMR specimens from patients with BE were treated with 2-NBDG, and confocal imaging was performed using pCLE and a hand-held probe related to eCLE called the Five-1. The images acquired by each endomicroscopy system were then evaluated by three investigators using the Mainz eCLE classification system, Miami pCLE classification, and a new simplified classification system, the fluorescence intensity criteria classification. The fluorescence intensity criteria includes features of normal mucosa (organized cellular architecture with no intracellular fluorescence); nondysplastic BE (organized cellular architecture and minimal intracellular fluorescence); and dysplasia (heterogeneous cell size with intense intracellular fluorescence, and disorganized cellular architecture). Using these criteria for identifying dysplasia, the fluorescence intensity criteria had an interobserver agreement that was almost perfect, with a kappa of 0.87, whereas the Mainz criteria showed substantial agreement (k = 0.68) and Miami pCLE criteria showed slight agreement (k = 0.17). Accuracy for identification of neoplasia was highest with the fluorescence intensity criteria (79%). Further investigation of 2-NBDG as a contrast agent and evaluation of the fluorescence intensity criteria should be considered, and in vivo evaluation of the fluorescence intensity criteria is needed before it can be used widely for in vivo BE image interpretation.

Another approach to identifying neoplasia in BE is to use a targeting antibody or peptide. An anti-EGFR antibody has been developed that binds to colonic neoplasia, but no targeting antibodies have been developed for BE neoplasia.[32] A small fluorescent-labeled peptide specific for neoplastic BE has also been developed and tested in EMR specimens.[33] The fluorescence intensity was measured for each specimen and was found to be highest in neoplastic BE tissue and lowest in squamous and gastric mucosa. Fluorescent-bound lectins, applied topically, have also been found to bind preferentially to dysplasia in BE in biopsy specimens and in esophagus specimens removed during esophagectomy.[34] These new contrast agents specific for neoplasia have the potential to help better identify dysplasia in patients with BE.

New types of endomicroscopy are also in development. Reflectance confocal microscopy, also known as "spectrally encoded confocal microscopy," has been used in ex vivo studies to image the GI mucosa, including the esophagus.[35] This technique uses scattered light to create images of the GI mucosa and no contrast agent is needed. This technique is an ex vivo research tool, but could potentially be developed for in vivo use in the future.

A low-cost endomicroscope probe, called high-resolution microendoscopy (HRME), has been developed and can be used with topical contrast agents, such as acriflavine or proflavine. The HRME probe can pass through the biopsy channel of an endoscope, provides 400-fold magnification, a field of view of 720 μm, and a resolution of 4.4 μm. Initially tested on biopsy and EMR specimens, and now used in research studies of patients with BE and other GI disorders, HRME provides visualization of microscopic histopathology, with clear differentiation between dysplastic and normal tissue.[36,37] With new endomicroscopes and advent of contrast agents that selectively target dysplasia, endomicroscopy will continue to develop as a tool for assessment of BE.

SUMMARY

BE presents a challenge for the endoscopist, because neoplasia can be subtle and difficult to detect, requiring numerous biopsies of nondysplastic BE. CLE, whether endoscope- or probe-based, can identify changes of early neoplasia in BE, and has the potential to improve care of patients with BE. The role of CLE in management of patients with BE is evolving, but there are several potential benefits for patients. Real-time histopathology results could lead to immediate treatment of dysplasia, such as same-session EMR or ablative therapy. The potential to avoid biopsy of normal or nondysplastic BE is also possible using CLE. Improved technology and contrast agents that better highlight dysplasia are also a focus of research. These factors will help establish the role of CLE in the care of patients with BE.

REFERENCES

1. Spechler SJ, Sharma P, Souza RF, et al. American Gastroenterological Association medical position statement on the management of Barrett's esophagus. Gastroenterology 2011;140:1084–91.
2. Wang KK, Sampliner RE. Updated guidelines 2008 for the diagnosis, surveillance and therapy of Barrett's esophagus. Am J Gastroenterol 2008;103:788–97.
3. Hirota WK, Zuckerman MJ, Adler DG, et al. ASGE guideline: the role of endoscopy in the surveillance of premalignant conditions of the upper GI tract. Gastrointest Endosc 2006;63:570–80.
4. Cameron AJ, Carpenter HA. Barrett's esophagus, high-grade dysplasia, and early adenocarcinoma: a pathological study. Am J Gastroenterol 1997;92:586–91.
5. Konda VJ, Ross AS, Ferguson MK, et al. Is the risk of concomitant invasive esophageal cancer in high-grade dysplasia in Barrett's esophagus overestimated? Clin Gastroenterol Hepatol 2008;6:159–64.
6. Curvers WL, van Vilsteren FG, Baak LC, et al. Endoscopic trimodal imaging versus standard video endoscopy for detection of early Barrett's neoplasia: a multicenter, randomized, crossover study in general practice. Gastrointest Endosc 2011;73:195–203.
7. Kiesslich R, Gossner L, Goetz M, et al. In vivo histology of Barrett's esophagus and associated neoplasia by confocal laser endomicroscopy. Clin Gastroenterol Hepatol 2006;4:979–87.
8. Sharma P, Meining AR, Coron E, et al. Real-time increased detection of neoplastic tissue in Barrett's esophagus with probe-based confocal laser

endomicroscopy: final results of an international multicenter, prospective, randomized, controlled trial. Gastrointest Endosc 2011;74:465–72.

9. Dunbar KB, Okolo P III, Montgomery E, et al. Confocal laser endomicroscopy in Barrett's esophagus and endoscopically inapparent Barrett's neoplasia: a prospective, randomized, double-blind, controlled, crossover trial. Gastrointest Endosc 2009;70:645–54.

10. Gaddam S, Mathur SC, Singh M, et al. Novel probe-based confocal laser endomicroscopy criteria and interobserver agreement for the detection of dysplasia in Barrett's esophagus. Am J Gastroenterol 2011;106:1961–9.

11. Wallace MB, Sharma P, Lightdale C, et al. Preliminary accuracy and interobserver agreement for the detection of intraepithelial neoplasia in Barrett's esophagus with probe-based confocal laser endomicroscopy. Gastrointest Endosc 2010; 72:19–24.

12. Wallace MB, Meining A, Canto MI, et al. Review article: safety of intravenous fluorescein for confocal laser endomicroscopy in the gastrointestinal tract. Aliment Pharmacol Ther 2010;31(5):548–52.

13. Lipson BK, Yannuzzi LA. Complications of intravenous fluorescein injections. Int Ophthalmol Clin 1989;29:200–5.

14. Sanduleanu S, Driessen A, Gomez-Garcia E, et al. In vivo diagnosis and classification of colorectal neoplasia by chromoendoscopy-guided confocal laser endomicroscopy. Clin Gastroenterol Hepatol 2010;8:371–8.

15. Kiesslich R, Burg J, Vieth M, et al. Confocal laser endoscopy for diagnosing intraepithelial neoplasias and colorectal cancer in vivo. Gastroenterology 2004;127:706–13.

16. Goetz M, Toermer T, Vieth M, et al. Simultaneous confocal laser endomicroscopy and chromoendoscopy with topical cresyl violet. Gastrointest Endosc 2009;70:959–68.

17. Meining A, Saur D, Bajbouj M, et al. In vivo histopathology for detection of gastrointestinal neoplasia with a portable, confocal miniprobe: an examiner blinded analysis. Clin Gastroenterol Hepatol 2007;5:1261–7.

18. Landis JR, Koch GG. An application of hierarchical kappa-type statistics in the assessment of majority agreement among multiple observers. Biometrics 1977; 33:363–74.

19. Pohl H, Rosch T, Vieth M, et al. Miniprobe confocal laser microscopy for the detection of invisible neoplasia in patients with Barrett's oesophagus. Gut 2008; 57:1648–53.

20. Wallace M, Lauwers GY, Chen Y, et al. Miami classification for probe-based confocal laser endomicroscopy. Endoscopy 2011;43:882–91.

21. Bajbouj M, Vieth M, Rosch T, et al. Probe-based confocal laser endomicroscopy compared with standard four-quadrant biopsy for evaluation of neoplasia in Barrett's esophagus. Endoscopy 2010;42:435–40.

22. Bertani H, Frazzoni M, Dabizzi E, et al. Improved detection of incident dysplasia by probe-based confocal laser endomicroscopy in a Barrett's esophagus surveillance program. Dig Dis Sci 2013;58(1):188–93.

23. Leung KK, Maru D, Abraham S, et al. Optical EMR: confocal endomicroscopy-targeted EMR of focal high-grade dysplasia in Barrett's esophagus. Gastrointest Endosc 2009;69:170–2.

24. Diamantis G, Bocus P, Realdon S, et al. Role of confocal laser endomicroscopy in detection of residual Barrett's esophagus after radiofrequency ablation. Case Rep Gastrointest Med 2011;2011:593923.

25. Konda VJ, Chennat JS, Hart J, et al. Confocal laser endomicroscopy: potential in the management of Barrett's esophagus. Dis Esophagus 2010;23:E21–31.

26. Johnson EA, De Lee R, Agni R, et al. Probe-based confocal laser endomicroscopy to guide real-time endoscopic therapy in Barrett's esophagus with dysplasia. Case Rep Gastroenterol 2012;6:285–92.

27. Jayasekera C, Taylor AC, Desmond PV, et al. Added value of narrow band imaging and confocal laser endomicroscopy in detecting Barrett's esophagus neoplasia. Endoscopy 2012;44:1089–95.

28. Canto M, Anandasabapathy S, Brugge WR, et al. In vivo endoscope-based confocal laser endomicroscopy (eCLE) improves detection of unlocalized Barrett's esophagus-related neoplasia over high resolution white light endoscopy: an international multicenter randomized controlled trial. Gastrointest Endosc 2012; 75:AB174.

29. Wallace MB, Crook JE, Saunders M, et al. Multicenter, randomized, controlled trial of confocal laser endomicroscopy assessment of residual metaplasia after mucosal ablation or resection of GI neoplasia in Barrett's esophagus. Gastrointest Endosc 2012;76:539–547.e1.

30. Thekkek N, Maru DM, Polydorides AD, et al. Pre-clinical evaluation of fluorescent deoxyglucose as a topical contrast agent for the detection of Barrett's-associated neoplasia during confocal imaging. Technol Cancer Res Treat 2011;10:431–41.

31. Gorospe EC, Leggett CL, Sun G, et al. Diagnostic performance of two confocal endomicroscopy systems in detecting Barrett's dysplasia: a pilot study using a novel bioprobe in ex vivo tissue. Gastrointest Endosc 2012;76:933–8.

32. Liu J, Zuo X, Li C, et al. In vivo molecular imaging of epidermal growth factor receptor in patients with colorectal neoplasia using confocal laser endomicroscopy. Cancer Lett 2013;330(2):200–7.

33. Li M, Anastassiades CP, Joshi B, et al. Affinity peptide for targeted detection of dysplasia in Barrett's esophagus. Gastroenterology 2010;139:1472–80.

34. Bird-Lieberman EL, Neves AA, Lao-Sirieix P, et al. Molecular imaging using fluorescent lectins permits rapid endoscopic identification of dysplasia in Barrett's esophagus. Nat Med 2012;18:315–21.

35. Kang D, Suter MJ, Boudoux C, et al. Comprehensive imaging of gastroesophageal biopsy samples by spectrally encoded confocal microscopy. Gastrointest Endosc 2010;71:35–43.

36. Muldoon TJ, Anandasabapathy S, Maru D, et al. High-resolution imaging in Barrett's esophagus: a novel, low-cost endoscopic microscope. Gastrointest Endosc 2008;68:737–44.

37. Pierce MC, Vila PM, Polydorides AD, et al. Low-cost endomicroscopy in the esophagus and colon. Am J Gastroenterol 2011;106:1722–4.

Red-Flag Technologies in Gastric Neoplasia

Susana Gonzalez, MD

KEYWORDS

- Gastric cancer • Narrow-band imaging • Magnification narrow-band imaging
- Chromoendoscopy

KEY POINTS

- The early detection and diagnosis of gastric cancer continues to be a focus of intense research.
- Magnification narrow-band imaging has shown increased sensitivity and specificity for the detection of gastric neoplasia, and has also demonstrated promising results when combined with chromoendoscopy.
- Further imaging enhancing techniques, such as flexible spectral imaging color enhancement and autofluorescence endoscopic imaging, have also yielded results superior to those obtained by white-light endoscopy in the detection of gastric neoplasia.
- The common clinical use of these imaging techniques is limited by a lack of widespread availability.
- A major challenge to be overcome in the screening for gastric cancer is the large surface area of the gastric lumen and the need to perform image-enhanced wide-field imaging that can highlight small abnormal mucosal areas, which can be further targeted with imaging-enhancing techniques such as endomicroscopy.

 A video of image-enhanced endoscopy technology accompanies this article at http://www.geriatric.theclinics.com/

INTRODUCTION

Gastric cancer remains a leading cause of morbidity and mortality. Worldwide, gastric cancer is the fourth most commonly diagnosed cancer in males and the fifth in females, with the highest incidence rates in Eastern Asia, the Middle East, and Latin America.[1,2] Five-year survival rates are a dismal 15% to 20% primarily because of diagnosis at a late, less curable stage.[3] Gastric cancer is subdivided into 2 main histopathologic subtypes, intestinal type and diffuse type.[4] The diffuse type is poorly differentiated, is associated with hereditary diffuse gastric cancer, and has been linked to a molecular abnormality in the cell adhesion protein E-cadherin (CDH1). The

Henry D. Janowitz Division of Gastroenterology, Mount Sinai School of Medicine, One Gustave L. Levy Place, Box 1069, New York, NY 10029, USA
E-mail address: susana.gonzalez@mssm.edu

Gastrointest Endoscopy Clin N Am 23 (2013) 581–595
http://dx.doi.org/10.1016/j.giec.2013.03.012
1052-5157/13/$ – see front matter © 2013 Published by Elsevier Inc.

intestinal type, the major subtype, is well differentiated and common in high-risk populations, is more often sporadic, and its development is usually also related to environmental factors. Early detection with screening endoscopy has been used in countries with high-risk populations, such as Japan, Chile, and Korea.[5–7] Given that the prognosis of gastric cancer depends on the stage of the cancer at the time of diagnosis, early detection and treatment is the only way to reduce mortality. The incidence of early gastric cancer, that is, gastric cancer that invades the mucosa and submucosa irrespective of lymph node metastasis, has an incidence in Japan from 15% to 57%, following the implementation of screening programs.[8–10] However, despite these screening methods, the sensitivity of endoscopy in detecting gastric cancer has been reported to range from 77% to 84%.[11] Therefore, recent research in gastric cancer screening has focused on improving endoscopic detection with magnification endoscopy, narrow-band imaging, autofluorescence imaging, and chromoendoscopy. This review focuses on these endoscopic imaging techniques and their potential usefulness in the detection and management of early gastric cancer.

WHO TO SCREEN

The major histopathologic subtype of gastric cancer, the intestinal type, progresses through various histologic stages before developing into adenocarcinoma. An accepted model for the development of gastric adenocarcinoma, the Correa cascade, consists of the development of nonatrophic gastritis into multifocal atrophic gastritis followed by intestinal metaplasia, and finally dysplasia and the development of carcinoma.[12] Intestinal metaplasia is a frequently identified histologic finding in the gastric biopsies of high-risk populations for gastric cancer, such as Asians and Latin Americans.[13] In the United States, endoscopic surveillance is not routinely recommended in patients with gastric intestinal metaplasia, and is reserved for patients at high risk because of family history or ethnic background.[14] Recently, several European societies of experts convened to propose guidelines for the diagnosis and management of patients with precancerous conditions of the stomach. The panel concluded that because gastric atrophy and intestinal metaplasia are part of the pathway of the development of intestinal-type gastric cancer, these lesions should be considered precancerous, and that patients with extensive atrophy and/or extensive intestinal metaplasia should therefore be offered surveillance endoscopy every 3 years (**Fig. 1**).[15] Further studies will be needed to determine the cost-effectiveness of this surveillance strategy. In addition, surveillance has been recommended in other patients at high risk for developing gastric cancer, which includes patients with adenomatous gastric polyps, familial adenomatous polyposis, and hereditary nonpolyposis colorectal cancer.[14]

ENDOSCOPIC DETECTION
White-Light Endoscopy

With the advent of the flexible gastroscope and the flexible gastric-biopsy tube, researchers found that there was little correlation between the endoscopist's impression of gastritis or atrophy and the histologic findings present on biopsy. In 1956, Atkins and Benedict[16] attempted to correlate gross endoscopic findings with histologic findings on biopsy. In cases with presumed chronic gastritis at gastroscopy, 76.7% were normal microscopically, and in cases of suspected acute gastritis 61.5% were microscopically normal. Despite continued advancements in the instruments used for endoscopy since this study, there is little evidence that high-resolution endoscopes have improved the correlation between gastroscopic and microscopic findings. A recent study attempted to classify the mucosal patterns of *Helicobacter pylori*–related

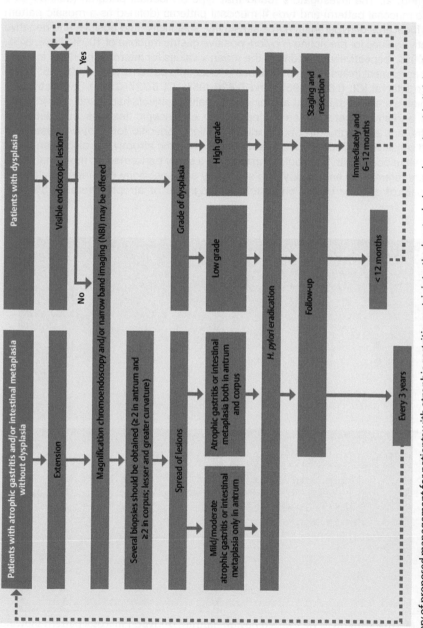

Fig. 1. Summary of proposed management for patients with atrophic gastritis, gastric intestinal metaplasia, and gastric epithelial dysplasia. Asterisk indicates that further management was not covered by the referenced guideline. (*From* Dinis-Ribeiro M, Areia M, de Vries AC, et al. Management of precancerous conditions and lesions in the stomach (MAPS): guideline from the European Society of Gastrointestinal Endoscopy (ESGE), European Helicobacter Study Group (EHSG), European Society of Pathology (ESP), and the Sociedade Portuguesa de Endoscopia Digestiva (SPED). Endoscopy 2012;44:77; with permission.)

gastritis in the gastric body with standard endoscopy and evaluate its reproducibility. One hundred twelve patients with dyspepsia had examinations with upper endoscopy, and the observed mucosal morphology in the gastric body was categorized into 4 types (**Fig. 2**). The investigators found that type 3 mucosal patterns (defined as a mosaic mucosal pattern) and type 4 mucosal patterns (defined as a mosaic pattern with a focal area of hyperemia) had a sensitivity, specificity, and positive and negative predictive values for predicting *H pylori*–positive gastric mucosa of 100%, 86%, 94%, and 100%, respectively. In addition, the mean κ values for interobserver and intraobserver agreement in assessing the various endoscopic patterns were 0.808 (95% confidence interval [CI] 0.678–0.938) and 0.826 (95% CI 0.727–0.925), respectively.[17] However, a previous study that examined 52 healthy subjects had found poor interobserver agreement between endoscopists for endoscopic features suggestive of gastritis, and although antral nodularity was highly specific for *H pylori* gastritis, it lacked sensitivity.[18] Endoscopic determination of gastric atrophy has also been found to correlate poorly with histologic diagnosis. In a study performed on more than 1300 subjects referred for endoscopy, the sensitivity and specificity of endoscopy for the diagnosis of atrophy based on histologic diagnosis of atrophy were 61.5% and

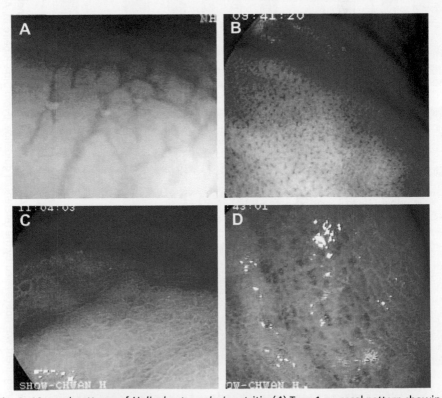

Fig. 2. Mucosal patterns of *Helicobacter pylori* gastritis. (*A*) Type 1 mucosal pattern showing cleft-like appearance. (*B*) Type 2 mucosal pattern showing regular arrangement of red dots. (*C*) Type 3 mucosal pattern showing mosaic appearance. (*D*) Type 4 mucosal pattern showing mosaic appearance with focal area of hyperemia. (*From* Yan SL, Wu ST, Chen CH, et al. Mucosal patterns of *Helicobacter pylori*-related gastritis without atrophy in the gastric corpus using standard endoscopy. World J Gastroenterol 2010;16:498; with permission.)

57.7% in the antrum and 46.8% and 76.4% in the body of the stomach.[19] Several studies have also found that gastric cancer is missed on initial endoscopic examinations. Sensitivity of endoscopy in detecting gastric cancer has ranged from 77% to 93%, with researchers suggesting that a high threshold for performing biopsies of lesions that appear benign as a possible cause of missed early gastric cancer (**Fig. 3**).[11,20-23]

Narrow-Band Imaging and Magnification Endoscopy

Narrow-band imaging (NBI) enhances the imaging of mucosal and glandular changes and the visualization of abnormal vascular patterns without using dyes. NBI uses optical filters that can be enabled or disabled during endoscopy and allow limited wavelengths of light, specifically blue light at 390 to 445 bandwidth and green light at 530 to 550 nm bandwidth. These wavelengths can only penetrate superficially and therefore enhance the visualization of the superficial mucosa and vasculature, aiding in the detection of cancer and precancerous lesions.[24] An advantage of NBI is its ease of use and wide availability. In a study of patients with known intestinal metaplasia or dysplasia undergoing surveillance endoscopy, NBI without magnification increased the diagnostic yield for the detection of advanced premalignant gastric lesions in comparison with routine white-light endoscopy (WLE).[25] The sensitivity, specificity, and positive and negative predictive values for the detection of premalignant lesions were 71%, 58%, 65% and 65% for NBI and 51%, 67%, 62% and 55% for WLE, respectively. However, several researchers have noted that a limitation of NBI without magnification is that, owing to the large gastric lumen, it produces dark images that are not meaningful for investigation. Recently a consensus of experienced endoscopists in the Asia-Pacific region convened, and agreed that it is often difficult to survey the whole gastric lumen by NBI; therefore almost all participants thought that NBI alone was not useful for detection of early gastric cancer.[26] By contrast, magnification endoscopy with NBI (M-NBI) was found to be useful in distinguishing gastric neoplasia from nonneoplasia, and in determining tumor margins but not tumor depth.

The use of M-NBI, which enhances color differences with magnified views, has shown increased accuracy for the detection of premalignant lesions. However, a major limitation of M-NBI is its limited availability. The LUCERA system (Olympus Medical Systems Co. Inc, Tokyo, Japan) is a red/green/blue (RGB) sequential system that uses a monochromatic charge-coupled device (CCD) and is available in Japan, Korea, China, Taiwan, and the United Kingdom. The EXERA system (Olympus Medical Systems) is a nonsequential system that uses a color CCD, and is available in the rest of

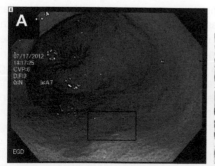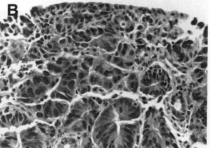

Fig. 3. Missed gastrointestinal cancers. (*A*) Subtle depressed lesion in the gastric mucosa with unclear borders. (*B*) Biopsies of the lesion revealed intramucosal adenocarcinoma (hematoxylin-eosin, original magnification ×40).

the world.[26] Nevertheless, multiple studies performed using both platforms have demonstrated an increased accuracy for the detection of cancerous and precancerous lesions. Bansal and colleagues[27] used the EXERA system with M-NBI, and found that the endoscopic finding of a ridge/villous pattern when correlated with histology had sensitivity of 80% and specificity of 100% for the detection of gastric intestinal metaplasia. Similarly, Tahara and colleagues[28] found that the endoscopic appearance of tubulovillous pits had very high sensitivity for intestinal metaplasia, and Uedo and colleagues[29] found that the endoscopic appearance of light blue crests, defined as a fine, blue-white line on the crests of the epithelial surface/gyri, correlated with histologic evidence of intestinal metaplasia with a sensitivity of 89%. Although these studies found improved diagnostic accuracy with M-NBI, there was variability in the NBI classification systems. A recent, multicenter study was performed to describe and estimate the accuracy and reliability of a classification system for NBI in the diagnosis of gastric lesions (**Table 1**).[30] Consecutive patients undergoing NBI endoscopy at 2 reference centers (N = 85, 33% with dysplasia) were included. In total, 224 different areas were biopsied and recorded onto video. Pattern A, defined as regular vessels with circular mucosa, was associated with normal histology (accuracy 83%; 95% CI 75%–90%). Pattern B, tubulovillous mucosa, was associated with intestinal metaplasia (accuracy 84%; 95 CI 77%–91%). Pattern C, irregular vessels and mucosa, was associated with dysplasia (accuracy 95%; 95 CI 90%–99%). Furthermore, the reproducibility of these patterns was high ($\kappa = 0.62$).

M-NBI has been further studied in the detection of early gastric cancer. Yao and colleagues[31] developed a comprehensive diagnostic system called the "VS (vessel plus surface) classification system," which takes into account vascular patterns and surface patterns. According to the VS system, the characteristic M-NBI findings of early gastric cancer include an irregular microvascular pattern with a demarcation line and an irregular microsurface pattern with a demarcation line. If either finding or both are fulfilled, the diagnosis of gastric cancer can be made, with 97% of early gastric cancers fitting these criteria. Recently, Ezoe and colleagues[32] performed a multicenter, prospective, randomized controlled trial of patients with undiagnosed depressed lesions 10 mm or less in diameter, identified by esophagogastroduodenoscopy. Patients were randomly assigned to groups that were analyzed by WLE (n = 176) or M-NBI (n = 177) immediately after detection; the WLE group received M-NBI after WLE. Overall, 40 gastric cancers (20 in each group) were identified. The median diagnostic values for M-NBI and WLE were as follows: accuracy, 90.4% and 64.8% ($P \leq .001$); sensitivity, 60.0% and 40.0% ($P = .34$); and specificity, 94.3% and 67.9% ($P \leq .001$), respectively. The combination of M-NBI with WLE significantly enhanced performance when compared with WLE alone; accuracy increased from (median) 64.8% to 96.6% ($P \leq .001$), sensitivity increased from 40.0% to 95.0% ($P \leq .001$), and specificity increased from 67.9% to 96.8% ($P \leq .001$).[32] In addition, M-NBI has been used to differentiate gastric low-grade adenoma from early gastric cancer. Yao and colleagues[33] investigated whether a white opaque substance (WOS) morphology could be a useful optical sign for discriminating between adenoma and carcinoma. When they examined the prevalence and the morphology of WOS as visualized using M-NBI according to histologic type (adenoma vs carcinoma), WOS was more frequently present in adenomas than in carcinomas. In addition, the WOS morphology in 100% of adenomas with WOS showed a regular distribution; by contrast, 83% of carcinomas with WOS showed an irregular WOS distribution.[33] For superficial elevated-type tumors with either WOS with a regular distribution or a regular microvascular pattern, the sensitivity and specificity for differentiating adenoma from carcinoma were 94% and 96%, respectively.[34]

Table 1
Proposed classification for gastric lesions on narrow-band imaging

	A	B	HP+	C
Mucosal Pattern	Regular circular	Regular ridge/tubulovillous Light blue crest	Regular	Irregular/absent White opaque substance
Vascular Pattern	Regular thin/peripheric or thick/central vessels	Regular	Regular with variable vascular density	Irregular
Expected Outcome	Normal	Intestinal metaplasia	Helicobacter pylori infection	Dysplasia
Accuracy (95% confidence interval)	83% (75%–90%)	84% (77%–91%)	70% (59%–80%)	95% (90%–99%)

Chromoendoscopy

Chromoendoscopy is a technique whereby a dye, such as indigo carmine or methylene blue, is sprayed on the gastric mucosa to highlight mucosal irregularities. A recent study from Korea used acetic acid in combination with indigo carmine to determine how accurately the lateral extent of differentiated and undifferentiated gastric adenocarcinomas could be assessed. This aspect is particularly important in clinical practice for determining the margin of a carcinoma before endoscopic resection. Although this combination improved the identification of the border of differentiated gastric adenocarcinoma in comparison with conventional endoscopy (89.8% vs 68.5%; *P*<.001), the border differentiation for undifferentiated adenocarcinomas did not differ between conventional endoscopy and acetic acid–indigo carmine chromoendoscopy (62.8% vs 70%; *P* = .494) (**Fig. 4**).[35] Furthermore, studies have compared chromoendoscopy with M-NBI and have shown some of the limitations of chromoendoscopy. A study of 110 patients undergoing endoscopic submucosal

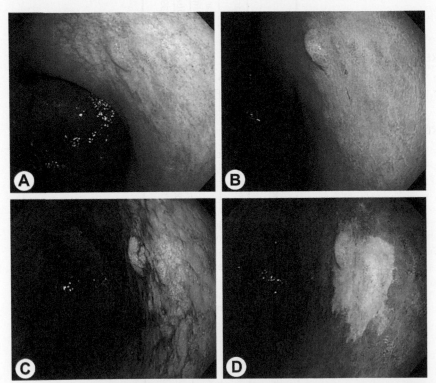

Fig. 4. Acetic acid chromoendoscopy of a differentiated adenocarcinoma. (*A*) A combined flat and elevated lesion with an unclear border at the lower body of the stomach. (*B*) Endoscopic view after acetic acid was sprinkled. (*C*) Endoscopic view after indigo carmine was additionally sprinkled. (*D*) Endoscopic view after the lesion was washed with clean water. After chromoendoscopy with indigo carmine dye added to acetic acid, the lesion's borders became distinct and the clarity of the image is high. The lesion was resected by endoscopic submucosal dissection and was shown to be a differentiated adenocarcinoma. (*From* Lee BE, Kim GH, Park do Y, et al. Acetic acid-indigo carmine chromoendoscopy for delineating early gastric cancers: its usefulness according to histological type. BMC Gastroenterol 2010;10:3; with permission.)

dissection for gastric tumors randomized the patients into M-NBI or indigo carmine chromoendoscopy to determine tumor margins. The rate of accurate marking of the M-NBI group was significantly higher than that of the indigo carmine chromoendoscopy group (97.4% vs 77.8%; P = .009).[36] Zhang and colleagues[37] performed a retrospective study to compare the accuracy and sensitivity of M-NBI endoscopy with conventional endoscopy and chromoendoscopy for the diagnosis of precancerous lesions and early gastric cancer. The study reviewed the images and pathology of 122 cases ultimately diagnosed on pathology or surgical specimens as early gastric cancer or precancerous lesions. The investigators found that the accuracy, sensitivity, and specificity for the diagnosis of early gastric cancer and precancerous gastric lesions were 68.9%, 95.1%, and 63.1% for conventional endoscopy, 93.6%, 92.7%, and 94.5% for M-NBI, and 91.3%, 88.6%, and 93.2% for magnifying chromoendoscopy, respectively. When assessing image resolution, M-NBI and magnifying chromoendoscopy were significantly superior to magnifying conventional endoscopy in morphology, pit pattern, and blood capillary form (P<.01), and M-NBI was significantly superior to magnifying chromoendoscopy in blood capillary form (P<.01).[37] Therefore, while chromoendoscopy is superior to conventional endoscopy, it appears to have limitations versus M-NBI in determining lesion margins. These data are promising in regard to improving early detection of gastric cancer as well as accurately determining resection margins before the treatment of early gastric cancers. However, an argument against its extended use is the increase in endoscopic procedure time and the lack of widespread availability of the M-NBI system; therefore, it currently remains limited to centers experienced in using this technique.

FLEXIBLE SPECTRAL IMAGING COLOR ENHANCEMENT

Flexible spectral imaging color enhancement (FICE; Fujifilm Corp, Tokyo, Japan) is a spectral estimation technique that enhances the contrast of mucosal surfaces without dyes. It performs arithmetical processing of a white-light image captured by a video endoscope and sends it to a spectral estimation matrix processing circuit. FICE processes the image into spectral images composed from a single wavelength and then displays them in real time. The digital processing system is able to switch between a white-light image and the FICE image by simply pushing a button on the endoscope (**Fig. 5**).[38] Preliminary studies with the FICE system have yielded promising results. Early validation studies showed a 46% improvement in the detection of early gastric cancer with the application of FICE.[38] When examining early gastric cancers with WLE versus the FICE system, greater median color differences between malignant lesions and the surrounding mucosa are seen in the FICE images, resulting in images with better contrast (27.2 vs 18.7, P<.001) (**Fig. 6**).[39] Researchers have also observed that the diagnostic accuracy of the extent of gastric cancer using FICE is superior to that using conventional white-light imaging, and that diagnosis of early gastric cancer with the FICE system can be performed even with nonmagnified images and half-magnified images. FICE can yield higher color contrast between a cancerous lesion and the surrounding area, and reveal an irregular structural pattern in cancerous lesions without magnification. In addition, FICE can also produce microvascular patterns with magnification.[40]

AUTOFLUORESCENCE IMAGING

Autofluorescence endoscopic imaging (AFI) uses the detection of natural tissue fluorescence emitted by endogenous molecules (fluorophores) such as collagen, flavins, and porphyrins. After excitation of the fluorophores by a short-wavelength light

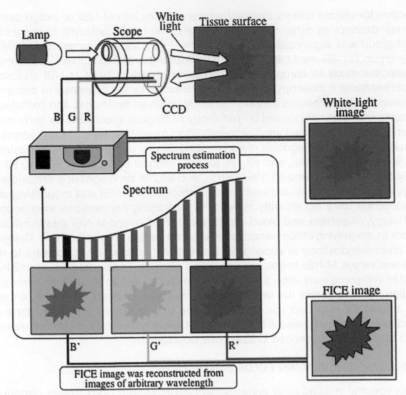

Fig. 5. Schematic diagram of the flexible spectral imaging color enhancement (FICE) system. (*From* Mouri R, Yoshida S, Tanaka S, et al. Evaluation and validation of computed virtual chromoendoscopy in early gastric cancer. Gastrointest Endosc 2009;69:1054; with permission.)

source, they emit light of longer wavelengths (fluorescence).[41] The overall fluorescence emission differs among normal tissue and neoplastic tissue. The color differences in fluorescence emission are captured during real-time endoscopy and are used for lesion detection or characterization. RGB-based video endoscopes with AFI capability (EVIS LUCERA Spectrum; Olympus Medical Systems) are commercially available in Asia and Europe. The integration of AFI technology is currently not feasible in conventional color CCD video endoscopes that are marketed for use in the United States (EVIS EXERA II; Olympus America Inc, Center Valley, PA).[42] Kato and colleagues[43] performed a prospective feasibility study to compare WLE with AFI for the detection of early gastric neoplasia. Although AFI detected 10% more neoplasias than were not identified by WLE, the sensitivity of WLE and AFI were comparable and the specificity of AFI was lower than WLE owing to a high number of false positives; therefore, AFI was considered to be of limited clinical value. However, the same investigators[44] recently performed a feasibility study of trimodal imaging endoscopy (TME) combining WLE, AFI, and NBI for superficial gastric neoplasia. A higher diagnostic accuracy of TME over WLE was found: on a per-lesion analysis the sensitivity of TME (89.4%) was higher than that of WLE (76.6%) and AFI (68.1%), and the specificity of TME (98.0%) was higher than that of WLE (84.3%) and AFI (23.5%). By a per-patient analysis, the sensitivity of TME (90.9%) was higher than that of WLE (75%) and AFI (68.2%), and the specificity of TME (100%) was higher than that of WLE (72.2%)

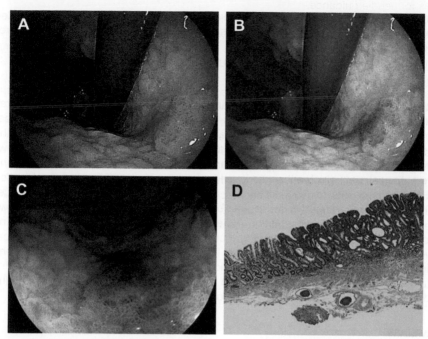

Fig. 6. FICE imaging of early gastric cancer. (*A*) Conventional image with small-caliber endoscope (EG530-NW) reveals a slightly reddish mucosal change in the lesser curvature of the upper body. (*B*) FICE image with small-caliber endoscope enhances a reddish cancerous lesion, and can determine with precision a clear line of demarcation between cancer and the yellowish surrounding mucosa. (*C*) FICE image with low magnification (EG590-ZW) also detects a much clearer demarcation line. (*D*) Specimen after endoscopic submucosal dissection shows a high density of glandular structure and an apparently irregular microvessel in intervening parts between crypts, which may cause a reddish mucosal change in depressed area. (*From* Osawa H, Yamamoto H, Miura Y, et al. Diagnosis of extent of early gastric cancer using flexible spectral imaging color enhancement. World J Gastrointest Endosc 2012;4:358; with permission.)

and AFI (44.4%). Whereas AFI alone had lower sensitivity and specificity than WLE, the combined modalities yielded significant improvement in diagnostic sensitivity and specificity. Therefore in TME, M-NBI shows high specificity for the diagnosis of early gastric neoplasia and correctly diagnoses the false-positive lesions obtained with WLE and AFI. An autofluorescence video endoscopy system created by Pentax called the SAFE 3000 was recently investigated to assess its effectiveness in diagnosing superficial gastric neoplasia. Ordinary WLE, AFI, and chromoendoscopy were used to diagnose the existence and extent of tumor in 14 patients with gastric adenoma, 40 patients with intestinal-type early gastric cancer (10 protruded and 30 depressed), and 9 patients with diffuse-type early gastric cancer. The diagnostic accuracies of the 3 imaging modalities were evaluated by comparing with histopathology of resected specimens. The diagnostic accuracy between AFI and WLE did not differ significantly, and for protruded intestinal-type early gastric cancers and diffuse-type early gastric cancers the diagnostic accuracy did not differ significantly between any of the imaging modalities. For depressed intestinal-type early gastric cancers, the diagnostic accuracy of AFI tended to be higher than that of the WLE images ($P<.05$), but was not significantly different from that of the chromoendoscopy images.[45] Although the SAFE 3000 system showed promise for diagnosing depressed intestinal-type early gastric cancers, it did not seem to have additional value over chromoendoscopy alone.

I-SCAN TECHNOLOGY

i-Scan is a newly developed image-enhanced endoscopy technology from Pentax (Tokyo, Japan). The system has 3 modes of image enhancement: surface enhancement, which enhances light/dark contrast and allows for detailed imaging of the mucosal surface structure; contrast enhancement, which adds blue color in low-density areas and enhances depressed areas and subtle surface irregularities; and tone enhancement, which enhances individual organs by modifying the combination of RGB components for each pixel.[46,47] Switching between the various enhancements, which are arranged in series, can be done by pushing a button, which allows for efficient endoscopic observation (Video 1). Although formal studies comparing i-Scan with other endoscopic imaging techniques in the detection of gastric cancer have not yet been published, case reports have highlighted its usefulness in detecting lesion boundaries and in highlighting gastric lesions to allow for targeted biopsies.[46,48] Future comparative studies are needed to determine whether this imaging technique adds value in the detection of early gastric cancers.

SUMMARY

The early detection and diagnosis of gastric cancer continues to be a focus of intense research. Chromoendoscopy has been shown to be superior to conventional endoscopy and M-NBI has shown an increased sensitivity and specificity for the detection of gastric neoplasia. Further imaging-enhancing techniques such as FICE and AFI have also yielded results that have been superior to those of WLE in the detection of gastric neoplasia. However, the common clinical use of these imaging techniques is limited by a lack of widespread availability. In addition, a major challenge to be overcome in the screening for gastric cancer is the large surface area of the gastric lumen, and the need to perform image-enhanced wide-field imaging that can highlight small abnormal mucosal areas, which can be further targeted with imaging-enhancing techniques such as endomicroscopy. It is unlikely that one single imaging technique alone will be able to overcome this challenge and most likely combined imaging modalities will need to be used within an endoscopic session for an extensive examination of the entire stomach followed by a detailed investigation of abnormal areas.

SUPPLEMENTARY DATA

Supplementary data related to this article can be found online at http://dx.doi.org/10.1016/j.giec.2013.03.012.

REFERENCES

1. Jemal A, Bray F, Center MM, et al. Global cancer statistics. CA Cancer J Clin 2011;61:69–90.
2. Ferlay J, Shin HR, Bray F, et al. Estimates of worldwide burden of cancer in 2008: GLOBOCAN 2008. Int J Cancer 2010;127:2893–917.
3. Siegel R, Naishadham D, Jemal A. Cancer statistics, 2012. CA Cancer J Clin 2012;62:10–29.

4. Lauren P. The two histological main types of gastric carcinoma: diffuse and so-called intestinal-type carcinoma. An attempt at a histo-clinical classification. Acta Pathol Microbiol Scand 1965;64:31–49.
5. Tashiro A, Sano M, Kinameri K, et al. Comparing mass screening techniques for gastric cancer in Japan. World J Gastroenterol 2006;12:4873–4.
6. Llorens P. Gastric cancer mass survey in Chile. Semin Surg Oncol 1991;7: 339–43.
7. Hamashima C, Shibuya D, Yamazaki H, et al. The Japanese guidelines for gastric cancer screening. Jpn J Clin Oncol 2008;38:259–67.
8. Gotoda T. Endoscopic resection of early gastric cancer: the Japanese perspective. Curr Opin Gastroenterol 2006;22:561–9.
9. Shimizu S, Tada M, Kawai K. Early gastric cancer: its surveillance and natural course. Endoscopy 1995;27:27–31.
10. Noguchi Y, Yoshikawa T, Tsuburaya A, et al. Is gastric carcinoma different between Japan and the United States? Cancer 2000;89:2237–46.
11. Nam JH, Choi IJ, Cho SJ, et al. Association of the interval between endoscopies with gastric cancer stage at diagnosis in a region of high prevalence. Cancer 2012;118:4953–60.
12. Correa P. Human gastric carcinogenesis: a multistep and multifactorial process—First American Cancer Society Award Lecture on Cancer Epidemiology and Prevention. Cancer Res 1992;52:6735–40.
13. Wu X, Chen VW, Andrews PA, et al. Incidence of esophageal and gastric cancers among Hispanics, non-Hispanic whites and non-Hispanic blacks in the United States: subsite and histology differences. Cancer Causes Control 2007;18:585–93.
14. Hirota WK, Zuckerman MJ, Adler DG, et al. ASGE guideline: the role of endoscopy in the surveillance of premalignant conditions of the upper GI tract. Gastrointest Endosc 2006;63:570–80.
15. Dinis-Ribeiro M, Areia M, de Vries AC, et al. Management of precancerous conditions and lesions in the stomach (MAPS): guideline from the European Society of Gastrointestinal Endoscopy (ESGE), European Helicobacter Study Group (EHSG), European Society of Pathology (ESP), and the Sociedade Portuguesa de Endoscopia Digestiva (SPED). Endoscopy 2012;44:74–94.
16. Atkins L, Benedict EB. Correlation of gross gastroscopic findings with gastroscopic biopsy in gastritis. N Engl J Med 1956;254:641–4.
17. Yan SL, Wu ST, Chen CH, et al. Mucosal patterns of *Helicobacter pylori*-related gastritis without atrophy in the gastric corpus using standard endoscopy. World J Gastroenterol 2010;16:496–500.
18. Laine L, Cohen H, Sloane R, et al. Interobserver agreement and predictive value of endoscopic findings for *H. pylori* and gastritis in normal volunteers. Gastrointest Endosc 1995;42:420–3.
19. Eshmuratov A, Nah JC, Kim N, et al. The correlation of endoscopic and histological diagnosis of gastric atrophy. Dig Dis Sci 2010;55:1364–75.
20. Voutilainen ME, Juhola MT. Evaluation of the diagnostic accuracy of gastroscopy to detect gastric tumours: clinicopathological features and prognosis of patients with gastric cancer missed on endoscopy. Eur J Gastroenterol Hepatol 2005;17: 1345–9.
21. Suvakovic Z, Bramble MG, Jones R, et al. Improving the detection rate of early gastric cancer requires more than open access gastroscopy: a five year study. Gut 1997;41:308–13.
22. Amin A, Gilmour H, Graham L, et al. Gastric adenocarcinoma missed at endoscopy. J R Coll Surg Edinb 2002;47:681–4.

23. Hosokawa O, Tsuda S, Kidani E, et al. Diagnosis of gastric cancer up to three years after negative upper gastrointestinal endoscopy. Endoscopy 1998;30: 669–74.
24. Kuznetsov K, Lambert R, Rey JF. Narrow-band imaging: potential and limitations. Endoscopy 2006;38:76–81.
25. Capelle LG, Haringsma J, de Vries AC, et al. Narrow band imaging for the detection of gastric intestinal metaplasia and dysplasia during surveillance endoscopy. Dig Dis Sci 2010;55:3442–8.
26. Uedo N, Fujishiro M, Goda K, et al. Role of narrow band imaging for diagnosis of early-stage esophagogastric cancer: current consensus of experienced endoscopists in Asia-Pacific region. Dig Endosc 2011;23(Suppl 1):58–71.
27. Bansal A, Ulusarac O, Mathur S, et al. Correlation between narrow band imaging and nonneoplastic gastric pathology: a pilot feasibility trial. Gastrointest Endosc 2008;67:210–6.
28. Tahara T, Shibata T, Nakamura M, et al. Gastric mucosal pattern by using magnifying narrow-band imaging endoscopy clearly distinguishes histological and serological severity of chronic gastritis. Gastrointest Endosc 2009;70:246–53.
29. Uedo N, Ishihara R, Iishi H, et al. A new method of diagnosing gastric intestinal metaplasia: narrow-band imaging with magnifying endoscopy. Endoscopy 2006; 38:819–24.
30. Pimentel-Nunes P, Dinis-Ribeiro M, Soares JB, et al. A multicenter validation of an endoscopic classification with narrow band imaging for gastric precancerous and cancerous lesions. Endoscopy 2012;44:236–46.
31. Yao K, Anagnostopoulos GK, Ragunath K. Magnifying endoscopy for diagnosing and delineating early gastric cancer. Endoscopy 2009;41:462–7.
32. Ezoe Y, Muto M, Horimatsu T, et al. Magnifying narrow-band imaging versus magnifying white-light imaging for the differential diagnosis of gastric small depressive lesions: a prospective study. Gastrointest Endosc 2010;71:477–84.
33. Yao K, Iwashita A, Tanabe H, et al. White opaque substance within superficial elevated gastric neoplasia as visualized by magnification endoscopy with narrow-band imaging: a new optical sign for differentiating between adenoma and carcinoma. Gastrointest Endosc 2008;68:574–80.
34. Maki S, Yao K, Nagahama T, et al. Magnifying endoscopy with narrow-band imaging is useful in the differential diagnosis between low-grade adenoma and early cancer of superficial elevated gastric lesions. Gastric Cancer 2013;16(2): 140–6.
35. Lee BE, Kim GH, Park do Y, et al. Acetic acid-indigo carmine chromoendoscopy for delineating early gastric cancers: its usefulness according to histological type. BMC Gastroenterol 2010;10:97.
36. Kiyotoki S, Nishikawa J, Satake M, et al. Usefulness of magnifying endoscopy with narrow-band imaging for determining gastric tumor margin. J Gastroenterol Hepatol 2010;25:1636–41.
37. Zhang J, Guo SB, Duan ZJ. Application of magnifying narrow-band imaging endoscopy for diagnosis of early gastric cancer and precancerous lesion. BMC Gastroenterol 2011;11:135.
38. Mouri R, Yoshida S, Tanaka S, et al. Evaluation and validation of computed virtual chromoendoscopy in early gastric cancer. Gastrointest Endosc 2009;69: 1052–8.
39. Osawa H, Yamamoto H, Miura Y, et al. Diagnosis of depressed-type early gastric cancer using small-caliber endoscopy with flexible spectral imaging color enhancement. Dig Endosc 2012;24:231–6.

40. Osawa H, Yamamoto H, Miura Y, et al. Diagnosis of extent of early gastric cancer using flexible spectral imaging color enhancement. World J Gastrointest Endosc 2012;4:356–61.
41. Filip M, Iordache S, Saftoiu A, et al. Autofluorescence imaging and magnification endoscopy. World J Gastroenterol 2011;17:9–14.
42. Song LM, Banerjee S, Desilets D, et al. Autofluorescence imaging. Gastrointest Endosc 2011;73:647–50.
43. Kato M, Kaise M, Yonezawa J, et al. Autofluorescence endoscopy versus conventional white light endoscopy for the detection of superficial gastric neoplasia: a prospective comparative study. Endoscopy 2007;39:937–41.
44. Kato M, Kaise M, Yonezawa J, et al. Trimodal imaging endoscopy may improve diagnostic accuracy of early gastric neoplasia: a feasibility study. Gastrointest Endosc 2009;70:899–906.
45. Imaeda H, Hosoe N, Kashiwagi K, et al. Autofluorescence videoendoscopy system using the SAFE-3000 for assessing superficial gastric neoplasia. J Gastroenterol Hepatol 2010;25:706–11.
46. Kodashima S, Fujishiro M. Novel image-enhanced endoscopy with i-Scan technology. World J Gastroenterol 2010;16:1043–9.
47. Cho WY, Jang JY, Lee DH. Recent advances in image-enhanced endoscopy. Clin Endosc 2011;44:65–75.
48. Hancock S, Bowman E, Prabakaran J, et al. Use of i-Scan endoscopic image enhancement technology in clinical practice to assist in diagnostic and therapeutic endoscopy: a case series and review of the literature. Diagn Ther Endosc 2012;2012:1–9.

Endomicroscopy and Targeted Imaging of Gastric Neoplasia

Martin Goetz, MD, PhD

KEYWORDS

- Endomicroscopy • Gastric cancer • Helicobacter pylori • Gastric adenoma
- Intestinal metaplasia • Molecular imaging

KEY POINTS

- Confocal laser endomicroscopy (CLE) is an endoscopic ultrahigh magnification technique that allows microscopic analysis of the mucosa during ongoing endoscopy.
- Multiple studies have demonstrated the ability of gastroenterologists to obtain microscopic tissue analysis of gastric pathologies in real time by CLE.
- Intravital analysis by CLE is used to target biopsies in large or diffuse lesions ("smart biopsies") and to guide and survey endoscopic resection.
- Translational research and molecular imaging with CLE enables visualization of microscopic events in their natural micromilieu virtually free of artifact.

INTRODUCTION

Confocal laser endoscopy (CLE) enables the endoscopist to obtain an in vivo microscopic evaluation of the mucosa. The first studies using CLE in gastrointestinal (GI) endoscopy established the feasibility of such an approach, demonstrating that endoscopists are able to read microscopic images by relying on simplified classification systems. These initial studies more or less followed a proof-of-principle strategy in different GI indications, but the advantage of obtaining in vivo microscopy over ex vivo histology after biopsy sampling was not clearly defined. However, follow-up trials used CLE in a more precise and complementary fashion to random biopsy protocol. This included *targeting* real biopsies by using multiple optical biopsies in conditions in which white light endoscopy alone was unreliable to identify the areas of interest, such as in intestinal metaplasia of the stomach. This "smart biopsy" concept was soon supplemented by using CLE to guide endoscopic resection. This is of advantage for mucosal alterations that are difficult to relocate macroscopically when detected by random biopsies (such as intraepithelial neoplasia in Barrett's esophagus). In such a situation, diagnosis by CLE can be followed by immediate endoscopic resection within the same endoscopic session without the time lag of

Deptartment of Medicine I, University of Tübingen, Otfried-Müller-Str. 10, 72076 Tübingen, Germany
E-mail address: martin.goetz@med.uni-tuebingen.de

Gastrointest Endoscopy Clin N Am 23 (2013) 597–606
http://dx.doi.org/10.1016/j.giec.2013.03.004
1052-5157/13/$ – see front matter © 2013 Elsevier Inc. All rights reserved.

waiting for histopathology results.[1] Guidance of endoscopic therapy is also important before endoscopic resection, where multiple biopsies may induce fibrosis and interfere with subsequent resection, or after endoscopic resection when margins cannot be completely surveyed with real biopsies, but with multiple optical biopsies, to guide re-resection. In a next step, it was shown that CLE did not only imitate histopathology in real time, but it was appreciated that CLE, by its intravital nature, could provide information that was both *complementary* and *different* from histopathology. CLE is virtually free of artifacts, such as from sampling, fixation, cutting, or staining. This offers a unique option to observe (sub)cellular mechanisms in real time and allows functional imaging instead of a static snapshot. Last, because CLE relies on fluorescent imaging, molecular targets have been labeled in experimental settings. Such molecular imaging is currently studied in 2 main indications, the first being detection of lesions (which may not be a major domain of a microscopic point technique, such as CLE), and the second being exact intravital characterization for prediction of response to molecular targeted therapy.

TECHNIQUE OF ENDOMICROSCOPY

For CLE, 2 systems are currently available for clinical use[2–4] that use monochrome blue laser light at 488 nm for excitation. The first system uses a miniaturized confocal scanner integrated into the tip of an otherwise conventional endoscope (endoscope-integrated CLE [eCLE]; Pentax, Tokyo, Japan). Imaging plane depth is adaptable from surface to 250 μm in 4-μm steps. Image acquisition rate is about 1 frame per second at high resolution. The other system in clinical use is probe-based (pCLE; MaunaKea-Technology, Paris, France) and has the advantage of compatibility with most conventional endoscopes. Frame-rate is faster, but with the compromise of a somewhat lower resolution and a fixed imaging plane depth. Optical biopsies by both systems represent optical sections parallel to the mucosal surface (ie, 90° to histopathological sections). A formal head-to-head comparison between the 2 systems has not been performed. For animal and bench-top research, confocal systems are available with similar scanners as for in-patient use that significantly ease translational approaches.

CLE relies on the application of fluorescent contrast agents. Most studies have used fluorescein, which shows a favorable safety profile.[5] Fluorescein is injected intravenously at 5 mL 10%, and imaging becomes possible after a few seconds and lasts for up to 60 minutes. Patients notice a slight yellowish discoloration of their skin for about 1 hour, and a discoloration of the urine (predominant renal clearance of fluorescein). Fluorescein does not result in a staining of cell nuclei; therefore, other contrast options have been evaluated, such as acriflavine[6] or cresyl violet,[7,8] which yield direct or indirect nuclear visualization after topical application. For CLE, the confocal imaging window that is protruding from the distal tip in eCLE, or the probe, has to be in direct contact with the tissue of interest. In the stomach, mucus sometimes has to be cleared off to provide good contact, and peristalsis may be reduced using butylscopolamine. Tissue sampling should be performed only after CLE imaging because blood (containing fluorescein) may blur the microscopic view.

As in every advanced endoscopy technique, CLE has a learning curve. Both handling of the endoscope (positioning, motion artifacts) and image interpretation require training. For Barrett's esophagus and associated neoplasia it has been demonstrated that adequate diagnosis can be obtained after initial training and 100 cases of CLE.[9] For gastric pathology, experienced endoscopists in CLE had greater accuracy in the diagnosis of intestinal metaplasia.[10] In early clinical applications of CLE, close collaboration with an expert GI pathologist should be sought for feedback.

CLINICAL APPLICATIONS
Healthy Stomach

Normal gastric epithelium in the absence of metaplasia or inflammation shows a cobblestone appearance with polygonal columnar cells (**Fig. 1**).[11] Goblet cells cannot be found in the epithelium. Deep aspects of the gastric pits are usually not visible even when the full range of z-axis adaptation in eCLE is exploited, and laser penetration to deeper sections seems to be compromised compared with other areas of the GI mucosa for ill-defined reasons. Differentiation of cell types, such as chief and parietal cells, is not possible with CLE.[12] The gastric epithelium is darker than the epithelium in the rest of the GI tract even when same laser settings and fluorescein doses are applied, probably due to the acidic gastric milieu and the pH-dependent fluorescence intensity of fluorescein. This can be used, for example, for better delineation of intestinal metaplasia, which is brighter than the normal gastric epithelium (see later in this article). Although cardiac and antral mucosa shows slitlike opening of gastric pits, corpus and fundus pits are roundish and cryptlike. Vasculature is usually well

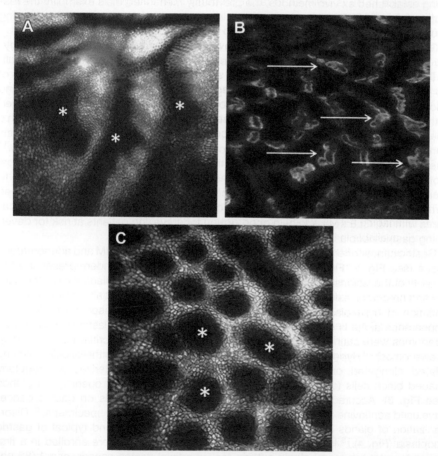

Fig. 1. (*A*) In the normal gastric antrum, pit openings are slitlike (*asterisks*). The epithelium has a cobblestonelike appearance. (*B*) In deeper sections, the regular vasculature can be visualized (*arrows*). (*C*) The corpus mucosa is honeycombed by roundish pit openings (*asterisks*), resembling colonic crypts. The cobblestone appearance is visible (original magnification ×1000).

delineated in the antrum in subepithelial optical sections, but less clearly visible in the corpus (see **Fig. 1**).

Gastric Pathology

In gastritis, endoscopic suspicion is usually confirmed by histopathologic analysis that includes differentiation of the inflammatory cells (eg, lymphocyte vs granulocyte infiltration). Such differentiation is difficult to obtain with CLE when nuclei cannot be stained with fluorescein; therefore, grading/staging of gastritis has not been an area of major clinical research of CLE. On the other hand, an early feasibility study has demonstrated that *Helicobacter pylori* can be visualized with eCLE as tiny rods in close association with the gastric epithelium owing to its active uptake of topical acriflavine in a background of fluorescein-stained imaging of gastritis.[13] In follow-up studies, CLE was able to predict *H pylori* infection with 93% accuracy in 103 patients in vivo[14] and to accurately visualize the histologic severity of *H pylori*–associated gastritis in 118 patients.[15] Although *H pylori* diagnosis is well and reliably standardized using established ex vivo methods, the previously mentioned trials exemplify the resolution power of CLE and its ability to visualize live oncogenic bacteria during ongoing endoscopy.

Gastric atrophy and intestinal metaplasia (IM) are well-recognized sequelae of *H pylori* infection and carry a risk of gastric neoplasia on their own. Surveillance is difficult, as IM is not reliably visible using white light endoscopy alone. Microscopic features of IM include the presence of goblet cells, high prismatic cells with brush border, and villous transformation of the mucosa (**Fig. 2**). These features can be readily visualized with CLE.[16] In 53 patients and 267 optical biopsies, IM was correctly diagnosed with a specificity of 95% and a sensitivity of 98%. Interobserver agreement for IM diagnosis during endoscopy was 0.94.[17] Gastric atrophy was visualized with similar results.[11] The advantage of CLE in these settings is the ability to rapidly obtain multiple optical biopsies from different gastric regions. Real specimens can be targeted by CLE to areas that show the highest grade of mucosal alterations. Although it has not been formally studied that a CLE endoscopy protocol results in better surveillance of patients with IM, CLE seems to be a good option for surveying patients at risk for developing gastric neoplasia at multiple sites.

Gastric cancer often arises within precursor lesions that harbor IM and adenomatous tissue (see **Fig. 2**; **Fig. 3**), and untargeted biopsies may be underrepresenting the severity of the lesions (sampling error). CLE has been shown to diagnose gastric cancer and precursor lesions with high accuracy in most,[18–20] but not all,[21] studies. Differentiation of hyperplastic from adenomatous gastric polyps based on endoscopic appearance alone is often unreliable. In 66 patients, 60 hyperplastic polyps and 27 adenomas were stained with systemic fluorescein and topical acriflavine (for grading of adenomas).[20] Hyperplastic polyps showed regular columnar epithelial cells covering dilated, elongated, or branchlike pits. Adenomas were characterized by irregularly shaped black cells forming ridges or villi with focally distorted openings of glands (see **Fig. 3**). Accuracy of CLE prediction was 90%. Early trials on gastric cancer have used acriflavine staining for ex vivo confocal microscopy on specimens.[22] Disorganization of glands after fluorescein injection in vivo were found typical of gastric neoplasia (**Fig. 4**).[18] In the largest study so far, 182 patients were enrolled in a first phase to establish morphologic criteria for superficial gastric cancer, and 1786 patients were prospectively evaluated for validation.[19] Criteria indicative for gastric cancer were loss of gland polarity and disorganized or destroyed glands, irregular cell size, and irregular vessels with increased diameter. Using these criteria, real-time accuracy was 98% for the definition of high-grade intraepithelial neoplasia/gastric cancer.

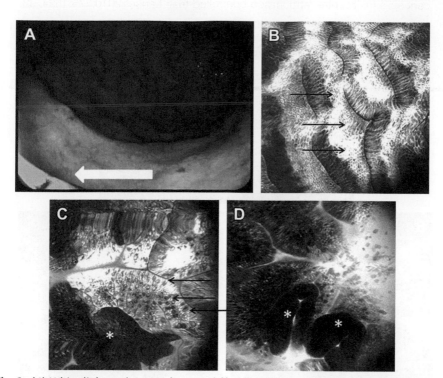

Fig. 2. (*A*) White light endoscopy shows a diffusely irregular surface pattern of the gastric mucosa. The confocal imaging window can be seen protruding from the 7 o'clock position (*arrow*). (*B*) Significant extravasation of fluorescein (*arrows*) brightly stains the lamina propria and the interstitium, indicating gastritis. The epithelium is fairly uncompromised at this site. (*C*) A sudden break of darker gastric mucosa (*asterisk*) to brighter mucosa harboring goblet cells (characterized by their dark mucin inclusion, *arrows*) can be identified by CLE. This clearly defines intestinal metaplasia. The double lining at the surface of the metaplastic tissue corresponds to the brush border. (*D*) Similarly, only 2 residual normal gastric glands (*asterisks*) can be found within an area of intestinal metaplasia. Cell shedding and leakage of fluorescein into the lumen indicate associated gastritis ([*B, C, D*] original magnification ×1000).

Guidance of Endoscopic Therapy

Asian countries have a high incidence of gastric cancer, and screening programs result in a higher frequency of detection at an early stage. Endoscopic submucosal dissection (ESD) has become the treatment of choice for such early lesions, but requires adequate staging. CLE can be combined with endoscopic ultrasound within the same session.[23] Usually, multiple biopsies are then obtained before resection to establish the diagnosis. However, they are prone to sampling error underestimating the grade of dysplasia, and may limit subsequent dissection by fibrosis from scarring. In a single-center study on 31 patients with 35 lesions, endoscopic and optical biopsies were compared for diagnosis and differentiation of gastric adenomas and adenocarcinomas.[24] The accuracy of CLE was significantly higher at 94% (vs 86% for histologic diagnosis on biopsies), with post-ESD histopathology as the reference standard. There was also a trend for better CLE diagnosis to grade adenocarcinomas. This may limit the need for pre-ESD biopsy, facilitating submucosal dissection. After resection, residual tumor at the deep margin is generally considered an indication

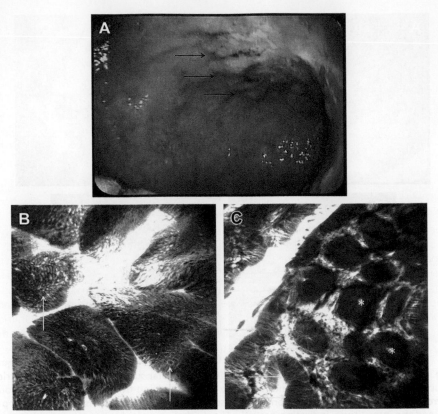

Fig. 3. (A) In the same patient, white light endoscopy identifies a suspicious type 0-IIa lesion (*arrows*). (B) In the periphery of the lesions, typical aspects of a gastric adenoma can be seen. The pattern is villous, cell size is irregular (*arrows*), and significant extravasation of fluorescein indicates enhanced vessel leakiness. (C) In adjacent areas, tubular structures can be identified with regular basal membrane (*asterisks*). Epithelial height is variable in some glands (*arrows*) ([B, C] original magnification ×1000).

for surgery, whereas a positive lateral margin can be retreated endoscopically. In 24 patients, eCLE was performed 2 weeks after endoscopic resection.[25] In 5 patients, indefinite lateral margins were suspected by CLE. Immediate retreatment was performed under endomicroscopic guidance, and accuracy of CLE to predict incomplete resection was 92%.

Functional and Translational Imaging

CLE not only aims at imitating histopathology, but is also unique in its ability to visualize functional microscopic details within the natural micromilieu. This feature was exploited by a recent translational study demonstrating that fluorescein leakage through intercellular spaces was a predominant functional feature of H pylori–associated gastritis in 42 patients.[26] Eradication of H pylori reversed this increased leakage to normal values. In contrast, leakiness persisted once morphologic sequelae, such as intestinal metaplasia, was present, despite successful eradication therapy. eCLE was used in this setting to demonstrate the impaired mucosal barrier function in vivo that may contribute to carcinogenesis in these patients.

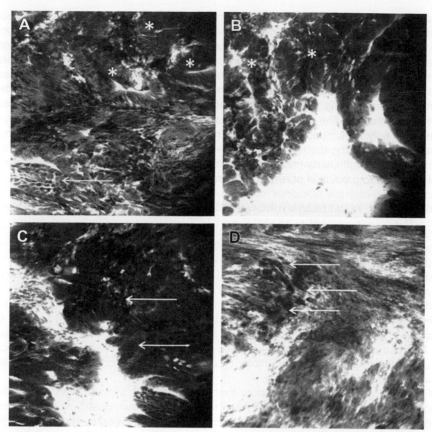

Fig. 4. When scanning the complete lesion from **Fig. 3** by CLE, different aspects of gastric cancer can be found. In (*A*) areas of diffusely irregular cells (*arrow*) are surrounded by glandular structures only incompletely contained by basal membranes (*asterisks*). Glands become more and more disorganized and ragged in (*B*) (*asterisks*), and the lumen is completely filled with malignant cells in (*C*) (*arrows*). The subepithelial space seems to be completely filled with irregular cells. In (*D*), the tissue structure is lost, and only single dark cells (but no more glands) are found within areas of necrosis (*arrows*). In (*A–D*), leakage of fluorescein to the tissue and to the lumen is evident (original magnification ×1000).

A different approach was followed in a feasibility trial for imaging of myenteric neurons and muscle cells.[27] After endoscopic tunneling through mucosa and submucosa in live pigs, neurons or smooth muscle cells were selectively stained at 9 gastric sites using molecular probes, and imaged after introduction of a CLE probe. Although disease models were not yet studied, such an approach could represent an interesting tool to study gastro-motoric malfunction that is otherwise not accessible by our current diagnostic methods.

Molecular Imaging

Molecular imaging is followed with growing interest in the field of translational GI endoscopy, but has not yet entered clinical practice.[28] In a proof-of-principle study, fluorescein isothiocyanate (FITC)-labeled antibodies targeting epidermal growth factor receptor (EGFR) and survivin were topically applied onto the healthy gastric mucosa or administered via submucosal injection, and imaging performed with pCLE in pigs to study expression patterns in vivo.[29] Our group recently used a human-mouse xenograft model for specific staining of EGFR on human gastric cancer cells. In vivo fluorescence after injection of FITC-labeled antibodies could be captured in vivo and quantified against the healthy background,[30] demonstrating that human cancer cells can be specifically labeled and visualized by CLE. MG7, a marker for gastric cancer, has been another target for molecular imaging with CLE of gastric cancer. After demonstrating labeling of human xenografts in a mouse model, MG7 also stained 96% of human gastric cancer specimens ex vivo, whereas healthy mucosa was stained in only 22%.[31] In vivo molecular imaging of gastric cancer has been further investigated by using therapeutic antibodies against EGFR, such as cetuximab, as molecular probes.[30] Current studies aim to link fluorescence intensity after therapeutic drug labeling to prediction of response to targeted therapy.[32]

CURRENT CONTROVERSIES/FUTURE CONSIDERATIONS

Endomicroscopy of the stomach has evolved considerably during the past years. Starting from an initial role of "real-time" histopathology, new applications have arisen. Especially with the advent of new resection techniques, the need for an exact microscopic staging, ideally without the risk of submucosal fibrosis after multiple biopsies, becomes evident. In this regard, the study by Jeon and colleagues[24] is important in showing that 10% of patients would have undergone surgery instead of ESD if CLE classification would have been used (showing undifferentiated cancer) instead of biopsies. Thus, reduction of sampling error before resection may be a good indication for CLE of the stomach, and further studies are needed, as well as for the surveillance of patients with diffuse gastric pathology carrying a risk for neoplasia, such as intestinal metaplasia or gastric atrophy.

For such indications, it is essential that a reproducible classification system be applied. Most of the trials cited previously have used their own classification systems. Especially in countries with a high prevalence of early gastric lesions, efforts should be undertaken to join and unify these classification systems. Most of the studies have used eCLE for gastric imaging. Because the system comes with a more rigid tip, full inversion is compromised, and the cardia and fundus are sometimes difficult to image.[18] Whether pCLE is of advantage in this setting has not been shown, and many trials with pCLE in other regions of the GI tract have used a transparent cap on the endoscope to stabilize the probe. Head-to-head comparisons of the different systems are not available to date and need to be performed.

Most studies on molecular imaging with CLE have been performed in the context of colorectal cancer for enhanced detection and characterization of lesions, and only a few imaging agents have successfully accomplished transition into clinical studies. There is a strong clinical need for early detection of gastric cancer with such advanced methods of detection, and early prediction of response to targeted chemotherapy (personalized cancer therapy) could significantly lower the burden on the patient and health care systems.

SUMMARY

Endomicroscopy enables microscopic tissue analysis of the gastric mucosa at real time during endoscopy. This not only aims at imitation of histopathology, but is used to target few biopsies to regions of interest by multiple optical biopsies, and to guide endoscopic interventions. Here, follow-up studies are awaited after encouraging initial trials that have shown superiority over untargeted biopsies. CLE furthermore provides a powerful tool for translational studies to unravel the pathophysiology of diseases in vivo virtually free of artifact. Molecular imaging may help to detect suspicious lesions and to predict response to targeted therapy. With this, CLE significantly affects patient care and translational science.

REFERENCES

1. Dunbar KB, Canto MI. Confocal laser endomicroscopy in Barrett's esophagus and endoscopically inapparent Barrett's neoplasia: a prospective, randomized, double-blind, controlled, crossover trial. Gastrointest Endosc 2010;72:668.
2. Goetz M, Watson A, Kiesslich R. Confocal laser endomicroscopy in gastrointestinal diseases. J Biophotonics 2011;4:498–508.
3. Kiesslich R, Goetz M, Neurath MF. Confocal laser endomicroscopy for gastrointestinal diseases. Gastrointest Endosc Clin N Am 2008;18:451–66, viii.
4. De Palma GD, Wallace MB, Giovannini M. Confocal laser endomicroscopy. Gastroenterol Res Pract 2012;2012:216209.
5. Wallace MB, Meining A, Canto MI, et al. The safety of intravenous fluorescein for confocal laser endomicroscopy in the gastrointestinal tract. Aliment Pharmacol Ther 2010;31:548–52.
6. Polglase AL, McLaren WJ, Skinner SA, et al. A fluorescence confocal endomicroscope for in vivo microscopy of the upper- and the lower-GI tract. Gastrointest Endosc 2005;62:686–95.
7. George M, Meining A. Cresyl violet as a fluorophore in confocal laser scanning microscopy for future in-vivo histopathology. Endoscopy 2003;35:585–9.
8. Goetz M, Toermer T, Vieth M, et al. Simultaneous confocal laser endomicroscopy and chromoendoscopy with topical cresyl violet. Gastrointest Endosc 2009;70: 959–68.
9. Dunbar K, Montgomery EA, Canto MI. The learning curve for in vivo confocal laser endomicroscopy for prediction of Barrett's esophagus. Gastroenterology 2008;134:A62–3.
10. Lim LG, Yeoh KG, Salto-Tellez M, et al. Experienced versus inexperienced confocal endoscopists in the diagnosis of gastric adenocarcinoma and intestinal metaplasia on confocal images. Gastrointest Endosc 2011;73:1141–7.
11. Zhang JN, Li YQ, Zhao YA, et al. Classification of gastric pit patterns by confocal endomicroscopy. Gastrointest Endosc 2008;67:843–53.
12. Vieth M, Kiesslich R, Thomas S, et al. Microarchitecture of the normal gut seen with conventional histology and endomicroscopy. In: Kiesslich R, Galle PR, Neurath MF, editors. Atlas of endomicroscopy. Heidelberg (Germany): Springer; 2008. p. 39–54.
13. Kiesslich R, Goetz M, Burg J, et al. Diagnosing Helicobacter pylori in vivo by confocal laser endoscopy. Gastroenterology 2005;128:2119–23.
14. Ji R, Li YQ, Gu XM, et al. Confocal laser endomicroscopy for diagnosis of Helicobacter pylori infection: a prospective study. J Gastroenterol Hepatol 2010;25: 700–5.
15. Wang P, Ji R, Yu T, et al. Classification of histological severity of Helicobacter pylori-associated gastritis by confocal laser endomicroscopy. World J Gastroenterol 2010;16:5203–10.
16. Goetz M, Hoffman A, Kiesslich R. Confocal endomicroscopy of the stomach: gastritis, intestinal metaplasia, adenoma and gastric cancer (with video). Video Journal of Gastrointestinal Endoscopy, in press.
17. Guo YT, Li YQ, Yu T, et al. Diagnosis of gastric intestinal metaplasia with confocal laser endomicroscopy in vivo: a prospective study. Endoscopy 2008;40:547–53.

18. Kitabatake S, Niwa Y, Miyahara R, et al. Confocal endomicroscopy for the diagnosis of gastric cancer in vivo. Endoscopy 2006;38:1110–4.

19. Li WB, Zuo XL, Li CQ, et al. Diagnostic value of confocal laser endomicroscopy for gastric superficial cancerous lesions. Gut 2011;60:299–306.

20. Li WB, Zuo XL, Zuo F, et al. Characterization and identification of gastric hyperplastic polyps and adenomas by confocal laser endomicroscopy. Surg Endosc 2010;24:517–24.

21. Li Z, Yu T, Zuo XL, et al. Confocal laser endomicroscopy for in vivo diagnosis of gastric intraepithelial neoplasia: a feasibility study. Gastrointest Endosc 2010;72: 1146–53.

22. Yeoh KG, Salto-Tellez M, Khor CJ. Confocal laser endoscopy is useful for in-vivo rapid diagnosis of gastric neoplasia and preneoplasia. Gastroenterol 2005;128: A27.

23. Gheorghe C, Iacob R, Dumbrava M, et al. Confocal laser endomicroscopy and ultrasound endoscopy during the same endoscopic session for diagnosis and staging of gastric neoplastic lesions. Chirurgia (Bucur) 2009;104:17–24.

24. Jeon SR, Cho WY, Jin SY, et al. Optical biopsies by confocal endomicroscopy prevent additive endoscopic biopsies before endoscopic submucosal dissection in gastric epithelial neoplasias: a prospective, comparative study. Gastrointest Endosc 2011;74:772–80.

25. Ji R, Zuo XL, Li CQ, et al. Confocal endomicroscopy for in vivo prediction of completeness after endoscopic mucosal resection. Surg Endosc 2011;25(6): 1933–8.

26. Ji R, Zuo XL, Yu T, et al. Mucosal barrier defects in gastric intestinal metaplasia: in vivo evaluation by confocal endomicroscopy. Gastrointest Endosc 2012;75: 980–7.

27. Ohya TR, Sumiyama K, Takahashi-Fujigasaki J, et al. In vivo histologic imaging of the muscularis propria and myenteric neurons with probe-based confocal laser endomicroscopy in porcine models (with videos). Gastrointest Endosc 2012;75: 405–10.

28. Goetz M. Molecular imaging in GI endoscopy. Gastrointest Endosc 2012;76: 1207–9.

29. Nakai Y, Shinoura S, Ahluwalia A, et al. Molecular imaging of epidermal growth factor-receptor and survivin in vivo in porcine esophageal and gastric mucosae using probe-based confocal laser-induced endomicroscopy: proof of concept. J Physiol Pharmacol 2012;63:303–7.

30. Hoetker MS, Kiesslich R, Diken M, et al. Molecular in vivo imaging of gastric cancer in a human-murine xenograft model: Targeting epidermal growth factor receptor (EGFR). Gastrointest Endosc 2012;76:612–20.

31. Li Z, Zuo XL, Li CQ, et al. In vivo molecular imaging of gastric cancer by targeting MG7 antigen with confocal laser endomicroscopy. Endoscopy 2013;45:79–85.

32. Goetz M, Hoetker MS, Diken M. In vivo molecular imaging with cetuximab, an anti-EGFR antibody, for prediction of response in xenograft models of human colorectal cancer. Endoscopy, in press.

Advanced EUS Imaging for Early Detection of Pancreatic Cancer

Sunil Amin, MD, MPH, Christopher J. DiMaio, MD,
Michelle Kang Kim, MD, MSc*

KEYWORDS

- Endoscopic ultrasound • Elastography • Contrast-enhanced endoscopic ultrasound
- Confocal endomicroscopy • Three-dimensional endoscopic ultrasound
- Optical coherence tomography • High-resolution microendoscopy

KEY POINTS

- Endoscopic ultrasound (EUS)-fine needle aspiration remains the gold standard for diagnosing pancreatic malignancy. However, in a subset of patients, limitations remain in regard to image quality and diagnostic yield of biopsies.
- Several new devices and processors have been developed that allow for enhancement of the EUS image.
- Initial studies of these modalities do show promise. However, cost, availability, and overall incremental benefit to EUS-fine needle aspiration have yet to be determined.

INTRODUCTION

Endoscopic ultrasound (EUS) was initially developed in the 1980s to aid in the diagnosis of abdominal pathologic abnormality. By generating transgastric and transduodenal images, EUS represented a significant advance over traditional transabdominal ultrasound or computer tomography (CT) imaging.[1] With its ability to assess tumor size and depth, detect regional lymph node involvement and distant metastases, and also perform fine needle aspiration (EUS-FNA) to acquire tissue confirmation, EUS is now a routine part of the initial staging evaluation of a patient with suspected gastrointestinal cancer.

EUS plays an especially prominent role in pancreatic cancer. Not only does EUS provide real-time, high-resolution imaging, but it also complements imaging modalities such as helical CT and magnetic resonance imaging. EUS is particularly helpful in the evaluation of tumor resectability and the detection of vascular invasion.[2–9] EUS is also exquisitely able to detect small tumors.[9] Furthermore, the sensitivity

Financial Disclosures: None.
Funding: None.
Division of Gastroenterology, Department of Medicine, Mount Sinai School of Medicine, 5 East 98th Street, 11th Floor, New York, NY 10029, USA
* Corresponding author.
E-mail address: michelle.kim@mountsinai.org

and specificity of EUS-FNA for confirming a diagnosis of suspected pancreatic cancer have been reported as high as 92% and 96%, respectively.[10–12] Pancreatic cyst fluid carcinoembryonic antigen values obtained by EUS-FNA can also be helpful in differentiating between mucinous and nonmucinous cysts.[13]

Today, the clinical impact of EUS in patients with suspected pancreatic cancer is significant, with its use resulting in a change in diagnosis in 26% of patients and a change in management in 48% of patients undergoing an examination, including the avoidance of unnecessary surgeries.[14] Most recently, Canto and colleagues[15,16] have identified EUS as a preferred modality of initial screening for patients with an increased risk of familial pancreatic cancer and confirmed the superiority of EUS over CT for the detection of small pancreatic cysts including premalignant lesions, such as pancreatic intraepithelial neoplasia and intraductal papillary mucinous neoplasms, among asymptomatic high-risk individuals.

Despite the progressively increased use of EUS to detect and stage pancreatic lesions over the last 3 decades, limitations remain. Most notably, EUS depends significantly on the skill of the endosonographer.[17] Moreover, although on-site cytopathology has been shown to improve diagnostic yield from the FNA procedure, most centers do not have the resources to provide an on-site cytopathologist or cytotechnician to confirm sample adequacy consistently.[18] It is particularly helpful to have an onsite cytologist because obtaining a diagnosis may require as many as 5 to 7 passes in a patient with a pancreatic mass. In addition, the presence of chronic pancreatitis has been shown to limit the accuracy of EUS considerably,[19–21] which is especially important, because patients with chronic pancreatitis are at increased risk for pancreatic cancer and the symptoms and imaging findings of chronic pancreatitis may closely mimic those of pancreatic cancer, engendering even more difficulty in distinguishing the 2 conditions.

As such, several general, initial improvements were developed to improve EUS as an imaging technique. The first such improvement was the development of the electronic radial echoendoscope, which studies have now confirmed provides superior image quality over the mechanical radial echoendoscope for both solid and cystic pancreatic lesions.[22,23] Furthermore, unlike the initial mechanical radial echoendoscopes, the electronic echoendoscopes are compatible with the same processors as the linear echoendoscopes.

Using this electronic platform, more advanced techniques of image enhancement have been developed (**Box 1**). This review discusses each of these advanced techniques.

Box 1
Advanced EUS image-enhancement techniques

Elastography

Contrast-enhanced EUS

Contrast harmonic-enhanced EUS

Three-dimensional EUS

Needle-based confocal laser-induced endomicroscopy

High-resolution microendoscopy

Optical coherence tomography

Trans-needle pancreatic cystoscopy

ADJUNCTIVE IMAGING TECHNIQUES
Elastography

EUS elastography has emerged as a potentially valuable adjunctive technique in the evaluation of the solid pancreatic mass. Although traditional EUS-FNA has a high sensitivity and specificity for the detection of pancreatic cancer (92% and 96%, respectively),[10–12] the yield is significantly lower in the presence of chronic pancreatitis (73.9% vs 91.3% and 54% vs 85%).[19–21] This decreased yield is explained by the great difficulty endosonographers have in differentiating the inflammation of chronic pancreatitis from a discrete neoplasm. Elastography is based on the premise that malignant tissue is generally firmer than adjacent benign tissue.[24] As such, measuring the strain generated in response to compression or vibration may be a reliable way of distinguishing benign from malignant tissues. Benign tissues would be expected to generate a larger amount of strain.[25] Elastography has also been used extensively to evaluate the degree of liver fibrosis as well as to evaluate cervical, prostate, thyroid, and breast lesions.[26–30]

Several studies have been published investigating the accuracy of EUS elastography to evaluate pancreatic masses. In their initial series of 49 patients and subsequent multicenter follow-up study of 222 patients, Giovannini and colleagues[31,32] reported a sensitivity of 92.3% and a specificity of 80% of elastography to detect malignant pancreatic lesions compared with 92.3% and 68.9%, respectively, for traditional B-mode imaging. Specifically, the authors characterized elastographic images based on color and hardness, assigning each a score of 1 to 5. Although a score of 1 represented green, homogenous, soft tissue and was interpreted as normal, 5 represented blue, hard, heterogeneous tissue and was interpreted as malignancy. EUS-FNA and surgical pathologic abnormality were used to obtain the final diagnosis. Iglesias and colleagues[33] studied 130 consecutive patients with solid pancreatic masses and 20 controls. The authors also categorized patients by specific elastographic patterns. Using a hue color map (red-green-blue), where dark blue represents hard tissue, green represents intermediate tissue, and red represents soft tissue, the 4 following groups were created: (1) green predominant, homogenous; (2) green predominant, heterogeneous; (3) blue predominant, homogenous; and (4) blue predominant, heterogeneous. Their group reported a sensitivity, specificity, and overall accuracy of EUS elastography for the diagnosis of malignancy of 100%, 85.5%, and 94%, respectively (**Fig. 1**).

Despite these promising results, first-generation elastography has been criticized for its subjective nature. By generating a color map of tissue elastography (with blue representing the hardest tissue and red representing the softest tissue) that is superimposed on traditional gray-scale B-mode EUS images, the technique is inherently subjective; interpretation may vary between endosonographers.[34] As such, quantitative methods, such as the strain ratio (ratio of the elasticity of a reference region in the adjacent tissue to elasticity of a given mass), hue histogram analysis, and most recently, artificial neural networks, have been developed.[25,35,36] With regard to strain ratio, initial reports have been conflicting. Iglesias-Garcia and colleagues[37] reported an improved specificity (92.9% vs 85.7%) and overall accuracy (97.7% vs 95.35%) of quantitative elastography over qualitative elastography for the diagnosis of malignancy among 86 patients with solid pancreatic masses; however, in the largest single-center study to date, Dawwas and colleagues[25] showed that the area under the receiver operator curve for the detection of pancreatic malignancy using the strain ratio was only 0.69 with an associated sensitivity of 100% and a specificity of 16.7%. In terms of hue-histogram analysis, Săftoiu and colleagues[35] have published encouraging results in a large, multicenter prospective study. By applying postprocessing

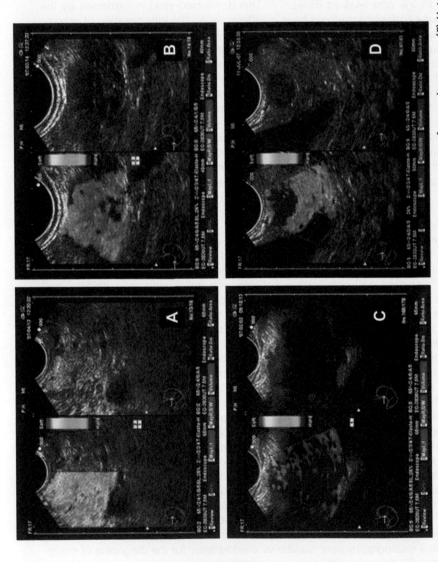

Fig. 1. Different elastographic patterns of solid pancreatic masses. (A) Homogeneous green pattern of normal pancreas. (B) Heterogeneous green-predominant pattern with slight yellow lines of a pancreatic inflammatory mass. (C) Heterogeneous blue-predominant pattern with green and red lines and geographic appearance of a ductal pancreatic adenocarcinoma. (D) Homogeneous blue pattern of a pancreatic neuroendocrine tumor. (*From* Iglesias-Garcia J, Larino-Noia J, Abdulkader I, et al. EUS elastography for the characterization of solid pancreatic masses. Gastrointest Endosc 2009;70(6):1101–8; with permission.)

software analysis to the traditional color distribution of hardness (hue histogram), the authors were able to create a quantitative scale of elasticity from 0 (softest) to 255 (hardest). Using an average hue histogram value of 175, the authors were able to show a sensitivity of 93.4%, specificity of 66.0%, and overall accuracy of 85.4% for the technique. Finally, a recent study with neural networks using artificial intelligence methodology also appears encouraging.[36]

In an attempt to define the diagnostic accuracy of EUS elastography better, 2 recent meta-analyses were published. Mei and colleagues[38] selected 13 studies of both qualitative (color pattern) and quantitative (strain ratio, hue histogram analysis) elastography with 1042 patients and calculated a pooled sensitivity of 95% and specificity of 67% of EUS elastography in differentiation of benign from malignant solid pancreatic masses. The area under the summary receiver operatic characteristic curve (sROC) was 0.8872, suggesting good validity of elastography as a diagnostic test. Pei and colleagues[39] published almost identical results, with a sensitivity, specificity, and area under the sROC of 95%, 69%, and 0.8695, respectively.

In summary, EUS elastography may be a valuable adjunctive diagnostic technique in the evaluation of the solid pancreatic mass. To date, usage has been limited by its subjectivity and the need for compatible processors. Further studies will need to be performed to delineate more clearly the role of elastography in EUS and EUS-FNA.

Contrast-enhanced EUS and Contrast Harmonic-enhanced EUS

Intravenous contrast agents have long been used in transabdominal ultrasound; however, their use has only recently been applied to endoscopic ultrasound. Contrast-enhanced EUS (CE-EUS) uses either color/power Doppler EUS or dedicated contrast harmonic-enhanced EUS (CHE-EUS) as a signal intensifier. The technology is based on the finding that lesions associated with pancreatic adenocarcinoma are hypoenhancing compared with neuroendocrine or cystic neoplasms.[40] Although a first attempt to differentiate ductal carcinoma from chronic pancreatitis and neuroendocrine tumors was published more than 15 years ago,[41] traditional contrast agents were too large to cross the lung bed. Newer gas-filled lipid microsphere contrast agents that are able to do so have only recently been produced.[42]

Power Doppler EUS is a technique used to analyze the vascular abnormalities associated with pancreatic disease. By displaying the integrated power of the Doppler signal as opposed to the mean Doppler frequency shift, it is able to overcome some of the drawbacks of traditional color Doppler EUS.[43] Even in the absence of contrast enhancement, power Doppler has been shown to be an accurate test to discriminate between pancreatic cancer and chronic pancreatitis. Săftoiu and colleagues[44] reported an accuracy of 88% with a negative predictive value of 83% (compared with 93% and 81% for EUS-FNA) for the absence of power Doppler signals inside a mass in predicting pancreatic cancer. Furthermore, when the presence or absence of collateral vessels as detected by the power Doppler signal was factored into the analysis, the accuracy and negative predictive value improved to 95% and 92%, respectively.

The addition of intravenous ultrasound contrast agents has proved useful in conjunction with color/power Doppler in certain specific clinical contexts. First, with regards to using hypovascularity to differentiate ductal adenocarcinoma from other lesions, Dietrich and colleagues[45] published a series of 93 patients with undetermined, solitary, and predominantly solid lesions. Using CE-EUS (color Doppler) in conjunction with the first-generation contrast agent Levovist (Bayer AG, Leverkusen, Germany), they were able to report a sensitivity and specificity for hypovascularity as a marker for malignancy in CE-EUS as 92% and 100%, respectively. All other lesions in their series (neuroendocrine tumors, serous microcystic adenomas, and 1 teratoma) revealed an either isovascular or hypervascular pattern. CE-EUS has also shown promise in differentiating chronic pancreatitis from pancreatic cancer. Hocke and colleagues[46,47] published 2 studies suggesting that the addition of contrast agent SonoVue (Bracco, Amsterdam, Netherlands) to power Doppler enhances the differentiation between chronic pancreatitis and pancreatic adenocarcinoma. In their larger series of 194 patients, CE-EUS increased the sensitivity of diagnosing pancreatic cancer from 79% to 92% and the sensitivity of detecting chronic pancreatitis from 82% to 96% compared with EUS alone. Finally, in a series of 41 patients from Japan, Ishikawa and colleagues[48] showed a higher sensitivity for CE-EUS in preoperative localization of pancreatic endocrine tumors (95.1%) compared with either multidetector CT (80.6%) and conventional transabdominal ultrasound (45.2%). On multivariable logistic regression analysis, heterogeneous ultrasonographic texture seemed to be the strongest predictor of malignancy (odds ratio 53.33, 95% confidence interval 10.79–263.58) (Fig. 2).

Limitations of conventional EUS however include Doppler-related artifacts such as "overpainting" (ie, vessel and tumor size appear larger than actual secondary to larger pixel sizes) and "blooming" (ie, decreased vessel delineation secondary to overamplification of Doppler signals). As such, tissue harmonic EUS (CHE-EUS) was subsequently developed for use with ultrasound contrast agents to minimize these effects. Even without the addition of a contrast agent, tissue harmonic imaging appears to generate images that are significantly clearer than traditional EUS imaging for both cystic and solid lesions.[49] Not surprisingly, with the addition of contrast agents, tissue harmonic imaging has shown even more promising results. Unlike power Doppler, harmonic imaging is able to display the microcirculation accurately. Napoleon and colleagues[50] used the second-generation contrast agent SonoVue in conjunction with harmonic imaging and reported a sensitivity, specificity, and accuracy of 89%, 88%, and 88.5%, respectively, of harmonic imaging to detect pancreatic adenocarcinoma based on hypointensity compared with 72%, 100%, and 86% for EUS-FNA alone. A second group, in their series of 277 patients, reported similar results; however, they also compared CHE-EUS to multidetector row CT, and showed that CHE-EUS was significantly better than multidetector row CT in diagnosing small (less than or equal to 2 cm) carcinomas.[51] Interestingly, Fusaroli and colleagues[52] also reported the utility of CHE-EUS in detecting malignancy and guiding EUS-FNA in small lesions with uncertain EUS findings due to either biliary stents or chronic pancreatitis. Finally, Romagnuolo and colleagues[42] used a second-generation perflutren lipid microsphere contrast agent to assess the accuracy of contrast-enhanced harmonic EUS. Although the positive and negative predictive values of CHE-EUS were similar to that of EUS-FNA (80.0%/100% vs 84.6%/100%), they found that in 2 of 30 cases, management changed significantly—by avoiding FNA in a liver hemangioma and a mediastinal cyst confirmed as solid.

Similar to EUS elastography, however, CE-EUS and CHE-EUS have been criticized for their qualitative nature. As such, several quantitative methods have been proposed to improve reliability. Seicean and colleagues[53] used the index of the contrast uptake ratio to discriminate between pancreatic adenocarcinoma and chronic pancreatitis. Although both types of lesions were hypo-enhancing after standard injection with SonoVue, the index of the contrast uptake ratio was significantly lower in adenocarcinoma. Their cutoff uptake ratio index of 0.17 yielded a sensitivity of 80% and a specificity of 92%. In similar fashion, 2 groups have used the "time intensity curve" of contrast uptake and showed that the peak intensity and maximum intensity gain of lesions associated with pancreatitis were significantly higher than those associated with carcinoma.[54,55]

Several prospective studies have since been published attempting to assess the diagnostic accuracy of both CE-EUS and CHE-EUS with sensitivities and specificities ranging from 92%–96% and 93%–96%, respectively, for CE-EUS[47,55] to 80%–100% and 88%–99%, respectively, for CHE-EUS.[50–53] In a recent meta-analysis including 1139 patients who underwent CE-EUS or CHE-HUS, the authors reported a pooled sensitivity of 94%, specificity of 89%, and area under the sROC curve of 0.9732 for assessing the accuracy of CE-EUS in diagnosing pancreatic adenocarcinoma.[56]

In review, the addition of ultrasound contrast agents to power/color Doppler EUS is useful in certain clinical contexts. Studies have confirmed the utility of both CE-EUS and CHE-EUS in helping to differentiate pancreatic malignancy from chronic pancreatitis as well as to guide FNA in small lesions with uncertain EUS findings. As quantitative methods continue to improve and newer contrast agents continue to be developed, the use of CE-EUS may become more widespread. However, similar to elastography, CE-EUS currently remains an adjunctive technique to EUS-FNA.

Three-Dimensional EUS

Three-dimensional EUS (3D-EUS) is an emerging technique that allows for the accurate calculation of volumes by digitizing and reconstructing traditional 2-dimensional (2D) images. Each 2D image is placed into its correct location in a 3D grid, which subsequently creates a volume in cubic form.[57] In doing so, 3D-EUS facilitates an improved understanding of spatial relationships between lesions of interest and surrounding structures.[40] Furthermore, by allowing for the acquisition of multiplanar images, 3D-EUS may facilitate preoperative planning of particular surgical approaches. Although the data are most robust for 3D-EUS in conjunction with endorectal ultrasound in the assessment of rectal cancer[58–60] and for the evaluation of anorectal fistulas,[61,62] one study has shown utility with regard to pancreaticobiliary imaging. In a series of 22 patients with solid pancreatic lesions, Fritscher-Ravens and colleagues[63] compared 3D linear EUS to conventional linear EUS to differentiate between vascular compression and vascular involvement. Using surgical histology as the gold standard, 3D-EUS proved more accurate than 2D-EUS in the evaluation of vascular involvement, particularly in patients with chronic pancreatitis. Nevertheless, given the limited amount of published data, prospective studies still must be performed to investigate the utility of 3D-EUS further in clinical pancreatic imaging.

Needle-based Confocal Laser-induced Endomicroscopy

Confocal laser-induced endomicroscopy (CLE) is an optical technique that produces images at the cellular and subcellular level, enabling the user to perform targeted, "smart biopsies," rather than random biopsies.[64] With adjustable imaging of plane depth, CLE yields sequential high-resolution sections through the mucosal layer. To obtain confocal images, fluorescent contrast agents are applied to a sample.[65,66] An optical fiber acts as both illumination source and detection pinhole, producing high spatial resolution. The created gray-scale image is an optical section representing one focal plane within the examined specimen. Although intravenous fluoroscein is used most commonly, topical agents such as acriflavine have also been used.

The utility of CLE has been shown most widely in an array of mucosal gastrointestinal diseases such as Barrett's esophagus, ulcerative colitis, and colorectal cancer.[67–71] CLE has demonstrated the ability to differentiate neoplastic from normal tissue, and even to differentiate low-grade from high-grade dysplasia. This technology has

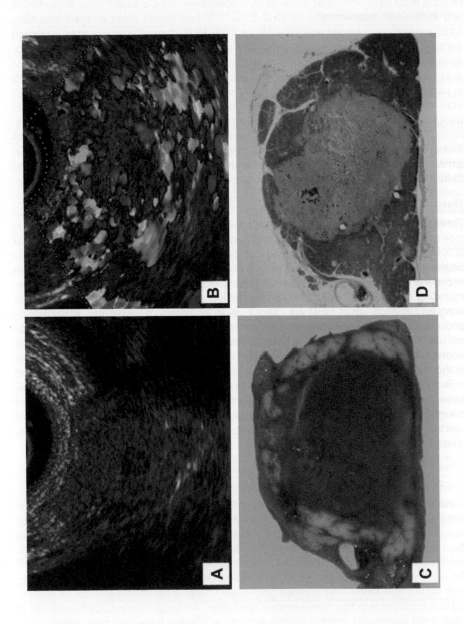

recently become miniaturized; a new confocal miniprobe now exists (Cellvizio; Mauna Kea Technology, Paris, France), enabling easier, in vivo real-time histopathologic imaging without need for a confocal endoscope. Although probe-based CLE gives lower resolution and a fixed imaging plane depth, it has the advantage of faster image acquisition.

Recently, a needle-based miniaturized probe has broadened the potential applications to nonmucosal surfaces such as intra-abdominal viscera. The feasibility of needle-based confocal endomicroscopy (nCLE) has been evaluated in multiple animal models. Becker and colleagues[72] first demonstrated feasibility of this needle-based system in a porcine model. Imaging was performed in 10 pigs with a confocal miniprobe inserted through a 22-gauge needle and intravenous fluorescein. Real-time images were obtained and correlated with biopsy specimens. Pancreatic imaging was deemed to be more complicated than hepatic imaging because of anatomic positioning; 8 of 10 attempts were successful. This study demonstrated that it is feasible to extend imaging into the lesion of interest and possibly enable targeted biopsy. This targeted biopsy could lead to improved yield or fewer passes during EUS-FNA; in the best scenario, it could reduce the need for onsite cytology. Similar findings were demonstrated in an EUS-guided needle-based confocal laser-induced endomicroscopy study published in abstract form.[73] EUS-guided nCLE was again shown to be feasible. In addition, images appeared to correlate with histology.

The first study looking at the feasibility of nCLE during EUS-FNA of the pancreas in humans was authored by Konda and colleagues.[74] The prototype was based on the CholangioFlex miniprobe (Mauna Kea Technologies). The study population included 16 cysts and 2 masses. A 19-gauge FNA needle was used to puncture the lesion. The authors report technical challenges with several features: postloading (probe loaded into needle after stylet removed), longer ferules (metallic tip at distal end of probe, protecting the device from the beveled tip of the needle), and a transduodenal FNA approach. One drawback is that this nCLE fiber required a 19-gauge needle. In another multicenter, international study by the same investigators, the authors looked at nCLE in vivo in pancreatic cysts and presented their work in abstract form. Endosonographers in 8 centers performed nCLE in 67 patients with pancreatic cysts during EUS-FNA with a 19-gauge needle. Although this study demonstrated feasibility, 2 adverse events of pancreatitis and 3 cases of bleeding occurred.[75] Although nCLE seems promising, its current safety profile is unlikely to be acceptable to the EUS community at large.

High-resolution Microendoscopy

The authors' group recently demonstrated the potential utility of a high-resolution microendoscope (HRME) device in pancreatic imaging.[76] Previous ex vivo and in vivo studies in the esophagus and colon have suggested this device may be able

---

Fig. 2. (A) EUS showed a 30-mm large hypoechoic tumor in the pancreatic tail. Heterogeneous hypoechoic area was seen in the center of the tumor. (B) Contrast-enhanced EUS revealed obvious enhancement in the tumor, but no enhancement in the central hypoechoic area on EUS (type B). (C) Photograph of the gross specimen contains severe hemorrhage inside the tumor. (D) H&E stain of the resected specimen shows necrosis with hemorrhage in the center of the tumor and invasive growth to surrounding fat tissue. The tumor was diagnosed as a well-differentiated endocrine tumor, "uncertain" behavior. (From Ishikawa T, Itoh A, Kawashima H, et al. Usefulness of EUS combined with contrast-enhancement in the differential diagnosis of malignant versus benign and preoperative localization of pancreatic endocrine tumors. Gastrointest Endosc 2010;71(6):951–9; with permission.)

to provide guidance to aid in performing targeted biopsy and potentially increase diagnostic yield. Although it does not have the optical sectioning ability of confocal endomicroscopy, it has demonstrated good image quality and offers the advantage of a cost-effective (less than $2500) and reusable probe. Their study demonstrated the feasibility of this new imaging technology in an in vivo swine model. Delivery of the contrast agent was straightforward and manipulation of the HRME probe was comparable to working with EUS-FNA alone. Experienced endosonographers with prior experience in HRME (over 50 cases) could achieve accuracy as high as 95% in the pancreas, indicating a relatively short learning curve. In addition, because the study coordinated the HRME images with ex vivo surgical specimens and coordinated tissue sections, an accurate pathologic diagnosis could be used as the gold standard (**Fig. 3**). Technical issues still needing to be addressed include timing and method of dye delivery.

Optical Coherence Tomography

Optical coherence tomography (OCT) is another adjunctive technique used to provide high-resolution optical imaging. It allows for imaging up to 2 mm, far beyond what CLE is able to perform. In one ex vivo study, investigators evaluated the OCT pattern of the main pancreatic duct in normal and various pathologies and compared these with histology from surgical specimens.[77] Using an OCT catheter, they assessed surgical specimens from 10 patients who had undergone the Whipple procedure for known adenocarcinoma. Although they noted poor agreement with histology for distinguishing normal pancreatic duct wall from inflammation, OCT was consistently able to distinguish neoplasm and agreed with histology in all cases where neoplasm was present. Another ex vivo study of 66 pancreatectomy specimens demonstrated that OCT could reliably differentiate between low-risk and high-risk cysts with greater than 95% sensitivity and specificity.[78] Using a training set from 20 tissue samples, OCT diagnostic criteria for pancreatic cysts was developed. These criteria were then validated by a separate validation set from 46 other tissue specimens. Feasibility of OCT was also demonstrated in an in vivo study of a dog model.[79]

Trans-Needle Pancreatic Cystoscopy

Trans-needle pancreatic cystoscopy uses a single-operator fiber optic visualization system originally introduced for cholangioscopy and pancreatoscopy (SpyGlass; Boston Scientific, Natick, MA, USA).[80] To date, 2 groups have reported its use in conjunction with EUS to visualize and biopsy pancreatic cystic lesions with nonspecific CT and EUS features. In the first case report by Antillon and colleagues,[81] although the cystic fluid was nondiagnostic, biopsy of the cyst wall was consistent with pseudocyst, and the lesion was irrigated and drained. In a subsequent series of 2 patients, Aparicio and colleagues[82] passed biopsy forceps through a 19-gauge EUS needle to obtain cyst wall biopsies where previous FNA did not obtain cells. Subsequent direct fiber optic intracystic visualization revealed normal mucosa in both patients, ruling out the possibility of pseudocysts. In both patients, biopsies were suggestive of mucinous cystadenomas. The forceps were able to be continuously visualized during EUS, optimizing its safety. The limitations of this procedure included limited accessibility because of the need for the 19-gauge needle and the small size of the biopsy samples. A prospective study using nCLE and Spyglass through a 19-gauge needle to evaluate pancreatic cysts is currently underway; results have been published in abstract form.[83] These pilot studies suggest that as image quality and therapeutic capabilities improve, the use of trans-needle pancreatic cystoscopy may become a more routine complement to nondiagnostic EUS examinations.

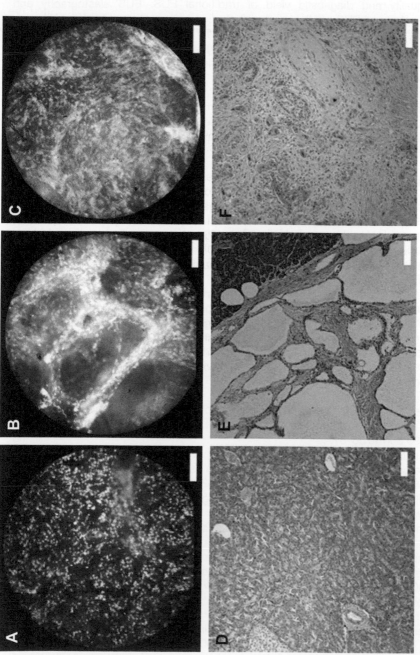

Fig. 3. (A–C) Representative HRME images of normal, benign, and malignant lesions of the pancreas. (D–F) Corresponding H&E-stained histology (original magnification, ×10). (A and D) Normal pancreas. Note the clustering of nuclei into acinar structures. (B and E) Microcystic adenoma, benign lesion. Note the cystic spaces of varying shapes and sizes. (C and F) Ductal adenocarcinoma, malignant lesion. Note the loss of normal architecture and infiltrating poorly formed glands amid desmoplastic stroma. Scale bars represent 100 μm. (*From* Regunathan R, Woo J, Pierce MC, et al. Feasibility and preliminary accuracy of high-resolution imaging of the liver and pancreas using FNA compatible microendoscopy (with video). Gastrointest Endosc 2012;76(2):293–300; with permission.)

SUMMARY

In summary, many promising techniques have now been developed to enhance the image quality and diagnostic yield of traditional EUS. EUS elastography and contrast-enhanced EUS are the most well-studied and most used to date. Although promising, issues of subjectivity and compatibility with current processors still need to be addressed for these technologies. Although well-designed prospective studies and meta-analyses show promising results, they remain adjunctive techniques to EUS-FNA rather than potential replacements at this point. 3D-EUS as well as needle-based techniques, such as confocal laser-induced endomicroendoscopy, high-resolution microendoscopy, optical coherence tomography, and trans-needle cystoscopy, remain mainly experimental, and the incremental benefit these technologies provide from a cost-benefit and practical standpoint above and beyond EUS-FNA is yet to be determined.

REFERENCES

1. Kaufman AR, Sivak MV Jr. Endoscopic ultrasonography in the differential diagnosis of pancreatic disease. Gastrointest Endosc 1989;35(3):214–9.
2. Agarwal B, Abu-Hamda E, Molke KL, et al. Endoscopic ultrasound-guided fine needle aspiration and multidetector spiral CT in the diagnosis of pancreatic cancer. Am J Gastroenterol 2004;99(5):844–50. http://dx.doi.org/10.1111/j.1572-0241.2004.04177.x.
3. Ahmad NA, Kochman ML, Lewis JD, et al. Endosonography is superior to angiography in the preoperative assessment of vascular involvement among patients with pancreatic carcinoma. J Clin Gastroenterol 2001;32(1):54–8.
4. Soriano A, Castells A, Ayuso C, et al. Preoperative staging and tumor resectability assessment of pancreatic cancer: prospective study comparing endoscopic ultrasonography, helical computed tomography, magnetic resonance imaging, and angiography. Am J Gastroenterol 2004;99(3):492–501. http://dx.doi.org/10.1111/j.1572-0241.2004.04087.x.
5. Gress FG, Hawes RH, Savides TJ, et al. Role of EUS in the preoperative staging of pancreatic cancer: a large single-center experience. Gastrointest Endosc 1999;50(6):786–91.
6. Aslanian H, Salem R, Lee J, et al. EUS diagnosis of vascular invasion in pancreatic cancer: surgical and histologic correlates. Am J Gastroenterol 2005;100(6):1381–5. http://dx.doi.org/10.1111/j.1572-0241.2005.41675.x.
7. Puli SR, Singh S, Hagedorn CH, et al. Diagnostic accuracy of EUS for vascular invasion in pancreatic and periampullary cancers: a meta-analysis and systematic review. Gastrointest Endosc 2007;65(6):788–97. http://dx.doi.org/10.1016/j.gie.2006.08.028.
8. Bao PQ, Johnson JC, Lindsey EH, et al. Endoscopic ultrasound and computed tomography predictors of pancreatic cancer resectability. J Gastrointest Surg 2008;12(1):10–6. http://dx.doi.org/10.1007/s11605-007-0373-y [discussion: 16].
9. DeWitt J, Devereaux BM, Lehman GA, et al. Comparison of endoscopic ultrasound and computed tomography for the preoperative evaluation of pancreatic cancer: a systematic review. Clin Gastroenterol Hepatol 2006;4(6):717–25. http://dx.doi.org/10.1016/j.cgh.2006.02.020.
10. Chen J, Yang R, Lu Y, et al. Diagnostic accuracy of endoscopic ultrasound-guided fine-needle aspiration for solid pancreatic lesion: a systematic review. J Cancer Res Clin Oncol 2012;138(9):1433–41. http://dx.doi.org/10.1007/s00432-012-1268-1.

11. Gress F, Gottlieb K, Sherman S, et al. Endoscopic ultrasonography-guided fine-needle aspiration biopsy of suspected pancreatic cancer. Ann Intern Med 2001; 134(6):459–64.

12. Harewood GC, Wiersema MJ. Endosonography-guided fine needle aspiration biopsy in the evaluation of pancreatic masses. Am J Gastroenterol 2002; 97(6):1386–91. http://dx.doi.org/10.1111/j.1572-0241.2002.05777.x.

13. Brugge WR, Lewandrowski K, Lee-Lewandrowski E, et al. Diagnosis of pancreatic cystic neoplasms: a report of the cooperative pancreatic cyst study. Gastroenterology 2004;126(5):1330–6.

14. Chong AK, Caddy GR, Desmond PV, et al. Prospective study of the clinical impact of EUS. Gastrointest Endosc 2005;62(3):399–405.

15. Canto MI, Harinck F, Hruban RH, et al. International Cancer of the Pancreas Screening (CAPS) Consortium summit on the management of patients with increased risk for familial pancreatic cancer. Gut 2012. http://dx.doi.org/10.1136/gutjnl-2012-303108.

16. Canto MI, Hruban RH, Fishman EK, et al. Frequent detection of pancreatic lesions in asymptomatic high-risk individuals. Gastroenterology 2012;142(4): 796–804. http://dx.doi.org/10.1053/j.gastro.2012.01.005 [quiz: e14–5].

17. Harewood GC, Wiersema LM, Halling AC, et al. Influence of EUS training and pathology interpretation on accuracy of EUS-guided fine needle aspiration of pancreatic masses. Gastrointest Endosc 2002;55(6):669–73.

18. Klapman JB, Logrono R, Dye CE, et al. Clinical impact of on-site cytopathology interpretation on endoscopic ultrasound-guided fine needle aspiration. Am J Gastroenterol 2003;98(6):1289–94. http://dx.doi.org/10.1111/j.1572-0241. 2003.07472.x.

19. Varadarajulu S, Tamhane A, Eloubeidi MA. Yield of EUS-guided FNA of pancreatic masses in the presence or the absence of chronic pancreatitis. Gastrointest Endosc 2005;62(5):728–36. http://dx.doi.org/10.1016/j.gie.2005.06.051 [quiz: 751, 753].

20. Bhutani MS, Gress FG, Giovannini M, et al. The No Endosonographic Detection of Tumor (NEST) Study: a case series of pancreatic cancers missed on endoscopic ultrasonography. Endoscopy 2004;36(5):385–9. http://dx.doi.org/10.1055/s-2004-814320.

21. Fritscher-Ravens A, Brand L, Knöfel WT, et al. Comparison of endoscopic ultrasound-guided fine needle aspiration for focal pancreatic lesions in patients with normal parenchyma and chronic pancreatitis. Am J Gastroenterol 2002; 97(11):2768–75. http://dx.doi.org/10.1111/j.1572-0241.2002.07020.x.

22. Anderson MA, Scheiman JM. Initial experience with an electronic radial array echoendoscope: randomized comparison with a mechanical sector scanning echoendoscope in humans. Gastrointest Endosc 2002;56(4):573–7. http://dx.doi.org/10.1067/mge.2002.127761.

23. Niwa K, Hirooka Y, Niwa Y, et al. Comparison of image quality between electronic and mechanical radial scanning echoendoscopes in pancreatic diseases. J Gastroenterol Hepatol 2004;19(4):454–9.

24. Frey H. Realtime elastography. A new ultrasound procedure for the reconstruction of tissue elasticity. Radiologe 2003;43(10):850–5. http://dx.doi.org/10.1007/s00117-003-0943-2.

25. Dawwas MF, Taha H, Leeds JS, et al. Diagnostic accuracy of quantitative EUS elastography for discriminating malignant from benign solid pancreatic masses: a prospective, single-center study. Gastrointest Endosc 2012;76(5):953–61. http://dx.doi.org/10.1016/j.gie.2012.05.034.

26. Friedrich-Rust M, Ong MF, Martens S, et al. Performance of transient elastography for the staging of liver fibrosis: a meta-analysis. Gastroenterology 2008; 134(4):960–74. http://dx.doi.org/10.1053/j.gastro.2008.01.034.

27. Sun L, Ning C, Liu Y, et al. Is transvaginal elastography useful in pre-operative diagnosis of cervical cancer? Eur J Radiol 2012;81(8):e888–92. http://dx.doi.org/10.1016/j.ejrad.2012.04.025.

28. Brock M, Von Bodman C, Palisaar RJ, et al. The impact of real-time elastography guiding a systematic prostate biopsy to improve cancer detection rate: a prospective study of 353 patients. J Urol 2012;187(6):2039–43. http://dx.doi.org/10.1016/j.juro.2012.01.063.

29. Azizi G, Keller J, Lewis Pa M, et al. Performance of elastography for the evaluation of thyroid nodules: a prospective study. Thyroid 2012. http://dx.doi.org/10.1089/thy.2012.0227.

30. Barr RG, Destounis S, Lackey LB 2nd, et al. Evaluation of breast lesions using sonographic elasticity imaging: a multicenter trial. J Ultrasound Med 2012;31(2): 281–7.

31. Giovannini M, Hookey LC, Bories E, et al. Endoscopic ultrasound elastography: the first step towards virtual biopsy? Preliminary results in 49 patients. Endoscopy 2006;38(4):344–8. http://dx.doi.org/10.1055/s-2006-925158.

32. Giovannini M, Thomas B, Erwan B, et al. Endoscopic ultrasound elastography for evaluation of lymph nodes and pancreatic masses: a multicenter study. World J Gastroenterol 2009;15(13):1587–93.

33. Iglesias-Garcia J, Larino-Noia J, Abdulkader I, et al. EUS elastography for the characterization of solid pancreatic masses. Gastrointest Endosc 2009;70(6): 1101–8. http://dx.doi.org/10.1016/j.gie.2009.05.011.

34. Saftoiu A, Vilman P. Endoscopic ultrasound elastography– a new imaging technique for the visualization of tissue elasticity distribution. J Gastrointestin Liver Dis 2006;15(2):161–5.

35. Săftoiu A, Vilmann P, Gorunescu F, et al. Accuracy of endoscopic ultrasound elastography used for differential diagnosis of focal pancreatic masses: a multicenter study. Endoscopy 2011;43(7):596–603. http://dx.doi.org/10.1055/s-0030-1256314.

36. Săftoiu A, Vilmann P, Gorunescu F, et al. Efficacy of an artificial neural network-based approach to endoscopic ultrasound elastography in diagnosis of focal pancreatic masses. Clin Gastroenterol Hepatol 2012;10(1):84–90.e1. http://dx.doi.org/10.1016/j.cgh.2011.09.014.

37. Iglesias-Garcia J, Larino-Noia J, Abdulkader I, et al. Quantitative endoscopic ultrasound elastography: an accurate method for the differentiation of solid pancreatic masses. Gastroenterology 2010;139(4):1172–80. http://dx.doi.org/10.1053/j.gastro.2010.06.059.

38. Mei M, Ni J, Liu D, et al. EUS elastography for diagnosis of solid pancreatic masses: a meta-analysis. Gastrointest Endosc 2012. http://dx.doi.org/10.1016/j.gie.2012.09.035.

39. Pei Q, Zou X, Zhang X, et al. Diagnostic value of EUS elastography in differentiation of benign and malignant solid pancreatic masses: a meta-analysis. Pancreatology 2012;12(5):402–8. http://dx.doi.org/10.1016/j.pan.2012.07.013.

40. Fusaroli P, Saftoiu A, Mancino MG, et al. Techniques of image enhancement in EUS (with videos). Gastrointest Endosc 2011;74(3):645–55. http://dx.doi.org/10.1016/j.gie.2011.03.1246.

41. Kato T, Tsukamoto Y, Naitoh Y, et al. Ultrasonographic and endoscopic ultrasonographic angiography in pancreatic mass lesions. Acta Radiol 1995;36(4):381–7.

42. Romagnuolo J, Hoffman B, Vela S, et al. Accuracy of contrast-enhanced harmonic EUS with a second-generation perflutren lipid microsphere contrast agent (with video). Gastrointest Endosc 2011;73(1):52–63. http://dx.doi.org/10.1016/j.gie.2010.09.014.

43. Koito K, Namieno T, Nagakawa T, et al. Pancreas: imaging diagnosis with color/power Doppler ultrasonography, endoscopic ultrasonography, and intraductal ultrasonography. Eur J Radiol 2001;38(2):94–104.

44. Săftoiu A, Popescu C, Cazacu S, et al. Power Doppler endoscopic ultrasonography for the differential diagnosis between pancreatic cancer and pseudotumoral chronic pancreatitis. J Ultrasound Med 2006;25(3):363–72.

45. Dietrich CF, Ignee A, Braden B, et al. Improved differentiation of pancreatic tumors using contrast-enhanced endoscopic ultrasound. Clin Gastroenterol Hepatol 2008;6(5):590–597.e1. http://dx.doi.org/10.1016/j.cgh.2008.02.030.

46. Hocke M, Schulze E, Gottschalk P, et al. Contrast-enhanced endoscopic ultrasound in discrimination between focal pancreatitis and pancreatic cancer. World J Gastroenterol 2006;12(2):246–50.

47. Hocke M, Schmidt C, Zimmer B, et al. Contrast enhanced endosonography for improving differential diagnosis between chronic pancreatitis and pancreatic cancer. Dtsch Med Wochenschr 2008;133(38):1888–92. http://dx.doi.org/10.1055/s-0028-1085571.

48. Ishikawa T, Itoh A, Kawashima H, et al. Usefulness of EUS combined with contrast-enhancement in the differential diagnosis of malignant versus benign and preoperative localization of pancreatic endocrine tumors. Gastrointest Endosc 2010;71(6):951–9. http://dx.doi.org/10.1016/j.gie.2009.12.023.

49. Ishikawa H, Hirooka Y, Itoh A, et al. A comparison of image quality between tissue harmonic imaging and fundamental imaging with an electronic radial scanning echoendoscope in the diagnosis of pancreatic diseases. Gastrointest Endosc 2003;57(7):931–6. http://dx.doi.org/10.1067/mge.2003.271.

50. Napoleon B, Alvarez-Sanchez MV, Gincoul R, et al. Contrast-enhanced harmonic endoscopic ultrasound in solid lesions of the pancreas: results of a pilot study. Endoscopy 2010;42(7):564–70. http://dx.doi.org/10.1055/s-0030-1255537.

51. Kitano M, Kudo M, Yamao K, et al. Characterization of small solid tumors in the pancreas: the value of contrast-enhanced harmonic endoscopic ultrasonography. Am J Gastroenterol 2012;107(2):303–10. http://dx.doi.org/10.1038/ajg.2011.354.

52. Fusaroli P, Spada A, Mancino MG, et al. Contrast harmonic echo-endoscopic ultrasound improves accuracy in diagnosis of solid pancreatic masses. Clin Gastroenterol Hepatol 2010;8(7):629–634.e1–2. http://dx.doi.org/10.1016/j.cgh.2010.04.012.

53. Seicean A, Badea R, Stan-Iuga R, et al. Quantitative contrast-enhanced harmonic endoscopic ultrasonography for the discrimination of solid pancreatic masses. Ultraschall Med 2010;31(6):571–6. http://dx.doi.org/10.1055/s-0029-1245833.

54. Imazu H, Kanazawa K, Mori N, et al. Novel quantitative perfusion analysis with contrast-enhanced harmonic EUS for differentiation of autoimmune pancreatitis from pancreatic carcinoma. Scand J Gastroenterol 2012;47(7):853–60. http://dx.doi.org/10.3109/00365521.2012.679686.

55. Matsubara H, Itoh A, Kawashima H, et al. Dynamic quantitative evaluation of contrast-enhanced endoscopic ultrasonography in the diagnosis of pancreatic diseases. Pancreas 2011;40(7):1073–9. http://dx.doi.org/10.1097/MPA.0b013e31821f57b7.

56. Gong T, Hu D, Zhu Q. Contrast-enhanced EUS for differential diagnosis of pancreatic mass lesions: a meta-analysis. Gastrointest Endosc 2012;76(2):301–9. http://dx.doi.org/10.1016/j.gie.2012.02.051.

57. Giovannini M. Contrast-enhanced and 3-dimensional endoscopic ultrasonography. Gastroenterol Clin North Am 2010;39(4):845–58. http://dx.doi.org/10.1016/j.gtc.2010.08.027.

58. Giovannini M, Bories E, Pesenti C, et al. Three-dimensional endorectal ultrasound using a new freehand software program: results in 35 patients with rectal cancer. Endoscopy 2006;38(4):339–43. http://dx.doi.org/10.1055/s-2005-870412.

59. Hünerbein M, Pegios W, Rau B, et al. Prospective comparison of endorectal ultrasound, three-dimensional endorectal ultrasound, and endorectal MRI in the preoperative evaluation of rectal tumors. Preliminary results. Surg Endosc 2000;14(11):1005–9.

60. Kim JC, Cho YK, Kim SY, et al. Comparative study of three-dimensional and conventional endorectal ultrasonography used in rectal cancer staging. Surg Endosc 2002;16(9):1280–5. http://dx.doi.org/10.1007/s00464-001-8277-5.

61. Buchanan GN, Bartram CI, Williams AB, et al. Value of hydrogen peroxide enhancement of three-dimensional endoanal ultrasound in fistula-in-ano. Dis Colon Rectum 2005;48(1):141–7.

62. Murad-Regadas SM, Regadas FS, Rodrigues LV, et al. The role of 3-dimensional anorectal ultrasonography in the assessment of anterior transsphincteric fistula. Dis Colon Rectum 2010;53(7):1035–40. http://dx.doi.org/10.1007/DCR.0b013e3181dce163.

63. Fritscher-Ravens A, Knoefel WT, Krause C, et al. Three-dimensional linear endoscopic ultrasound-feasibility of a novel technique applied for the detection of vessel involvement of pancreatic masses. Am J Gastroenterol 2005;100(6):1296–302. http://dx.doi.org/10.1111/j.1572-0241.2005.41681.x.

64. Goetz M, Watson A, Kiesslich R. Confocal laser endomicroscopy in gastrointestinal diseases. J Biophotonics 2011;4(7–8):498–508. http://dx.doi.org/10.1002/jbio.201100022.

65. Kiesslich R, Goetz M, Hoffman A, et al. New imaging techniques and opportunities in endoscopy. Nat Rev Gastroenterol Hepatol 2011;8(10):547–53. http://dx.doi.org/10.1038/nrgastro.2011.152.

66. Kiesslich R, Goetz M, Neurath MF. Virtual histology. Best Pract Res Clin Gastroenterol 2008;22(5):883–97. http://dx.doi.org/10.1016/j.bpg.2008.05.003.

67. Kiesslich R, Goetz M, Lammersdorf K, et al. Chromoscopy-guided endomicroscopy increases the diagnostic yield of intraepithelial neoplasia in ulcerative colitis. Gastroenterology 2007;132(3):874–82. http://dx.doi.org/10.1053/j.gastro.2007.01.048.

68. Sanduleanu S, Driessen A, Gomez-Garcia E, et al. In vivo diagnosis and classification of colorectal neoplasia by chromoendoscopy-guided confocal laser endomicroscopy. Clin Gastroenterol Hepatol 2010;8(4):371–8. http://dx.doi.org/10.1016/j.cgh.2009.08.006.

69. Li CQ, Li YQ. Endomicroscopy of intestinal metaplasia and gastric cancer. Gastroenterol Clin North Am 2010;39(4):785–96. http://dx.doi.org/10.1016/j.gtc.2010.08.023.

70. Canto MI. Endomicroscopy of Barrett's Esophagus. Gastroenterol Clin North Am 2010;39(4):759–69. http://dx.doi.org/10.1016/j.gtc.2010.08.032.

71. Neumann H, Kiesslich R, Wallace MB, et al. Confocal laser endomicroscopy: technical advances and clinical applications. Gastroenterology 2010;139(2):388–92. http://dx.doi.org/10.1053/j.gastro.2010.06.029, 392.e1–2.

72. Becker V, Wallace MB, Fockens P, et al. Needle-based confocal endomicroscopy for in vivo histology of intra-abdominal organs: first results in a porcine

model (with videos). Gastrointest Endosc 2010;71(7):1260–6. http://dx.doi.org/ 10.1016/j.gie.2010.01.010.

73. Shinoura S. EUS-guided needle-based confocal laser induced endomicroscopy (nCLE): a correlation study of "through the needle" imaging with normal histology in a porcine model. Gastrointest Endosc 2011;73:AB325–6.

74. Konda VJ, Aslanian HR, Wallace MB, et al. First assessment of needle-based confocal laser endomicroscopy during EUS-FNA procedures of the pancreas (with videos). Gastrointest Endosc 2011;74(5):1049–60. http://dx.doi.org/ 10.1016/j.gie.2011.07.018.

75. Jamil LH, Meining A, Wallace MB, et al. Safety Profile of Needle-Based Confocal Laser Endomicroscopy (nCLE) during EUS-FNA procedures of the pancreatic cystic lesions. Gastrointest Endosc 2012;75:AB188–9.

76. Regunathan R, Woo J, Pierce MC, et al. Feasibility and preliminary accuracy of high-resolution imaging of the liver and pancreas using FNA compatible microendoscopy (with video). Gastrointest Endosc 2012;76(2):293–300. http://dx.doi.org/10.1016/j.gie.2012.04.445.

77. Testoni PA, Mangiavillano B, Albarello L, et al. Optical coherence tomography compared with histology of the main pancreatic duct structure in normal and pathological conditions: an "ex vivo study". Dig Liver Dis 2006;38(9):688–95. http://dx.doi.org/10.1016/j.dld.2006.05.019.

78. Iftimia N, Cizginer S, Deshpande V, et al. Differentiation of pancreatic cysts with optical coherence tomography (OCT) imaging: an ex vivo pilot study. Biomed Opt Express 2011;2(8):2372–82. http://dx.doi.org/10.1364/BOE.2.002372.

79. Singh P, Chak A, Willis JE, et al. In vivo optical coherence tomography imaging of the pancreatic and biliary ductal system. Gastrointest Endosc 2005;62(6): 970–4. http://dx.doi.org/10.1016/j.gie.2005.06.054.

80. Chen YK. Preclinical characterization of the Spyglass peroral cholangiopancreatoscopy system for direct access, visualization, and biopsy. Gastrointest Endosc 2007;65(2):303–11. http://dx.doi.org/10.1016/j.gie.2006.07.048.

81. Antillon MR, Tiwari P, Bartalos CR, et al. Taking SpyGlass outside the GI tract lumen in conjunction with EUS to assist in the diagnosis of a pancreatic cystic lesion (with video). Gastrointest Endosc 2009;69(3 Pt 1):591–3. http://dx.doi.org/ 10.1016/j.gie.2008.05.003.

82. Aparicio JR, Martínez J, Niveiro M, et al. Direct intracystic biopsy and pancreatic cystoscopy through a 19-gauge needle EUS (with videos). Gastrointest Endosc 2010;72(6):1285–8. http://dx.doi.org/10.1016/j.gie.2010.08.036.

83. Nakai Y. Diagnosis of pancreatic cysts: endoscopic Ultrasound Through-the-needle confocal laser-induced Endomicroscopy and Cystoscopy Trial (DETECT Study). Gastrointest Endosc 2011;75(4S):AB145–6.

Advanced Techniques for Endoscopic Biliary Imaging
Cholangioscopy, Endoscopic Ultrasonography, Confocal, and Beyond

Charles Gabbert, MD[a], Matthew Warndorf, MD[a],
Jeffrey Easler, MD[a], Jennifer Chennat, MD[b],*

KEYWORDS

- Biliary imaging • Cholangioscopy • Endoscopic ultrasonography
- Malignant biliary strictures

KEY POINTS

- Cholangioscopy, endosonography, and confocal microscopy represent important technologies that expand biliary imaging beyond a level previously realized by noninvasive modalities (ultrasonography, computed tomography, and magnetic resonance cholangiopancreatography) and endoscopic retrograde cholangiopancreatography (ERCP).
- For the delineation of indeterminate bile duct strictures, cholangioscopy and confocal microscopy have shown a complimentary role to ERCP.
- Endoscopic ultrasonography (EUS) has shown efficacy for the evaluation of indeterminate biliary strictures; however, this modality seems most reliable for distal bile duct abnormalities and in the setting of a moderate to high pretest probability for malignancy.
- One advantage of EUS in this context is that it is a safe modality with a more favorable profile for risks of complications when compared with imaging techniques that rely on transpapillary access.
- Overall, major barriers for these techniques are linked to the need for substantial specialized training; with much of their efficacy in terms of image interpretation relying on the subjective gestalt of an experienced endoscopist.
- Further refinement of these technologies, validation of their respective diagnostic criteria, and study within the context of comparative, randomized trials are needed and will contribute greatly to expedient patient care.

[a] Division of Gastroenterology, Hepatology, & Nutrition, University of Pittsburgh Medical Center, 200 Lothrop Street, C Wing, Mezzanine Level, Pittsburgh, PA 15213, USA; [b] Division of Gastroenterology, Hepatology, & Nutrition, Liver-Pancreas Institute, University of Pittsburgh Medical Center, 200 Lothrop Street, C Wing, Mezzanine Level, Pittsburgh, PA 15213, USA
* Corresponding author.
E-mail address: chennatjs@upmc.edu

Gastrointest Endoscopy Clin N Am 23 (2013) 625–646
http://dx.doi.org/10.1016/j.giec.2013.03.009
1052-5157/13/$ – see front matter © 2013 Elsevier Inc. All rights reserved.

IMAGING THE BILIARY TREE: DIAGNOSTIC CHALLENGES AND DILEMMAS

Multiple modalities are in clinical use for noninvasive imaging of the biliary tree. Abdominal ultrasonography, computed tomography (CT), and magnetic resonance cholangiopancreatography (MRCP) are low-risk, widely available imaging modalities, which have been extensively studied for biliary disease. These modalities reliably identify ductal dilatation and, most notably with MRCP, can be excellent for the purpose of diagnosing clinically significant stone disease. However, evaluation of the biliary mucosal abnormalities can be challenging with noninvasive modalities. Also, rates of false-negative results for stone disease increase substantially by location and stone size (≤3 mm) with noninvasive imaging modalities.[1]

For 40 years, endoscopic retrograde cholangiopancreatography (ERCP) has been a well-established tool for both diagnosis and therapy for biliary ductal disease.[2] However, in the setting of advances in noninvasive imaging the role of diagnostic ERCP is diminishing. ERCP is now being changed to a predominantly therapeutic intervention. One notable exception to this trend is the continued use of diagnostic ERCP for the provision of index pathology. Yet as a stand-alone modality to establish a tissue diagnosis, ERCP remains hindered by poor sensitivity; reported between 54% and 71% even with combined brush cytology and intraductal biopsies.[3–5] Various adjunct techniques have been explored to improve the sensitivity of brush cytology obtained by ERCP, including fluorescence in situ hybridization (FISH) and immunohistochemical staining of specimens. FISH has been reported to improve sensitivity 10% to 20% when cytology is negative for malignancy; however, results are overall modest.[6,7] Other techniques, such as DNA methylation of tissue samples and p53 immunostaining of brushed specimens, have yet to show consistent benefit for routine practice despite initial promise.[8,9] Longer brushes with stiff bristles have failed to show a significant improvement in sensitivity and hence cancer detection rate.[10] Cytologic sampling both before and after endoscopic dilation of the bile duct showed a sensitivity around 30%, despite an improved diagnostic yield with repeat brushings.[11] Also, ERCP is not without risk of complications, principal of which is post-ERCP pancreatitis.[12] Hence, repetitive ERCP procedures are less than ideal.

Within the spectrum of biliary disease, one of the most challenging diagnostic dilemmas is the indeterminate stricture. The differential diagnosis for an undiagnosed biliary stricture encompasses both benign (primary sclerosing cholangitis [PSC], IgG4-related cholangitis, autoimmune pancreatitis) and malignant disease (cholangiocarcinoma, hepatocellular carcinoma, and metastatic disease). Cholangiocarcinoma is especially challenging to diagnose in this context. Frequently presenting as a biliary stricture, it may be found with or without a mass and its most common risk factor in Western countries is PSC, a benign fibroinflammatory disease that can independently cause benign biliary strictures.[13] Hilar lesions pose an additional diagnostic challenge. Hilar cholangiocarcinoma often has a relatively indolent course. Also, as many as 24% of patients with hilar strictures suspicious for cholangiocarcinoma based on abnormal tumor markers and imaging may have benign disease.[14,15] However, cholangiocarcinoma is the second most common primary hepatic malignancy, and emphasis is placed on early detection (before lymphatic involvement or extraluminal invasion), because patients may enjoy a favorable 5-year survival.[16,17]

In addition, biliary stone disease can be a diagnostic challenge. It is estimated that more than 20 million people in the United States have gallstone disease, leading to more than $6.2 billion dollars in annual costs.[18,19] Choledocholithiasis occurs in approximately 15% to 20% of patients with symptomatic cholelithiasis.[20] The potential for morbidity is high when untreated, with consequent complications of cholangitis, hepatic abscess, and acute pancreatitis.[21] American Society for Gastrointestinal Endoscopy guidelines[22] suggest that patients at intermediate risk of choledocholithiasis may benefit from additional biliary imaging before or during cholecystectomy. As mentioned earlier, noninvasive imaging has the potential for false-negative evaluations within this context.[1] ERCP also has diagnostic limitations. Small stones can be lost in the background of an undiluted contrast cholangiogram, and large stones can block ducts, preventing flow of contrast.[23] A multicenter study presented in abstract form[24] reported that almost 30% of patients who underwent ERCP for indications other than suspected choledocholithiasis had a false-negative cholangiogram for stone disease when followed and confirmed by cholangioscopy. Residual stone burden after mechanical lithotripsy was also found to be common in a similarly designed study.[25]

Overall, biliary imaging for the diagnosis of both benign and malignant disease remains a challenge for reliability and consistency. Consequently, a great deal of attention and research have been dedicated toward advanced modalities of biliary imaging, which are outlined in this article.

CHOLANGIOSCOPY

Cholangioscopy is a technique for direct endoscopic visualization of the bile ducts. Within this context, its use has been reported from expert centers, both for targeted tissue sampling and intraductal interventions. Common bile duct endoscopy was first reported in the form of intraoperative choledochoscopy. This technique was reported as early as 1941, used as a measure to exclude choledocholithiasis after cholecystectomy.[26] Twenty years later, this technology matured into a dedicated flexible choledochoscope, introduced via a percutaneous, transhepatic approach to diagnose biliary disease.[27,28] Transhepatic approaches are still in use; however, these are reserved for patients who cannot undergo a peroral intervention, such as in cases of altered anatomy or after peroral endoscopic failure. Peroral cholangioscopy was first reported in 1976 and is now the most common form of direct biliary endoscopy. Early techniques described the passage of a thin cholangioscope into the common bile duct (CBD) through the accessory port of a duodenoscope.[29,30] A single-scope direct peroral approach was described 1 year later; performed with an 8.8-mm fiberscope inserted into the biliary system after endoscopic papillotomy.[31]

Cholangioscopy has now evolved into a variety of systems used for multiple indications. However, its use continues to be largely realized at academic institutions and tertiary referral centers. Mother-baby cholangioscopy is a technique whereby a smaller, thinner cholangioscope (baby) is passed through the instrument channel of a larger duodenoscope (mother). Originally requiring 2 skilled endoscopists to manipulate a dual-endoscope system, early models were also limited by an absence of irrigation channel, fragile, small-caliber equipment, lack of tip deflection, and suboptimal image quality. SpyGlass Direct Visualization System (Boston Scientific, Natick, MA) is a late, single-operator system that attempted to address these early limitations (**Fig. 1**). Introduced in 2006, SpyGlass is a single-operator system, yet it is based on the original mother-baby platform.[32] An independent instrument, with an operator interface that allows 4-way tip defection, it attaches near the instrument channel of a duodenoscope. Using a flexible, 230-cm, 10-French access catheter, it is delivered into the biliary tract after papillary sphincterotomy or dilation, through the instrument channel of a duodenoscope or colonoscope (minimum channel diameter of 3.4 mm). The potential of the catheter for 4-way tip defection and its 3 ports (irrigation channel, a port for insertion of an optical probe able to provide 6000-pixel images, and a 1.2-mm accessory channel) represent advancement over early cholangioscopic systems.

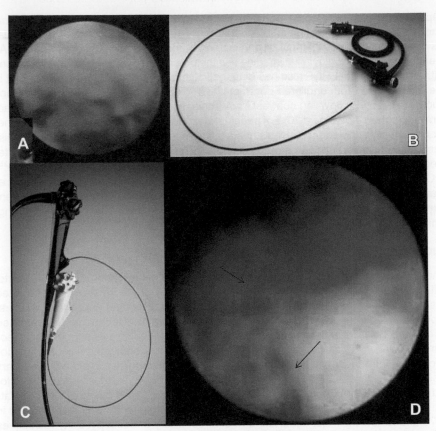

Fig. 1. (*A*) Nodular CBD mucosa on SpyGlass in the setting of cholangiocarcinoma, (*B*) Olympus CHF, BP30 transduodenal choledochofiberscope, (*C*) Boston Scientific SpyGlass system, Natick, MA (*D*) dilated CBD vessels on SpyGlass in the setting of cholangiocarcinoma (*arrows*).

Direct peroral video cholangioscopy is a recent system, which entails the insertion of an ultraslim endoscope into the biliary tree to achieve high-quality digital imaging. These endoscopes range from 5 to 6 mm in external diameter and can be fed over a stiff 0.89-mm (0.035-in) Jagwire (Boston Scientific, Natick, MA) to gain access to the bile duct.[33] Once the duodenoscope has been removed and fluoroscopic-guided wire exchange has been performed, the ultraslim endoscope is backloaded over the guidewire and advanced into the biliary system. A balloon-assisted anchoring system has also been reported to maintain stable access.[34] Direct peroral choledo-choscopes use video imaging, which despite formal comparative studies seems to be superior to many mother-baby systems.[35] In addition to being single-user system and providing high-quality images, models also provide a larger, 2-mm working channel for therapeutic interventions.

The safety profile of peroral cholangioscopy is still being defined. Overall, current data suggest a similar complication rate to that of ERCP alone, with some notable caveats. Chen and colleagues[36] report an incidence of serious adverse effects in 7.5% cases of diagnostic single-operator cholangioscopy and in 6.1% of patients undergoing directed stone fragmentation. A retrospective review[37] of 402 patients who underwent cholangiopancreatoscopy reported significantly higher rates of postcholangioscopy cholangitis (1.0%) when compared with 3475 patients who underwent ERCP alone (0.2%). There were no reported significant differences in the rates of pancreatitis or perforation. The investigators suggest that increased rates of cholangitis may be related to intraprocedural saline irrigation. Of additional concern is that cholangioscopy may more frequently induce episodes of cholangitis in patients with PSC or complex strictures.[38,39] For these reasons, prophylactic antibiotics with or without postprocedural biliary drainage are strongly recommended. Direct peroral video cholangioscopy has several reports of episodes of air embolism.[40]

Peroral cholangioscopy is now considered for a variety of diagnostic and therapeutic indications. This article focuses on (1) the evaluation of indeterminate bile duct strictures, (2) targeted tissue sampling to assist with the diagnosis or exclusion of malignancy, and (3) management of biliary stone disease.

Evaluation of Indeterminate and Malignant Biliary Strictures

As outlined earlier, efforts to improve the yield of diagnostic index pathology obtained during cholangiography has realized limited success. False-negative results remain unacceptably high, complicating and delaying timely patient care, especially in those with malignancy. Multiple studies have explored cholangioscopic systems to improve diagnostic accuracy in the evaluation of indeterminate strictures.

Current data suggest that cholangioscopy with and without biopsy is associated with an improved diagnostic yield when compared with ERCP alone. The SpyGlass system allows for direct visualization of biliary epithelium, targeting tissue sampling of previously undefined biliary lesions. Studies have reported adequate tissue sampling using the SpyBite biopsy forceps in 82% to 97% of cases.[36,41–43]

Single-operator cholangioscopy with biopsy has shown a possible, incremental accuracy as high as 85% for characterizing indeterminate strictures, when compared with cytology and transpapillary biopsy (34% and 54%, respectively). Sensitivity has been reported to be as high as 90% for this technique in diagnosing malignancy, with little impact on specificity and accuracy.[44–46]

Benefits of overall ERCP-cholangiography–directed index pathology have been reported to be related to: (1) direct visualization of epithelial features, some of which are now considered specific for malignancy, and (2) targeting biopsies for more meaningful specimens for histopathologic review. Unique to cholangioscopy is the added diagnostic usefulness of identifying various mucosal abnormalities suggestive of malignancy by an experienced biliary endoscopist. Mucosal neovascularization, manifested by irregular vasculature and dilated blood vessels, is reported as the most specific finding for malignancy (see Fig. 1).[47] In 1 study, detection of this abnormality endoscopically was reported to carry a sensitivity of nearly 100%[44] Nodularity and irregular patterns of luminal stenosis have also been appreciated within the context of malignant disease; however, these are believed to be lesser features with lower specificity (see Fig. 1). The significance of these findings within the context of malignancy and their association with benign disease is a major concern, and new modalities (ie, methylene blue-aided inspection) are being explored to further evaluate and validate these endoscopic characteristics.[48,49]

The diagnostic usefulness of both inspection in addition directed biopsies for indeterminate strictures was shown in a large multicenter prospective observational study that included 297 patients.[36] The investigators reported an overall sensitivity of 78% for visual inspection alone versus sensitivity of nearly 50% when directed biopsies were obtained. Clinical management was affected in 64% of patients undergoing cholangioscopy. The import of visual inspection has shown reproducibility across systems, with further supporting evidence from literature on the SpyGlass system. One study[42] reported a sensitivity of 85% and specificity of 79% when performing inspection alone using the SpyGlass system. Both sensitivity and specificity were noted to be 82%, respectively, with SpyBite miniforceps for targeted biopsies.

Cholangioscopy is also being explored for the classification of strictures in patient populations with fibroinflammatory biliary disease and anastomotic anatomy such as PSC, IgG4 cholangiopathy, and liver transplant recipients. A prospective study of 53 patients with a dominant stricture on imaging in the context of PSC showed superior efficacy for detecting malignancy when compared with ERCP alone.[50] Superior sensitivity (92% vs 66%), specificity (93% vs 51%), accuracy (93% vs 55%), and both positive (79% vs 29%) and negative predictive values (97% vs 84%) were observed in the cholangioscopy group. A diagnostic role for cholangioscopy in identifying IgG4-mediated disease in patients with a previous diagnosis of PSC is also being explored.[51] An observational study comprising 20 patients following orthotopic liver transplantation showed a role for cholangioscopy in diagnosing ischemic cholangiopathy, anastomotic ulceration, and even retained sutures.[52] Future considerations may further implicate a role for cholangioscopy in the mapping of intraductal tumor spread before surgical resection and even in the evaluation of recurrent pancreatitis of unknown cause.[46,53]

Adjunct imaging technologies are being paired with cholangioscopy as avenues for enhanced evaluation of biliary epithelium. These modalities include autofluorescence and narrow-band imaging (NBI). Autofluorescence technology highlights abnormal mucosa as black or dark green and is reported to increase the sensitivity of cholangioscopy to nearly 100%; however, this is at the expense of specificity and accuracy.[54] NBI achieves optical color separation by narrowing the bandwidth of transmitted images. Prototype models (Olympus, Center Valley, PA) have been used in various centers as attempts are made to validate its clinical usefulness. One study[55] evaluated both NBI and conventional white light cholangioscopy for 21 biliary lesions. Visualization of intraductal disease such as surface structures and vessel architecture was more often rated excellent when using NBI. These modalities add limited, incremental benefit. Major limitations include poor visualization in the setting of mucus and pus. Also, bile and blood appear similar with NBI. Although there is promise for these modalities in that they may enable the biliary endoscopist to detect early lesions that possess flat, minimally projecting architecture, technology that facilitates evaluation for submucosal abnormalities, proximal disease, and overall provides better magnification is desirable and yet to be realized.

Diagnosis and Management of Choledocholithiasis

Cholangioscopy has emerged as a useful nonsurgical method of achieving stone retrieval in difficult cases and has even been shown to detect residual stones in nearly 30% of patients who have previously undergone mechanical lithotripsy during conventional ERCP.[25]

Intraductal lithotripsy may be required in complicated choledocholithiasis in the setting of failed, traditional ERCP techniques. It is best performed under direct cholangioscopic visualization and the aim is to avoid the complications of bleeding or perforation. Cholangioscopy-directed lithotripsy has a reported success rate of 90% to 100% in various observational studies.[56,57] The precise technique of intervention varies by endoscopist and expert center. This variability begins even with the cholangioscopic system with SpyGlass, direct choledochoscopy and dual-operator systems reporting similar levels of success and often the need for only 1 session.[36,41,43,58] Universal to effective lithotripsy is a need for sufficient intraprocedural irrigation of the bile duct; late cholangioscopic systems offer the necessary working channels for technical success.

Specific techniques for intracorporeal stone fragmentation include laser ablation and shock wave (electrohydraulic) therapy. Laser lithotripsy is performed using a double-pulse yttrium aluminum garnet (YAG) or holmium laser, which can be directed at difficult stones for fragmentation.[59] A prospective, randomized trial reported that cholangioscopy-directed laser lithotripsy realized a significantly higher rate of stone clearance (97%) than conventional extracorporeal shock wave lithotripsy, with fewer sessions.[60] These findings have been validated in subsequent investigations.[56] No randomized data exist comparing laser lithotripsy and intraductal electrohydraulic lithotripsy under cholangioscopic guidance. Factors that affect the selection of a particular modality largely depend on the training and comfort of the biliary endoscopist with a certain technique. Laser lithotripsy may carry a higher cost and may be more time consuming.

Expanding Therapeutic Applications

Other emerging interventional applications for cholangioscopy include ablative therapy for the management of established, malignant biliary strictures. These applications include cholangioscopy-directed photodynamic therapy, YAG laser ablation, and argon plasma coagulation for management of intraductal tumor growth.[61–63] Cholangioscopy-assisted biliary access and drainage across complex stricture disease has also been described. In 1 report, intrahepatic duct stent placement was successfully achieved using a 5-mm ultraslim endoscope after repeated attempts during conventional ERCP had failed.[64] Cholangioscopy has also been reported as a modality to facilitate guidewire placement in the presence of severe, complex strictures in both malignant disease as well as in those with a history of liver transplantation.[65,66] Future considerations may also include a role for cholangioscopy in the assessment and treatment of hemobilia.[67]

ENDOSCOPIC ULTRASONOGRAPHY

Endoscopic ultrasonography (EUS) is an imaging modality that uses uniquely designed echo endoscopes that possess optical, sonographic, and mechanical properties beyond those of traditional ultrasound transducers and gastrointestinal endoscopes.[68–70] Since its inception around 30 years ago, EUS has played an important role in staging gastrointestinal and nongastrointestinal malignancies and diagnosing pancreaticobiliary disease and in recent years has been recognized as an important tool for the therapeutic endoscopist. The proximity of the stomach and duodenum to the extrahepatic biliary system has expanded EUS as a useful means of imaging biliary anatomy. The technique of fine-needle aspiration (FNA) offers the potential for tissue sampling to obtain index pathology.

Indeterminate Strictures and Cholangiocarcinoma

The role of EUS in the evaluation of indeterminate strictures is becoming increasingly prominent in the literature. However, there remains controversy regarding its efficacy and best use.

Several studies have reported EUS-guided FNA to be a reasonable modality for the evaluation of indeterminate biliary strictures. Retrospective cohort studies comprising fewer than 25 patients evaluated EUS-FNA for indeterminate strictures, reporting a sensitivity and specificity of 77% to 100% and 100%, respectively.[71,72] However, these studies stand in contrast to several, larger retrospective studies that show a sensitivity of 45% to 47%[73,74] Variable results are likely related to the anatomic location of the lesions within the extrahepatic biliary tree. This is best shown in a study by Rosch and colleagues,[3] in which they prospectively compared ERCP brush cytology/forceps biopsy versus EUS-guided FNA for biliary strictures. EUS-FNA was found to be inferior to ERCP in the subgroup of patients with proximal/hilar, biliary tumors (EUS 25% vs ERCP 75%); however, it was superior for distal malignant strictures in the setting of pancreatic mass (EUS 60% vs ERCP 38%).[3]

Promising results were found in a recent meta-analysis of 9 studies, comprising a total of 284 patients, that showed EUS-FNA to have a pooled sensitivity for the diagnosis of biliary strictures of 84% and specificity of 100%.[75] Moreover, significant rate of complications were not reported for EUS-FNA in this setting, suggesting that it is an overall safe modality.[75]

As is to be expected with many imaging modalities, when the pretest probability of malignancy is increased, EUS-FNA seems to have more consistent results. A large single-center prospective study of patients with cholangiocarcinoma showed that EUS (94%) was superior compared with triphasic CT (30%) and magnetic resonance imaging (42%) for tumor detection in patients with available imaging.[76] In terms of diagnostic histopathology, promising data are reported in prospective studies. Two studies with cohorts ranging from 28 to 42 patients found EUS-FNA to be both sensitive and specific for diagnosing suspicious biliary tree lesions, at greater than 86% and 100%, respectively.[77,78] Positive predictive value, negative predictive value, and diagnostic accuracy for this technique in the context of suspicious lesions for malignancy were 100%, 57%, and 88%.[78] In addition, EUS-FNA for proximal lesions in this context after a previous workup suggestive for malignancy have shown favorable results for yielding a confirmatory diagnosis. In one study,[79] 44 patients with potentially operable hilar strictures concerning for cholangiocarcinoma with previous inconclusive tissue diagnosis underwent EUS-guided FNA. Of these patients, 26 were found to have cholangiocarcinoma, 5 other malignancies, and 12 had benign findings. The accuracy, sensitivity, and specificity were reported as 91%, 89%, and 100%, respectively.[79] Moreover, in a case series of 10 patients with bile duct strictures at the hilum concerning for cholangiocarcinoma,[80] EUS-guided FNA provided adequate material for analysis in 9 patients.

Overall sensitivity of EUS-FNA for diagnosis of indeterminate strictures is variable. It seems that efficacy is greater for distal versus proximal lesions (81% vs 59%, respectively) and in the setting of lesions with higher pretest probability for malignancy.[76]

Choledocholithiasis

In contrast to evaluation of indeterminate strictures and malignant biliary disease, EUS is now established to be a reliable, safe modality for the diagnosis of biliary stone disease (Fig. 2).

In a prospective study of 64 consecutive patients referred for ERCP for suspected choledocholithiasis, Canto and colleagues[81] found the overall sensitivity and specificity of EUS for detecting choledocholithiasis to be 84% and 98%, compared with 95% and 98% for ERCP. There was no significant difference in terms of diagnostic accuracy for detecting choledocholithiasis between EUS and ERCP (94% and 97%, respectively).[81] Moreover, EUS had a significantly lower overall complication rate compared with diagnostic ERCP (1.6% vs 9.4%; $P<.05$).[81] The investigators suggest that EUS may be a useful technique for detecting or ruling out stones in patients at intermediate/moderate risk of choledocholithiasis, whereas ERCP is the preferred test in high-risk patients.[81]

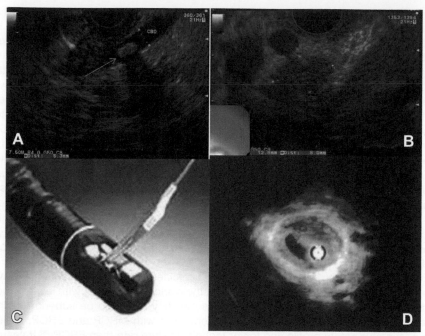

Fig. 2. (*A*) CBD stone (*arrow*). (*B*) Common hepatic duct mass (*green lines*). (*C*) UM-G20-29R IDUS miniprobe, Olympus. (*D*) Irregular bile duct wall on IDUS. ([*C, D*] *Courtesy of* Olympus America, Inc, Center Valley, PA; with permission.)

A multicenter prospective study of 36 patients with acute biliary pancreatitis assigned to undergo EUS before ERCP[82] was stopped after interim analysis reported the high accuracy of EUS in identifying absence of stones in the bile duct, because the researchers could not ethically justify performing ERCP in patients after normal EUS. The investigators reported sensitivity, specificity, diagnostic accuracy, positive predictive value, and negative predictive value of EUS for diagnosing choledocholithiasis as 91%, 100%, 97%, 100%, and 95%, respectively.[82] A systematic review of 4 studies comprising 420 patients comparing EUS-guided ERCP against diagnostic ERCP for the detection of choledocholithiasis reported that 143 ERCPs could be avoided when EUS did not detect choledocholithiasis. The investigators reported a significant relative risk reduction for overall complications of 0.35 (95% confidence interval [CI], 0.20–0.62) and, specifically, post-ERCP pancreatitis of 0.21 (95% CI, 0.06–0.83) when EUS was used before ERCP compared with diagnostic ERCP.[83] However, the drawback was that 38.5% of patients in the EUS-guided ERCP group required a second endoscopic procedure when a stone was identified compared with ERCP alone.[83]

The literature for EUS in evaluating choledocholithiasis has reached a critical mass to confidently assess its efficacy across large numbers of patients. A meta-analysis of 36 studies and more than 3500 patients[84] found that EUS had a pooled sensitivity of 88% and specificity of 90% for detecting biliary obstruction. Looking at choledocholithiasis, the investigators included 31 studies with 3075 patients, and found that EUS had a pooled sensitivity of 89% and specificity of 94% for detecting biliary obstruction.[84] Similarly, Tse and colleagues[85] conducted a meta-analysis of 27 studies and more than 2600 patients, and found pooled sensitivity and specificity of EUS for detecting choledocholithiasis of 94% and 95% respectively.

Numerous studies exist evaluating EUS compared with other imaging modalities for biliary stone disease. A prospective study of 45 patients with extrahepatic biliary dilatation by transabdominal ultrasonography found that EUS and MRCP had similar diagnostic accuracy (88.9% vs 93.3%), sensitivity (91.9% vs 97.3%, respectively), and equal specificity (75%) for evaluating the cause of ductal dilatation.[86] Nineteen of the 45 patients were found to have stones or sludge as the cause of their ductal dilatation, which was correctly identified by EUS in all 19 cases. However, MRCP identified biliary sludge in only 50% of cases. EUS in this study showed a sensitivity, specificity, diagnostic accuracy, positive predictive value, and negative predictive value of 100%, respectively.[86] A systematic review of 5 studies and more than 300 patients comparing EUS and MRCP for the detection of choledocholithiasis showed high diagnostic performance for both and no statistical difference between the 2 modalities.[87] This study reported aggregated sensitivities of EUS and MRCP to be 93% and 85%, with specificities of 96% and 93%, respectively.[87] Overall, it seems that EUS may be superior to MRCP, especially in detecting microlithiasis and sludge.

EUS seems to offer additional diagnostic usefulness over traditional noninvasive imaging modalities and diagnostic ERCP for the workup of patients with low to moderate suspicion for choledocholithiasis. This modality may also be superior for the identification of sludge and microlithiasis compared with MRCP and ERCP. It also has a favorable safety profile and lower technical failure rate than ERCP.[88] It seems to be an appropriate modality for excluding choledocholithiasis in patients being considered for ERCP with an intermediate pretest probability for biliary stone disease.

Intraductal Ultrasonography: Indeterminate Strictures and Choledocholithiasis

There are also multiple studies evaluating the usefulness of biliary endosonography with a transpapillary intraductal ultrasonography (IDUS) probe as an adjunct to ERCP.

Original designs incorporated large catheters, positioned without a guidewire, which were fragile and easily damaged by the duodenoscope elevator during biliary endoscopy.

Recent studies report results using probes smaller than 2.9 mm connected to a standard EUS processor. Passed over a guidewire in a monorail fashion, these probes provide radial scanned images perpendicular from their axis, at an ultrasound frequency of 20 to 30 MHz, with penetration of 2 cm with a resolution of 0.07 to 0.18 mm (see **Fig. 2**).[89] This technique is reported to add 5 to 10 minutes to ERCP in experienced hands.[6]

IDUS for the biliary system normally shows 3 layers: the hyperechoic mucosa and its interface with bile (innermost), the second hypoechoic fibromuscular layer, and the hyperechoic, subserosal fat (outermost).[89]

More than 10 years of literature exists for IDUS for indeterminate strictures. However, delineating asymmetric bile duct wall thickening in benign, inflammatory, and malignant strictures remains a challenge. The following criteria are considered concerning for malignancy in this context: hypoechoic strictures and irregular infiltrating margins. When only 1 of these features is present, abnormal stricture morphology (asymmetry, notching, or shelflike appearance) and suspicious lymph nodes assist with designating a stricture as malignant (see **Fig. 2**).[6,90–92] This criterion has been reported as 62% to 89% accurate depending on the clinical context.[90] Interruption of the bile duct, sessile tumors, and tumor size greater than 10 mm have also been reported as specific criteria.[93] However, despite what are becoming established criteria for this technology, endosonographer experience, clinical context of the examination, or general gestalt of the examiner have been shown to be important for IDUS when evaluating indeterminate strictures, especially within the context of such diseases as PSC.[6] In addition, previous stenting can hinder sonographic interpretation. This examination is best performed before biliary drainage at the time of index ERCP access.

Comparative studies have examined this technique against other modalities. Domagk and colleagues[91] evaluated 33 patients with biliary strictures who underwent ERCP, MRCP, and IDUS, correlating findings with surgical resection specimens. IDUS was successfully performed in all patients. ERCP/IDUS gave a correct diagnosis for malignancy in 88% of patients (29/33) versus ERCP alone (76% [25/33]). ERCP/IDUS had a greater accuracy than MRCP alone ($P = .0047$). Accuracy of IDUS in combination with various diagnostic approaches for biliary strictures approaches more than 90% in the literature.[91,93–97]

For established cholangiocarcinoma, IDUS may play a role in T staging and assessing longitudinal spread of malignancy within the biliary tree, with accuracy superior to that of EUS.[90,98] However, depth of penetration is limited to 2 cm, which may limit its role for fully staging nodal spread and assessing distant disease.

For stone disease, the role of IDUS in patient care remains unclear. Endo and colleagues[99] reported IDUS after a negative ERCP for suspected stone disease in 47 patients. Of these patients, 12 and 8 patients were found to have stones and sludge, respectively. Stones found in this group were smaller (5 mm vs 13 mm [$P<.001$]) and tended to have a CBD greater than 12 mm. The investigators found that sensitivity for ERCP was 74% for stones smaller than 8 mm and was affected by a CBD greater than 12 mm.

Overall, the role of IDUS as an advanced technique for biliary imaging is promising. As an adjunct to ERCP, it offers an interval increase in accuracy for the evaluation of biliary strictures and may have a role in identifying small stone disease and sludge. Also, miniprobes smaller than 2.9 mm may easily pass through tight strictures and a 2 cm depth of penetration, offering the ability to image lateral ducts. However, validation of diagnostic criteria for delineating benign and malignant indeterminate strictures requires further validation and is hindered by previous bile duct manipulation.

PROBE-BASED CONFOCAL LASER ENDOMICROSCOPY

Confocal microscopy captures direct, submillimeter images through optical sectioning of tissue in vivo.[100] Described as a laser-tipped endoscope system, image collection within the context of biliary disease occurs via an independent flexible miniprobe ranging from 0.9 to 2.5 mm in diameter.[100] Probe application for indeterminate strictures begins with standard-of-care biliary access using ERCP techniques. They can be positioned proximate to a stricture either through a catheter or using the cholangioscope system described earlier. Previously described catheters and cholangioscopic systems able to accommodate a probe-based confocal laser endomicroscopy (pCLE) probe are listed in **Table 1**.[101]

Real-time imaging is achieved through the projection of a coherent (488 nm, blue light) low-powered laser light. Light is passed through a confocal aperture as a focused, single point. The light emanating from this point is focused through a confocal aperture behind the lens to reduce both the scattering and detection of light of the focal plane.[15,100,101] Laser light is then detected by a photodetection device and transformed into electrical signals processed into grayscale images. Image collection

Table 1
Catheters and cholangioscopic systems able to accommodate pCLE catheters (1.2 mm channel or greater)

Devices (Cannulas and Cholangioscopy Systems), Alphabetical	Manufacturer
Catheters	
Cotton Graduate Dilation Catheter, T7.0	Cook Medical
Geenen Graduated Dilation Catheter	Cook Medical
Howell Biliary Introducer (H-BIN)	Cook Medical
Memory Dormia Basket (Rel MSB_35_2 × 4)	Cook Medical
Oasis One Action Stent Introduction System	Cook Medical
Swing Tip ERCP Cannula	Olympus Medical
Cholangioscopic Systems	
CHF-P20, T20	Olympus
CHF-BP-30[a]	Olympus
FCP-9P[a]	Pentax
SpyGlass catheter[a]	Boston Scientific

List does not include special order, rental program devices.
[a] Peroral devices.

occurs at 12 frames per second; with a field of 325 μm, a lateral resolution of 3.5 μm, and a depth of 40 to 70 μm.[100,101] Image processing occurs within a stand-alone computer unit with specialized software for image correction, stabilization, and real-time display for the endoscopist.

Intravenous fluorescein dye is administered at 1 to 5 mL, 10% solution before tissue imaging. A fluorophore, this dye binds to extracellular matrix in epithelium and the lamina propria. Cell nuclei and mucin are not stained and appear dark.[100] This dye facilitates a greater depth of imaging and helps delineate individual cells and their associated capillary network. A selective lack of uptake by neoplastic tissue gives it a contrasted, dark appearance. Proposed mechanisms include lack of uptake by vessels in neoplastic tissue, rapid excretion of contrast, or a greater degree of leak within diseased lamina propria.[15,101,102] Normal tissue has a white, netlike pattern.[15] Optimal timing for image collection after contrast injection is 10 minutes; however, imaging is possible as early as 10 seconds after dye injection and ideally occurs within 30 to 60 minutes of contrast administration.[103]

This technique for biliary imaging can be challenging to master. Optimal imaging necessitates substantial probe and patient stability and requires subtle, fine movements for probe placement. Logistic challenges include poor image quality with bleeding (which can be problematic when examining friable, previously instrumented strictures), perpendicular probe positioning (also difficult in narrow strictures), and small movements by the patient or the examiner, such as occur during respiration. Timing image collection with dye administration also makes this a time-dependent evaluation.[101]

This technology is indicated once an indeterminate stricture has already been detected via CT/MRCP or ERCP and is considered suspicious for malignancy.[100]

The miniprobe system was first reported in 2007 by Meining and colleagues[104]; it was used to evaluate gastrointestinal lesions outside the biliary tract. The first published study for indeterminate pancreaticobiliary strictures was also described by Meining and colleagues,[105] in 2008. A 0.94-mm confocal miniprobe introduced through a peroral cholangioscope (3.5 mm external diameter, 1.4 mm instrument channel) was reported. Continuous water flow was used during imaging, and the probe was placed under direct, cholangioscopic guidance. This study comprised 14 patients with hilar or CBD indeterminate strictures. Mean age was 61 years, 40% were female and 6 patients (40%) were diagnosed with malignancy. The investigators defined confirmed neoplasia for comparative purposes in the setting of positive tissue at surgery or if a malignant diagnosis was clearly confirmed by other forms of imaging, Strictures were considered benign if the aforementioned findings were absent after 9 months of follow-up. Lesions were reached and evaluated in all patients. Sensitivity, specificity, and overall accuracy were 50%, 100%, and 79%, respectively. Confocal microscopy findings correlated with a final diagnosis of malignancy on surgical pathology in 2 patients with negative endoscopic biopsies.

Further refinement and literature on this technique have now been reported by a pCLE working group. Criteria outlining neoplastic findings within pancreaticobiliary strictures are based on the Miami consensus working group. Suggestive criteria for malignancy include thick, dark bands larger than 40 μm, thick white bands larger than 20 μm with flow, dark clumps, abnormal visualized epithelial structures (villi, glands), and fluorescein leakage (**Fig. 3**). Criteria for benign strictures include thin, dark branching bands (<20 μm) without flow or thin, white bands. Acceptable interobserver agreement was shown in blinded, randomized fashion.[103]

This working group has published the largest study. In a multicenter study of 102 patients, the investigators reported data on 89 patients with evaluable findings. Mean age was 63 years, and 54% were male. Seventy percent were evaluated for an indeterminate pancreaticobiliary structure, followed by pancreaticobiliary mass on imaging and jaundice. Two-thirds of patients had previous biliary stent placement. Investigators were trained using a pCLE imaging dataset comprising confirmed benign and malignant strictures. A correlation of 90% with the correct diagnosis and the subsequent completion of 10 pCLE procedures independently were required before patients could participate in the study. The investigators reported sensitivity, specificity, positive predictive value, and negative predictive value of 98%, 67%, 71%, and 97%. This finding was in contrast to 45%, 100%, 100%, and 67% for index pathology samples. Overall accuracy for pCLE was 81% versus 75% when compared with index pathology sampling ($P \leq .001$). Use of cholangioscopic delivery rather than catheter delivery trended toward increased specificity; however, this was not

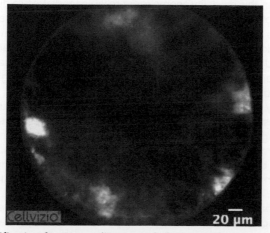

Fig. 3. Miami classification for CBD malignancy: dark clumps.

significant. When combined with standard ERCP technique, accuracy was reported to be 90% with pCLE (P = .001). Striking results include only 1 false-negative result for pCLE versus 22 for tissue sampling.[106]

Overall, pCLE represents a novel technology, showing a small, statistically significant improvement over index pathology for accuracy in diagnosis of a neoplastic tissue from indeterminate pancreaticobiliary strictures. Also, an added benefit of immediate diagnosis can affect medical decision making for biliary decompression (metal stent vs plastic) and expedite delivery of care for these patients. The most significant drawbacks include a learning curve (technical and image interpretation) for this technique, as with any new technology. Meining and colleagues[106] reported differences in specificity and ease of interpretation of images between early versus late cohorts of patients (0.55 vs 0.71). In addition, in 54% of patients, the investigators elected to wait for pathology results before establishing a diagnosis with therapeutic consequences. In addition, further studies are needed for confirmation of anatomic correlates with what are considered normal and abnormal features for pCLE in this context. This technology requires further study of indeterminate strictures in populations comprising patients with PSC, autoimmune cholangiopathy, and liver transplant.

DISCUSSION

Cholangioscopy, endosonography, and confocal microscopy represent important technologies that expand biliary imaging beyond a level previously realized by noninvasive modalities (ultrasonography, CT, and MRCP) and ERCP. The literature on these advanced modalities explores applications within the major challenges of biliary imaging, specifically, the evaluation of indeterminate strictures and reliable identification of biliary stone disease.

For the delineation of indeterminate bile duct strictures, cholangioscopy and confocal microscopy have shown a complementary role to ERCP. A limited, but significant, interval improvement in accuracy has been reported in multiple studies for these modalities for the evaluation of undifferentiated strictures and the diagnosis of cholangiocarcinoma. However, further validation of their respective diagnostic criteria, the need for subspecialized training, and the consequent significant barriers toward their wide dissemination throughout the medical community and in day-to-day practice limit their use. EUS has shown efficacy for the evaluation of indeterminate biliary strictures; however, this modality seems most reliable for distal bile duct abnormalities and in the setting of a moderate to high pretest probability for malignancy. One advantage of EUS in this context is that it is a safe modality with a more favorable profile for risks of complications when compared with imaging techniques that rely on transpapillary access. IDUS offers advantages in terms of a sensitive evaluation of strictures that have not been previously manipulated and access across tight strictures and possibly plays a role in tumor staging (**Table 2**).

Cholangioscopy and EUS have mature literature regarding their usefulness for the diagnosis or exclusion of biliary stone disease. EUS is now an established, reliable modality for evaluating patients at intermediate pretest probability for choledocholithiasis and those with diminutive stone disease, microlithiasis, and sludge. Cholangioscopy shows sensitivity beyond that of cholangiography and is becoming an established technique for the management of complex choledocholithiasis through intracorporeal lithotripsy.

Overall, major barriers for these techniques are linked to the need for substantial specialized training, with much of their efficacy in terms of image interpretation relying on the subjective gestalt of an experienced endoscopist. This observation is evident

Table 2
Advanced imaging techniques for the diagnosis of indeterminate biliary strictures

Imaging Technique	Types of Trials	Sensitivity (%)	Accuracy (%)	Limitations	Complications	Overall Role in Workup
Cholangioscopy	RC, PC, MA	78–100	~90	Requires ERCP for access Optical findings require further validation Limited access to peripheral/proximal lesions	Cholangitis, (above ERCP risk) Air embolism (case reports)	Adjunct to ERCP of proximal and distal strictures: Diagnosis Directing tissue biopsies
EUS-FNA	RC, PC, MA	Any 43–100 Hilar 25–67	70–91	Limited imaging and access to hilar/proximal lesions	Minimal beyond standard gastrointestinal endoscopy	Possible first test: especially for distal (CBD) strictures
IDUS	RC, PC	>87	76–92	Requires ERCP for access and tissue sampling Decreased accuracy after stenting Sonographic findings require further validation Limited stage for nodal and distant disease	None beyond ERCP	Adjunct to ERCP for diagnosis of proximal (hilar) lesions T staging in cholangiocarcinoma
pCLE	RC, PC	98	~80	Requires ERCP for access and tissue sampling Optical findings require further validation Timing with dye, technically challenging	Reaction to dye Otherwise None beyond ERCP	Adjunct to ERCP for diagnosis of proximal and distal lesions

Abbreviations: MA, meta-analysis; PC, prospective cohort; RC, retrospective cohort.

through the efficacy profiles of cholangioscopy, IDUS, and pCLE for the diagnosis of indeterminate strictures, which rely substantially on expert image interpretation beyond that of reported criteria.

Further refinement of these technologies, validation of their respective diagnostic criteria, and study within the context of comparative, randomized trials are needed and will contribute greatly to expedient patient care.

ACKNOWLEDGMENTS

Special thanks to Dr Kevin McGrath for supplying EUS pictures for **Fig. 2** and Dr Adam Slivka for supplying cholangioscopy images for **Fig. 2**.

REFERENCES

1. Yeh BM, Liu PS, Soto JA, et al. MR imaging and CT of the biliary tract. Radiographics 2009;29(6):1669–88.
2. Cohen S, Bacon BR, Berlin JA, et al. National Institutes of Health State-of-the-Science Conference Statement: ERCP for diagnosis and therapy, January 14-16, 2002. Gastrointest Endosc 2002;56(6):803–9.
3. Rosch T, Hofrichter K, Frimberger E, et al. ERCP or EUS for tissue diagnosis of biliary strictures? A prospective comparative study. Gastrointest Endosc 2004; 60(3):390–6.
4. Ponchon T, Gagnon P, Berger F, et al. Value of endobiliary brush cytology and biopsies for the diagnosis of malignant bile duct stenosis: results of a prospective study. Gastrointest Endosc 1995;42(6):565–72.
5. Schoefl R, Haefner M, Wrba F, et al. Forceps biopsy and brush cytology during endoscopic retrograde cholangiopancreatography for the diagnosis of biliary stenoses. Scand J Gastroenterol 1997;32(4):363–8.
6. Levy MJ, Baron TH, Clayton AC, et al. Prospective evaluation of advanced molecular markers and imaging techniques in patients with indeterminate bile duct strictures. Am J Gastroenterol 2008;103(5):1263–73.
7. Fritcher EG, Kipp BR, Halling KC, et al. A multivariable model using advanced cytologic methods for the evaluation of indeterminate pancreatobiliary strictures. Gastroenterology 2009;136(7):2180–6.
8. Parsi MA, Li A, Li CP, et al. DNA methylation alterations in endoscopic retrograde cholangiopancreatography brush samples of patients with suspected pancreaticobiliary disease. Clin Gastroenterol Hepatol 2008;6(11):1270–8.
9. Stewart CJ, Burke GM. Value of p53 immunostaining in pancreatico-biliary brush cytology specimens. Diagn Cytopathol 2000;23(5):308–13.
10. Fogel EL, deBellis M, McHenry L, et al. Effectiveness of a new long cytology brush in the evaluation of malignant biliary obstruction: a prospective study. Gastrointest Endosc 2006;63(1):71–7.
11. de Bellis M, Fogel EL, Sherman S, et al. Influence of stricture dilation and repeat brushing on the cancer detection rate of brush cytology in the evaluation of malignant biliary obstruction. Gastrointest Endosc 2003;58(2):176–82.
12. Anderson MA, Fisher L, Jain R, et al. Complications of ERCP. Gastrointest Endosc 2012;75(3):467–73.
13. Khan SA, Thomas HC, Davidson BR, et al. Cholangiocarcinoma. Lancet 2005; 366(9493):1303–14.
14. Koea J, Holden A, Chau K, et al. Differential diagnosis of stenosing lesions at the hepatic hilus. World J Surg 2004;28(5):466–70.

15. Parodi A, Fisher D, Giovannini M, et al. Endoscopic management of hilar chol-angiocarcinoma. Nat Rev Gastroenterol Hepatol 2012;9(2):105–12.
16. Klempnauer J, Ridder GJ, von Wasielewski R, et al. Resectional surgery of hilar cholangiocarcinoma: a multivariate analysis of prognostic factors. J Clin Oncol 1997;15(3):947–54.
17. Blechacz B, Gores GJ. Cholangiocarcinoma: advances in pathogenesis, diag-nosis, and treatment. Hepatology 2008;48(1):308–21.
18. Everhart JE, Khare M, Hill M, et al. Prevalence and ethnic differences in gall-bladder disease in the United States. Gastroenterology 1999;117(3):632–9.
19. Everhart JE, Ruhl CE. Burden of digestive diseases in the United States part I: overall and upper gastrointestinal diseases. Gastroenterology 2009;136(2): 376–86.
20. Hermann RE. The spectrum of biliary stone disease. Am J Surg 1989;158(3): 171–3.
21. Williams EJ, Green J, Beckingham I, et al. Guidelines on the management of common bile duct stones (CBDS). Gut 2008;57(7):1004–21.
22. Committee ASoP, Maple JT, Ben-Menachem T, et al. The role of endoscopy in the evaluation of suspected choledocholithiasis. Gastrointest Endosc 2010; 71(1):1–9.
23. Parsi MA. Peroral cholangioscopy in the new millennium. World J Gastroenterol 2011;17(1):1–6.
24. Chen YK, Parsi MA, Binmoeller KF, et al. Peroral cholangioscopy (POC) using a disposable steerable single operator catheter for biliary stone therapy and assessment of indeterminate strictures–a multicenter experience using SpyGlass. Gastrointest Endosc 2009;69:AB264–5.
25. Chen YK, Parsi MA, Binmoeller KF, et al. Peroral cholangioscopy using a dispos-able steerable single operator catheter for biliary stone therapy and assessment of indeterminate strictures – a multicenter experience using SpyGlass. Gastro-intest Endosc 2008;67:AB103.
26. McIver M. An instrument for visualizing the interior of the common duct at oper-ation. Surgery 1941;9:112–4.
27. Shore J, Lippman HN. A flexible choledochoscope. Lancet 1965;1(7397): 1200–1.
28. Takada T, Hanyu F, Kobayashi S, et al. Percutaneous transhepatic cholangial drainage: direct approach under fluoroscopic control. J Surg Oncol 1976;8(1): 83–97.
29. Nakajima M, Fukumoto K, Mitsuyoshi Y, et al. Peroral cholangiopancreatoscopy (PCPS): its development and clinical application. Nihon Shokakibyo Gakkai Zasshi 1976;73(11):1381–8 [in Japanese].
30. Rosch W, Koch H, Demling L. Peroral cholangioscopy. Endoscopy 1976;8: 172–5.
31. Urakami Y, Seifert E, Butke H. Peroral direct cholangioscopy (PDCS) using routine straight-view endoscope: first report. Endoscopy 1977;9(1):27–30.
32. Williamson JB, Judah JR, Gaidos JK, et al. Prospective evaluation of the long-term outcomes after deep small-bowel spiral enteroscopy in patients with obscure GI bleeding. Gastrointest Endosc 2012;76(4):771–8.
33. Larghi A, Waxman I. Endoscopic direct cholangioscopy by using an ultra-slim upper endoscope: a feasibility study. Gastrointest Endosc 2006;63(6):853–7.
34. Moon JH, Ko BM, Choi HJ, et al. Intraductal balloon-guided direct peroral chol-angioscopy with an ultraslim upper endoscope (with videos). Gastrointest En-dosc 2009;70(2):297–302.

35. Nguyen NQ, Binmoeller KF, Shah JN. Cholangioscopy and pancreatoscopy (with videos). Gastrointest Endosc 2009;70(6):1200–10.
36. Chen YK, Parsi MA, Binmoeller KF, et al. Single-operator cholangioscopy in patients requiring evaluation of bile duct disease or therapy of biliary stones (with videos). Gastrointest Endosc 2011;74(4):805–14.
37. Sethi A, Chen YK, Austin GL, et al. ERCP with cholangiopancreatoscopy may be associated with higher rates of complications than ERCP alone: a single-center experience. Gastrointest Endosc 2011;73(2):251–6.
38. Bogardus ST, Hanan I, Ruchim M, et al. "Mother-baby" biliary endoscopy: the University of Chicago experience. Am J Gastroenterol 1996;91(1):105–10.
39. Caldwell SH, Bickston SJ. Cholangioscopy to screen for cholangiocarcinoma in primary sclerosing cholangitis. Liver Transpl 2001;7(4):380.
40. Efthymiou M, Raftopoulos S, Antonio Chirinos J, et al. Air embolism complicated by left hemiparesis after direct cholangioscopy with an intraductal balloon anchoring system. Gastrointest Endosc 2012;75(1):221–3.
41. Chen YK, Pleskow DK. SpyGlass single-operator peroral cholangiopancreatoscopy system for the diagnosis and therapy of bile-duct disorders: a clinical feasibility study (with video). Gastrointest Endosc 2007;65(6):832–41.
42. Ramchandani M, Reddy DN, Gupta R, et al. Role of single-operator peroral cholangioscopy in the diagnosis of indeterminate biliary lesions: a single-center, prospective study. Gastrointest Endosc 2011;74(3):511–9.
43. Draganov PV, Lin T, Chauhan S, et al. Prospective evaluation of the clinical utility of ERCP-guided cholangiopancreatoscopy with a new direct visualization system. Gastrointest Endosc 2011;73(5):971–9.
44. Fukuda Y, Tsuyuguchi T, Sakai Y, et al. Diagnostic utility of peroral cholangioscopy for various bile-duct lesions. Gastrointest Endosc 2005;62(3): 374–82.
45. Shah RJ, Langer DA, Antillon MR, et al. Cholangioscopy and cholangioscopic forceps biopsy in patients with indeterminate pancreaticobiliary pathology. Clin Gastroenterol Hepatol 2006;4(2):219–25.
46. Kawakami H, Kuwatani M, Etoh K, et al. Endoscopic retrograde cholangiography versus peroral cholangioscopy to evaluate intraepithelial tumor spread in biliary cancer. Endoscopy 2009;41(11):959–64.
47. Kim HJ, Kim MH, Lee SK, et al. Tumor vessel: a valuable cholangioscopic clue of malignant biliary stricture. Gastrointest Endosc 2000;52(5):635–8.
48. Seo DW, Lee SK, Yoo KS, et al. Cholangioscopic findings in bile duct tumors. Gastrointest Endosc 2000;52(5):630–4.
49. Hoffman A, Kiesslich R, Bittinger F, et al. Methylene blue-aided cholangioscopy in patients with biliary strictures: feasibility and outcome analysis. Endoscopy 2008;40(7):563–71.
50. Tischendorf JJ, Kruger M, Trautwein C, et al. Cholangioscopic characterization of dominant bile duct stenoses in patients with primary sclerosing cholangitis. Endoscopy 2006;38(7):665–9.
51. Itoi T, Kamisawa T, Igarashi Y, et al. The role of peroral video cholangioscopy in patients with IgG4-related sclerosing cholangitis. J Gastroenterol 2012;48: 504–14.
52. Siddique I, Galati J, Ankoma-Sey V, et al. The role of choledochoscopy in the diagnosis and management of biliary tract diseases. Gastrointest Endosc 1999;50(1):67–73.
53. Parsi MA, Sanaka MR, Dumot JA. Iatrogenic recurrent pancreatitis. Pancreatology 2007;7(5-6):539.

54. Itoi T, Shinohara Y, Takeda K, et al. Improvement of choledochoscopy-chromoendoscopy, autofluorescence imaging, or narrow-band imaging. Dig Endosc 2007;19(Suppl 1):S95–104.
55. Itoi T, Sofuni A, Itokawa F, et al. Peroral cholangioscopic diagnosis of biliary-tract diseases by using narrow-band imaging (with videos). Gastrointest Endosc 2007;66(4):730–6.
56. Piraka C, Shah RJ, Awadallah NS, et al. Transpapillary cholangioscopy-directed lithotripsy in patients with difficult bile duct stones. Clin Gastroenterol Hepatol 2007;5(11):1333–8.
57. Parsi MA, Neuhaus H, Pleskow D, et al. Peroral cholangioscopy guided stone therapy–report of an international multicenter registry. Gastrointest Endosc 2008;67:AB102.
58. Maydeo A, Kwek BE, Bhandari S, et al. Single-operator cholangioscopy-guided laser lithotripsy in patients with difficult biliary and pancreatic ductal stones (with videos). Gastrointest Endosc 2011;74(6):1308–14.
59. Kim HI, Moon JH, Choi HJ, et al. Holmium laser lithotripsy under direct peroral cholangioscopy by using an ultra-slim upper endoscope for patients with retained bile duct stones (with video). Gastrointest Endosc 2011;74(5):1127–32.
60. Neuhaus H, Zillinger C, Born P, et al. Randomized study of intracorporeal laser lithotripsy versus extracorporeal shock-wave lithotripsy for difficult bile duct stones. Gastrointest Endosc 1998;47(5):327–34.
61. Choi HJ, Moon JH, Ko BM, et al. Clinical feasibility of direct peroral cholangioscopy-guided photodynamic therapy for inoperable cholangiocarcinoma performed by using an ultra-slim upper endoscope (with videos). Gastrointest Endosc 2011;73(4):808–13.
62. Park do H, Park BW, Lee HS, et al. Peroral direct cholangioscopic argon plasma coagulation by using an ultraslim upper endoscope for recurrent hepatoma with intraductal nodular tumor growth (with videos). Gastrointest Endosc 2007;66(1):201–3.
63. Brauer BC, Fukami N, Chen YK. Direct cholangioscopy with narrow-band imaging, chromoendoscopy, and argon plasma coagulation of intraductal papillary mucinous neoplasm of the bile duct (with videos). Gastrointest Endosc 2008;67(3):574–6.
64. Waxman I, Chennat J, Konda V. Peroral direct cholangioscopic-guided selective intrahepatic duct stent placement with an ultraslim endoscope. Gastrointest Endosc 2010;71(4):875–8.
65. Parsi MA, Guardino J, Vargo JJ. Peroral cholangioscopy-guided stricture therapy in living donor liver transplantation. Liver Transpl 2009;15(2):263–5.
66. Wright H, Sharma S, Gurakar A, et al. Management of biliary stricture guided by the SpyGlass Direct Visualization System in a liver transplant recipient: an innovative approach. Gastrointest Endosc 2008;67(7):1201–3.
67. Hayashi S, Baba Y, Ueno K, et al. Small arteriovenous malformation of the common bile duct causing hemobilia in a patient with hereditary hemorrhagic telangiectasia. Cardiovasc Intervent Radiol 2008;31(Suppl 2):S131–4.
68. DiMagno EP, Buxton JL, Regan PT, et al. Ultrasonic endoscope. Lancet 1980;1(8169):629–31.
69. Strohm WD, Phillip J, Hagenmuller F, et al. Ultrasonic tomography by means of an ultrasonic fiberendoscope. Endoscopy 1980;12(5):241–4.
70. Adler DG, Jacobson BC, Davila RE, et al. ASGE guideline: complications of EUS. Gastrointest Endosc 2005;61(1):8–12.

71. Ohshima Y, Yasuda I, Kawakami H, et al. EUS-FNA for suspected malignant biliary strictures after negative endoscopic transpapillary brush cytology and forceps biopsy. J Gastroenterol 2011;46(7):921–8.
72. DeWitt J, Misra VL, Leblanc JK, et al. EUS-guided FNA of proximal biliary strictures after negative ERCP brush cytology results. Gastrointest Endosc 2006; 64(3):325–33.
73. Lee JH, Salem R, Aslanian H, et al. Endoscopic ultrasound and fine-needle aspiration of unexplained bile duct strictures. Am J Gastroenterol 2004;99(6): 1069–73.
74. Byrne MF, Gerke H, Mitchell RM, et al. Yield of endoscopic ultrasound-guided fine-needle aspiration of bile duct lesions. Endoscopy 2004;36(8):715–9.
75. Wu LM, Jiang XX, Gu HY, et al. Endoscopic ultrasound-guided fine-needle aspiration biopsy in the evaluation of bile duct strictures and gallbladder masses: a systematic review and meta-analysis. Eur J Gastroenterol Hepatol 2011;23(2): 113–20.
76. Mohamadnejad M, DeWitt JM, Sherman S, et al. Role of EUS for preoperative evaluation of cholangiocarcinoma: a large single-center experience. Gastrointest Endosc 2011;73(1):71–8.
77. Meara RS, Jhala D, Eloubeidi MA, et al. Endoscopic ultrasound-guided FNA biopsy of bile duct and gallbladder: analysis of 53 cases. Cytopathology 2006;17(1):42–9.
78. Eloubeidi MA, Chen VK, Jhala NC, et al. Endoscopic ultrasound-guided fine needle aspiration biopsy of suspected cholangiocarcinoma. Clin Gastroenterol Hepatol 2004;2(3):209–13.
79. Fritscher-Ravens A, Broering DC, Knoefel WT, et al. EUS-guided fine-needle aspiration of suspected hilar cholangiocarcinoma in potentially operable patients with negative brush cytology. Am J Gastroenterol 2004;99(1):45–51.
80. Fritscher-Ravens A, Broering DC, Sriram PV, et al. EUS-guided fine-needle aspiration cytodiagnosis of hilar cholangiocarcinoma: a case series. Gastrointest Endosc 2000;52(4):534–40.
81. Canto MI, Chak A, Stellato T, et al. Endoscopic ultrasonography versus cholangiography for the diagnosis of choledocholithiasis. Gastrointest Endosc 1998; 47(6):439–48.
82. Chak A, Hawes RH, Cooper GS, et al. Prospective assessment of the utility of EUS in the evaluation of gallstone pancreatitis. Gastrointest Endosc 1999; 49(5):599–604.
83. Petrov MS, Savides TJ. Systematic review of endoscopic ultrasonography versus endoscopic retrograde cholangiopancreatography for suspected choledocholithiasis. Br J Surg 2009;96(9):967–74.
84. Garrow D, Miller S, Sinha D, et al. Endoscopic ultrasound: a meta-analysis of test performance in suspected biliary obstruction. Clin Gastroenterol Hepatol 2007;5(5):616–23.
85. Tse F, Liu L, Barkun AN, et al. EUS: a meta-analysis of test performance in suspected choledocholithiasis. Gastrointest Endosc 2008;67(2):235–44.
86. Palmucci S, Mauro LA, La Scola S, et al. Magnetic resonance cholangiopancreatography and contrast-enhanced magnetic resonance cholangiopancreatography versus endoscopic ultrasonography in the diagnosis of extrahepatic biliary pathology. Radiol Med 2010;115(5):732–46.
87. Verma D, Kapadia A, Eisen GM, et al. EUS vs MRCP for detection of choledocholithiasis. Gastrointest Endosc 2006;64(2):248–54.

88. Napoleon B, Alvarez-Sánchez MV, Markoglou C, et al. EUS in bile duct, gall-bladder, and ampullary lesions. In: Hawes RH, Fockens P, Varadarajulu S, editors. Endosonography. 2nd edition. Philadelphia: Elsevier Saunders; 2011. p. 178–200.

89. Tantau M, Pop T, Badea R, et al. Intraductal ultrasonography for the assessment of preoperative biliary and pancreatic strictures. J Gastrointestin Liver Dis 2008; 17(2):217–22.

90. Menzel J, Poremba C, Dietl KH, et al. Preoperative diagnosis of bile duct strictures–comparison of intraductal ultrasonography with conventional endosonography. Scand J Gastroenterol 2000;35(1):77–82.

91. Domagk D, Wessling J, Reimer P, et al. Endoscopic retrograde cholangiopancreatography, intraductal ultrasonography, and magnetic resonance cholangiopancreatography in bile duct strictures: a prospective comparison of imaging diagnostics with histopathological correlation. Am J Gastroenterol 2004;99(9): 1684–9.

92. Tamada K, Kanai N, Wada S, et al. Utility and limitations of intraductal ultrasonography in distinguishing longitudinal cancer extension along the bile duct from inflammatory wall thickening. Abdom Imaging 2001;26(6):623–31.

93. Tamada K, Tomiyama T, Wada S, et al. Endoscopic transpapillary bile duct biopsy with the combination of intraductal ultrasonography in the diagnosis of biliary strictures. Gut 2002;50(3):326–31.

94. Tamada K, Ueno N, Tomiyama T, et al. Characterization of biliary strictures using intraductal ultrasonography: comparison with percutaneous cholangioscopic biopsy. Gastrointest Endosc 1998;47(5):341–9.

95. Vazquez-Sequeiros E, Baron TH, Clain JE, et al. Evaluation of indeterminate bile duct strictures by intraductal US. Gastrointest Endosc 2002;56(3):372–9.

96. Stavropoulos S, Larghi A, Verna E, et al. Intraductal ultrasound for the evaluation of patients with biliary strictures and no abdominal mass on computed tomography. Endoscopy 2005;37(8):715–21.

97. Varadarajulu S, Eloubeidi MA, Wilcox CM. Prospective evaluation of indeterminate ERCP findings by intraductal ultrasound. J Gastroenterol Hepatol 2007; 22(12):2086–92.

98. Tamada K, Nagai H, Yasuda Y, et al. Transpapillary intraductal US prior to biliary drainage in the assessment of longitudinal spread of extrahepatic bile duct carcinoma. Gastrointest Endosc 2001;53(3):300–7.

99. Endo T, Ito K, Fujita N, et al. Intraductal ultrasonography in the diagnosis of bile duct stones: when and whom? Dig Endosc 2011;23(2):173–5.

100. De Palma GD. Confocal laser endomicroscopy in the "in vivo" histological diagnosis of the gastrointestinal tract. World J Gastroenterol 2009;15(46):5770–5.

101. Wallace M, Lauwers GY, Chen Y, et al. Miami classification for probe-based confocal laser endomicroscopy. Endoscopy 2011;43(10):882–91.

102. Chennat J, Konda VJ, Madrigal-Hoyos E, et al. Biliary confocal laser endomicroscopy real-time detection of cholangiocarcinoma. Dig Dis Sci 2011;56(12): 3701–6.

103. Meining A, Shah RJ, Slivka A, et al. Classification of probe-based confocal laser endomicroscopy findings in pancreaticobiliary strictures. Endoscopy 2012; 44(3):251–7.

104. Meining A, Saur D, Bajbouj M, et al. In vivo histopathology for detection of gastrointestinal neoplasia with a portable, confocal miniprobe: an examiner blinded analysis. Clin Gastroenterol Hepatol 2007;5(11):1261–7.

105. Meining A, Frimberger E, Becker V, et al. Detection of cholangiocarcinoma in vivo using miniprobe-based confocal fluorescence microscopy. Clin Gastroenterol Hepatol 2008;6(9):1057–60.

106. Meining A, Chen YK, Pleskow D, et al. Direct visualization of indeterminate pancreaticobiliary strictures with probe-based confocal laser endomicroscopy: a multicenter experience. Gastrointest Endosc 2011;74(5):961–8.

The New View of Colon Cancer Screening: Forwards and Backwards

Jerome D. Waye, MD

KEYWORDS

- Colon cancer screening • Colonoscopy • Sigmoidoscopy • Adenomas
- Computed tomographic colonography • Retroflexion • Third eye retroscope

KEY POINTS

- Many different techniques for colon cancer screening are available.
- The fecal immunochemical test is best for fecal-based screening, although the DNA investigation may be more specific when further developed.
- Computed tomographic colonography is as good as colonoscopy for detecting colon cancer and is almost as good as colonoscopy for detecting advanced adenomas, but it is poor for detecting small polyps (<5 mm in diameter), and its ability to recognize flat lesions such as sessile serrated polyps is limited.
- The flexible sigmoidoscopic examination markedly decreases the incidence of cancer in the visualized segments, but colonoscopy is currently the best procedure for evaluating the entire large bowel.
- However, colonoscopy has been shown to miss polyps and adenomas and has been criticized in its inability to protect against right colon cancer.
- Techniques for retroflexion or backward view of the colon have been investigated, with all showing increased polyp detection.

  Video of the inferior lip of the ileocecal valve as seen by a Third Eye Retroscope accompanies this article at http://www.giendo.theclinics.com/

SCREENING FOR COLORECTAL CANCER

Screening of asymptomatic individuals permits both prevention and early detection of colorectal cancer through discovery and removal of the precursor lesion, the adenomatous polyp. The current consideration is that colorectal cancer develops from a series of molecular changes that induce histopathologic abnormalities in benign adenomas, with increasingly deeper submucosal invasion, and eventually results in local, then distant spread of disease. If discovered in early phases of development, removal

Department of Medicine, Division of Gastroenterology, The Icahn School of Medicine at Mount Sinai, Mount Sinai Medical Center, 1 Gustave Levy Place, New York, NY 10029, USA
E-mail address: Jdwaye@aol.com

Gastrointest Endoscopy Clin N Am 23 (2013) 647–661
http://dx.doi.org/10.1016/j.giec.2013.03.013
1052-5157/13/$ – see front matter © 2013 Published by Elsevier Inc.
giendo.theclinics.com

of the adenoma/early cancer will interrupt the adenoma-to-cancer sequence and prevent the slow and staged progression of disease. Throughout the various stages of cancer development from a benign adenoma, the abnormal cellular tissue on the surface of the lesion sloughs, as does the entire normal mucosal lining of the colon. Both the incipient cancer and an established colon cancer sheds cells with abnormal DNA into the fecal stream. In the early stages, the lesion may have a benign appearance, but as abnormal cells proliferate, the morphology of the underlying adenoma changes and transforms its shape to have an abnormal contour with depression, friability, ulceration, and eventual replacement of the benign-appearing lesion with the contours typical of an established colon cancer. Blood is shed intermittently in small amounts from these progressive lesions, but as opposed to established cancer, benign adenomas only rarely lose enough blood for anemia to become manifest. Three types of screening tests are available: stool-based tests, radiologic procedures, and direct imaging examinations. All of these tests have positive and negative features, but the best screening test is the one that gets performed.

STOOL TESTING

Two types of screening procedures are based on stool testing. The most common is based on the tendency for large colon tumors or cancers to shed blood, and the finding of blood in the fecal effluent is a strong indicator of a lesion in the colon. The guaiac-based test (gFOBT) is not very sensitive, although it has a long history of being used to detect heme in the stool. If bleeding is from the proximal gastrointestinal tract, heme is broken down to basic constituents in the small bowel and will not trigger a positive test. The test is only sensitive for heme but not specific for heme from human or animal sources, and some food products may block the positive response to a reagent added to the developing paper used in this bedside or office-based test and cause a false-negative reaction. A restricted diet is usually prescribed before the patient collects 3 small stool smears from 3 different bowel evacuations. This test is intended to discover blood that is shed intermittently from tumors, which is more common with cancer or large adenomas than with smaller lesions. Multiple specimens are obtained because even malignant tumors do not bleed constantly but may do so intermittently, and obtaining multiple specimen tests increases the chance of finding a lesion if present. This test may be performed by patients themselves by dripping a reagent onto the specially prepared filter paper and watching for a blue (positive) color to develop. The alternative is to mail cards with 3 stool smears via postal service to a qualified laboratory technician or reference laboratory for development. A positive test, even in 1 of the 3 windows, mandates a colonoscopy to evaluate the entire large bowel to seek a tumor. Although the test is only positive in about 1% to 4% of examinations, the sensitivity of a positive test for colon cancer varies from 5% up to 20%. Because of the intermittent nature of bleeding from tumors causing the possibility of missing the time during which blood is shed into the lumen, the suggestion is that negative tests be repeated annually. The gFOBT screening test for colon cancer has been shown in multiple trials to result in a 16% relative risk reduction in colon cancer mortality. A more sensitive gFOBT is the Hemoccult SENSA, which detects more advanced adenomas than the gFOBT, but because of the nature of the test, it has a high rate of false-positive results.

FECAL IMMUNOCHEMICAL TEST

In contrast to the multispecimen gFOBT, which can be submitted by the patient on a folded card for activation/observation by adding a reagent drop by drop onto the smeared stool window, another test is the fecal immunochemical test (FIT), which is specific for human globin, not animal globin or blood, with no interference by drugs or diet. Because of the high sensitivity of a positive test for finding cancer (60%–85%) or for finding advanced adenomas (20%–50%), the FIT has been accepted as the best stool-based screening test for detecting advanced adenomas, which are larger than 1 cm or have high-grade dysplasia or villous features. This test involves sending whole stool specimens to a reference laboratory for quantitative testing and is a more complicated procedure than the FOBT stool smear examination.

The result is given numerically and the level of sensitivity for detecting a positive result can be set arbitrarily to capture the greatest number of cases. However, this must be balanced to exclude a large number of false-positive results, because a positive result requires referral for colonoscopy. The optimal level that triggers an invasive test must be finely adjusted to prevent colonoscopy being performed with little chance of finding a neoplasm.

THE DNA STOOL TEST

DNA shed from the surface of a neoplasm can signal its presence, and if the fingerprints of a tumor are found in the fecal stream, the positive result is equally effective for right- or left-sided lesions. Several markers for genetic abnormalities must be tested in the clinical laboratory, because no single gene can identify a colonic neoplasm. As with all stool-based procedures, the ability to detect a colonic neoplasia depends on several factors. The sensitivity and positive predictive value is directly dependent on the rate of exfoliation of DNA material from tumor tissue. This material has been estimated[1] to account for 20% of total human DNA in the stool of patients with colorectal cancer and up to 10% of those with large adenomas. The presence of a few methylated gene markers in the stool has been shown to allow differentiation of colorectal neoplasms from the normal DNA found in the stool. High analytical sensitivity is the key to stool DNA analysis, because human DNA represents only one part of up to 100,000 parts of total stool DNA derived from bacteria or ingested DNA. This DNA screening test is more specific than any stool test based on finding peripheral blood in the stool, because testing for blood in the stool is not a marker of tumors but is an indication that tumors shed blood through surface alterations or from trauma. Further test validations are currently under investigation for DNA stool testing.

IMAGING STUDIES: RADIOGRAPHIC
The Barium Enema

The barium enema was for many years the only method of total colon visualization. Before the advent of colonoscopy, rigid sigmoidoscopy was used to look for neoplasia in the rectum and occasionally in the distal sigmoid colon, after which the barium enema was performed. The barium enema uses a solution of barium, a radiologic contrast agent, and water to fill the colon through an enema under fluoroscopic control. Multiple radiographs are then taken with the patient in various positions with the colon filled with barium, and then another series of films are taken of the contracted colon after evacuation. Subsequently, air was often insufflated into the colon to provide contrast between the residual barium that coated the colon wall and the black image of air. Barium-coated polyps and tumors could be distinguished by their whitish outline. A more sensitive technique was developed called the *double-contrast barium enema* (DCBE), during which a small amount of barium was instilled into the rectum and air was then pumped in to push the barium through the entire colon and coat the wall with a thin layer. Although the barium enema was for many years the only method for total colonic visualization, its accuracy was low, with the sensitivity for lesions greater than 10 mm only approximately 50%.

Computed Tomographic Colonography

Computed tomographic colonography (CTC) produces a virtual view of the colon with computerized algorithmic programs reconstituting a luminal view by adding together a series of linear radiographic slices, with each slice through the abdomen giving the appearance of a movie frame. As the lumen is visualized sequentially at movie speed, the viewer is virtually inside the colon lumen as it twists and bends in the abdominal cavity. CTC has been shown to be accurate for detecting colon cancer and 90% accurate for detecting polyps larger than 1 cm in diameter. Polyps smaller than 6 mm are often not identified, and extremely flat lesions may not be seen. With recent advances in technology, several reports have been made of new developments concerning the performance of CTC without a colon cathartic preparation, an advance awaited by both patients and physicians. CTC is accurate in excluding colorectal cancer in patients who are at lower risk for colon cancer. The sensitivity of CTC for colorectal cancer was 94.3% in a study conducted in the Netherlands.[2] However, the sensitivity for flat lesions is poor, but improves with the increasing size of a lesion.[3]

A metanalysis[4] reviewed the performance of DCBE compared with CTC for detecting colon polyps greater than or equal to 6 mm, using colonoscopy as a gold standard. This comparison revealed that CTC markedly increased the ability to detect 6-mm polyps, and was also more sensitive than DCBE in detecting polyps of 6 to 9 mm. The conclusion was that DCBE has statistically lower sensitivity and specificity than CTC for detecting colorectal polyps greater than or equal to 6 mm.

In a retrospective report[5] reviewing findings of patients with colon cancer who had either a DCBE or CTC, only 21 of 33 patients had their malignant neoplasm detected using DCBE, whereas 32 of a similar cohort of 33 patients had the tumor detected on CTC.

In an editorial-type discussion, a radiologist[6] stated that, compared with DCBE radiographic examination of the colon, CTC is more accurate; is preferred by patients; has a shorter room time, fewer complications, and lower radiation exposure; and reveals therapeutically significant extracolonic lesions in 5% to 10% of cases. He states that it is "rather irresponsible to continue to offer routine DCBE examinations."

Magnetic Resonance Colonography

Magnetic resonance colonography (MRC) uses a strong magnetic force to change the axis of rotation of atoms, and this change can be detected by receiver coils to create an image of the affected tissue. This technique does not require ionizing radiation like CTC. MRC is currently under intense study, because MRI is able to detect polyps with a similar sensitivity as CTC without using x-rays.

ENDOSCOPIC TECHNIQUES
Sigmoidoscopy

The old rigid sigmoidoscope was a 25-cm open tube that could be advanced into the colon an average of approximately 15 cm before being impeded by the bends and angulations in the rectum. When flexible fiberoptics became available, flexible sigmoidoscopes were introduced and markedly decreased the amount of discomfort patients complained of when examined with the rigid tube. Although the procedure is called *sigmoidoscopy*, the tip of the flexible sigmoidoscope rarely reaches the end of the sigmoid colon because of angulation, infolding, and inability to straighten the instrument in the descending colon. Polyps and tumors may be removed through the flexible sigmoidoscope; however, a valid interpretation of intraluminal findings requires a competent endoscopist. The usual preparation for a flexible sigmoidoscopy is an enema. The flexible instruments are similar to those for colonoscopy but considerably shorter in length. However, air can be insufflated or aspirated, the instrument may be torqued to the right or left, and dial controls can direct the tip during a procedure. A large trial in the United Kingdom[7] demonstrated a mortality reduction associated with screening using the flexible sigmoidoscope. In a group of more than 40,000 persons who had flexible sigmoidoscopy screening, advanced adenomas or cancer was found in 5%, and a 23% reduction in colorectal cancer incidence was also reported during an 11-year follow-up interval. Opposite results were reported in a population-based flexible sigmoidoscopy study from Norway, with a 7-year follow-up that showed no decrease in colorectal cancer incidence or mortality.[8]

DIRECT IMAGING
Colonoscopy

Colonoscopy is performed using a flexible instrument with a length of approximately 160 or 180 cm that permits visualization of the entire colon and often the last few centimeters of the small intestine. It requires bowel preparation with a vigorous cathartic taken in 2 separate doses, with 1 taken approximately 4 to 6 hours before the procedure. During colonoscopy, the surface of the mucosa can be seen and biopsied and polyps can be removed. Colonoscopy is considered the gold standard for visualization of the colon, but some recent studies have shown flaws in its ability to detect all of the lesions in the large bowel.

The published literature contains several reports comparing CTC with colonoscopy when screening average- or high-risk populations for the presence of polyps or carcinoma. In several of these reports, a colonoscopic examination was performed after a full CTC examination, with the colonoscopist blinded to the results of the CTC. Because the contrast used for CTC has been found not to interfere with the colonoscopy procedure, such a blind comparison would seem to be the ideal method to identify whether the CTC missed any lesions, and conversely should also reveal whether lesions seen on CTC could have been missed by the subsequent colonoscopic examination. Most of these reports have adopted colonoscopy as the gold standard for evaluating CTC findings. Only a few articles have actually examined the possibility that colonoscopy may not find a true lesion that is found on the CTC examination. A meta-analysis[9] reported on 47 articles comparing CTC with colonoscopy, and all used colonoscopy as a gold standard to affirm or rule out the presence of a lesion found on CTC. Several comparative reports have stated that they used the technique of blind colonoscopy performed after the CTC examination; that is, after each segment was examined by the colonoscopist, the finding on the CTC was revealed. This type of study protocol was able to identify lesions missed by CTC, but most centers that used a "blind and then revealed" protocol did not report on the number of lesions that were found on CTC but missed on the first blind colonoscopic examination and then detected on a second pass after the finding on CTC examination was revealed.

The most effective and accurate method to ensure that both the CTC finding and the colonoscopy results were true positives has been addressed by Pickhardt and colleagues,[10] who enrolled 1253 asymptomatic adults to perform same-day CTC and colonoscopy. After interpretation of the CTC examination was available and reported, a colonoscopic examination was performed on the same day in all patients. Segmental unblinding of the CTC results was revealed to the colonoscopist after examining each area. If a reported polyp was not seen during the colonoscopy, that segment of the colon was viewed again with the intention to verify or completely exclude the presence of a polyp. Because CTC is not able to reliably find polyps that measure 5 mm or less, these polyps were excluded from both imaging analyses. A total of 511 polyps 5 mm or more in diameter were seen on CTC, with 55 (10.8%) found only on the second-look colonoscopy after segmental unblinding of the written CTC report. The adenoma miss rate on the initial blinded prospective colonoscopy examination was 10.0% (21 of 210 adenomas), measuring at or larger than 6 mm. The histology of these missed neoplasms found on the second-look colonoscopy after segmental unblinding showed that 17 were tubular adenomas, 3 were tubulovillous adenomas, and 1 was a small adenocarcinoma. During a review study of the CTC examinations, most of the nonrectal neoplasms (14 of 15) missed by the colonoscope were located on a fold, with 10 on the proximal aspect or the edge of folds. One adenoma was located on the inner aspect of an acute bend in the colon. The lesson from this study is that colonoscopy can overlook polyps in the colon, and that some reported lesions on CTC that are categorized as false-positive after subsequent negative colonoscopy may actually exist but can be overlooked on the colonoscopic examination. Areas that could be potentially blind to the colonoscopist are on the proximal side of folds, on the inner aspect of flexures, and in the rectum.

The recent comparison between imaging examinations were preceded by studies among colonoscopists that revealed missed lesions on same-day repeat colonoscopies. The first report of back-to-back colonoscopies immediately following each other was in 1991.[11] The next report of tandem colonoscopy appeared 6 years later,[12] and the most recent was in 2008.[13] The overall miss rates for adenomas in the earlier studies[11,12] were 15% to 24%. The large multicenter European study[13] found that the miss rates were 28% for all polyps, 31% for hyperplastic polyps, and 21% for adenomas. However, for those equal to or larger than 5 mm, the miss rates were 12% for all polyps and 9% for adenomas. In this study, which reported a 27% rate of missed adenomas for lesions less than 5 mm in diameter, the miss rate for lesions greater than 5 mm in diameter was 9%. In a previous study of 183 patients undergoing tandem colonoscopy, Rex and colleagues[12] reported a miss rate of 27% for polyps smaller than 6 mm in diameter, and only 6% for polyps larger than 9 mm. The 6% figure represented 2 patients whose polyps were detected on the repeat colonoscopic examination. Benson and colleagues[14] evaluated the polyp miss rate on repeat colonoscopic examinations with an interval between of 4 months, and then 1 year after the initial colonoscopic examination. A total of 15,000 colonoscopies were examined from multiple centers and the calculated miss rates were 17% for all polyps and 12% for neoplastic polyps. However, the percentage of missed neoplastic polyps greater than 9 mm was only 2%.

A meta-analysis[9] comparing the accuracy of CTC with colonoscopy reviewed 47 studies in which the findings on CTC were corroborated or not using conventional colonoscopy or surgery, and found the results were "highly heterogeneous." A report from Europe[15] compared CTC with segmental unblinding during colonoscopy, but no mention was made of any lesion missed by colonoscopy. In a more recent paper,[16] same-day colonoscopy with segmental unblinding was performed but did not reveal how many polyps found on CTC were actually missed by the colonoscopist after the CTC results were revealed. However, mention was made of 1 polyp detected on CTC that was missed at initial colonoscopy but found on repeat colonoscopy.

A study on the "Findings on Optical Colonoscopy After Positive CT Colonography Exam"[17] reported on the results of colonoscopy after a positive CTC examination in which a polyp or mass greater than 9 mm in diameter was seen or at least

2 medium-sized polyps (6–9 mm) were reported. Most patients in this prospective report underwent a colonoscopy within several hours of CTC or up to 30 days after the CTC procedure. In this study, the findings of colonoscopy examination were taken as the standard, and the colonoscopists were told exactly where the lesion was located. No attempt was made to perform a second colonoscopy if the first examination did not reveal an abnormality, and there was a false-positive CTC finding of 5% when the colonoscopy failed to locate a polyp.

In an early multicenter study[18] involving 600 participants, 9 clinical centers were recruited. Tandem colonoscopies were performed with endoscopists blinded to the CTC results, and the CTC finding was revealed after the colonoscopist examined each segment of the colon during scope withdrawal. In this study, conventional colonoscopy missed only one 7 mm lesion in the sigmoid colon and 19 lesions that ranged from 1 to 5 mm.

Colonoscopy was the reference standard in an article that evaluated CTC for the detection of advanced neoplasia in persons at high risk for colon cancer.[19] The authors noted that "colonoscopy itself may miss some lesions." In this study, which reported lesions smaller than 6 mm as negative, 93 cases had a positive CTC finding but lesions were not found on the subsequent reference colonoscopy performed approximately 3 hours after CTC. Each segment of the bowel was unblinded to the examiner once that area of the colon had been evaluated colonoscopically. In this study, a positive CTC result was recorded if the colonoscopic examination revealed at least one "advanced neoplasia 6 mm or larger," but if no polyp was seen on colonoscopy, the CTC was regarded as a false-positive. A total of 93 cases were classified as false-positive CTC findings when colonoscopy did not identify a polyp. In this study, blinded colonoscopy missed 2 advanced adenomas: a 13-mm pedunculated polyp in the cecum and an 18-mm flat lesion in the ascending colon. This article did not state the number of polyps that were missed on the first colonoscopy when a lesion was seen on CTC but subsequently found on the second colonoscopic examination.

In a comparison of miss rates on colonoscopy versus findings at surgical resection of an index lesion,[20] 16 more lesions were present on the surgical resection specimen in addition to all neoplasms detected at the presurgical colonoscopy. Most polyps were small, and only 1 polyp larger than 1 cm was missed, and that tumor was in the ascending colon. Comparison of findings with either CTC or colonoscopy would seem to be best served by examining a surgically resected specimen to truly ascertain the miss rate of CTC or colonoscopy.

Despite the greater sensitivity for polyp discovery with CTC over the DCBE, the US Preventive Services Task Force has not endorsed CTC as a diagnostic procedure for their guideline on screening recommendations.[21,22] The recommendation of the US Preventive Services Task Force "concludes that for CT colonography...there is insufficient evidence to permit a recommendation for colorectal cancer screening."[12] This guideline was developed to assess and recommend preventive care services for any patient without signs or symptoms of the target condition.

The most recent guideline on screening for colorectal cancer from the American College of Gastroenterology (ACG)[23] stated that colonoscopy every 10 years, beginning at age 50, is the preferred CRC screening strategy, but CTC every 5 years is an acceptable alternative when colonoscopy is not available or persons are unwilling to undergo colonoscopy. Another guideline has been issued by the American Cancer Society, the US Multisociety Task Force on Colorectal Cancer and the American College of Radiology.[24] This study group does recommend CTC for screening purposes; because of the "accumulation of evidence...the expert panel concludes that there are sufficient data to include CTC as an acceptable option for colorectal cancer screening."[24]

Colonoscopy and Lesion Detection

Characteristically, intubation of the colon is performed rather rapidly, for several reasons, one being to minimize patient discomfort by shortening the examination time. Another reason is to reduce spasm in the colon, which will occur if the procedure is prolonged, and to avoid overdistending the right colon with a slow intubation. The usual colonoscopic examination is best performed during withdrawal of the instrument, which must be carefully controlled. This technique of performing a rapid insertion with little or no emphasis on inspection, followed by inspection during the withdrawal phase, has not been scientifically proven to be an optimal approach for achieving maximum detection of adenomas or cancer.[25] Because most adenomas are found during extubation, careful withdrawal is of the utmost importance. In 2006, a combined task force of the ACG and the American Society for Gastrointestinal Endoscopy[26] recommended that the withdrawal phase of colonoscopy should last an average of 6 minutes. A private practice group scrutinized their data and found a strong correlation between withdrawal time and adenoma detection rate. In this study,[27] they reported that colonoscopists with an average withdrawal time of more than 6 minutes detected adenomas larger than 1 cm in 6.4% of screened patients compared with a 2.6% prevalence in colonoscopies performed by endoscopists whose withdrawal times averaged less than 6 minutes. The Mayo Clinic also validated the 6-minute withdrawal target as separating high from low adenoma detectors.[28] During the 6-minute withdrawal, the colonoscopist must make an assessment of each fold and try to visualize the area behind folds and on the inner aspect of angulations in the colon. The usual technique during withdrawal of the scope entails removal of air, which shortens the colon and moves the tip proximal to a fold, followed by tip angulation toward the fold while withdrawing the colonoscope, which pulls on the fold and bends the fold toward the examiner permitting increased visualization of the space behind the fold.

Whenever a fold or flexure is passed and a careful examination of its proximal aspect cannot be achieved, reinsertion, flexion of the tip, and repeat withdrawal is necessary. The angle of deflection is controlled with the left thumb on the major up/down control knob as the instrument is withdrawn, moving the tip toward the fold, while permitting visualization of its hidden portion. A retroflexion should be performed routinely in the rectum (**Fig. 1**).[29] Retroflexion of the instrument during the withdrawal phase at any location in the colon would seem be a worthwhile adjunct, but an article has stated that retroflexion in the right colon was not able to visualize any more of any additional abnormality than straight end-on colonoscopy.[30] Various techniques have been attempted to increase the ability to see portions of mucosa hidden during the withdrawal phase. One of these techniques is to use a cap on the end of the instrument, another is to use a wide-angle instrument. Studies[31–33] have not identified improved overall adenoma detection using these devices. Pickhardt and colleagues,[10] in comparing colonoscopy with CTC, developed a computer-simulated graphic representation of the area behind folds that cannot be seen with the straight end-on colonoscopic view during withdrawal of the instrument. Lieberman,[34] in an editorial, commented that "the data on colonoscopy accuracy (is) a humble reminder of the limitation of colonoscopy; nevertheless it remains the pre-eminent test for diagnosing and treating colonic neoplasia."

Despite the data concerning the ability of colonoscopists to find and remove polyps, recent literature[24] has pointed out that it is more protective against cancer in the left

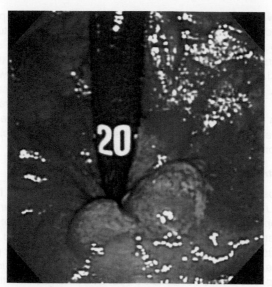

Fig. 1. Pediatric colonoscope in retroflexion at the rectum. Hemorrhoids are noted as 2 mounds. The white cap is related to prolapse through the anal sphincter.

colon than the right colon, perhaps because of poor colon cleansing, variability among endoscopists, flat lesions, or even perhaps a biologic difference in growth rate of right colon cancers. A recent report from the National Polyp Study[35] shows that death from colon cancer is markedly decreased after removal of adenomas.

Tandem Colonoscopy

The most recent back-to-back colonoscopy study for missed lesions was published in 2012.[36] The withdrawal time was more than 6 minutes in every case. The second colonoscopy was performed immediately after the first examination by the same examiner. A total of 149 patients completed all criteria for enrollment in this study, in which all polyps were removed during the initial examination. The miss rate (polyps found on the second examination) was 16.8% for all polyps and 7.2% for adenomas 6 to 9 mm. The location of polyps in the right or left colon did not significantly affect the miss rate, which was positively correlated with the size of the polyp.

Even in this study, the true adenoma miss rate is not known, because the second colonoscopy was used as the gold standard. The conclusion of the authors was that a significant number of adenomas (17%) was being missed during colonoscopy and that "development of new endoscopic techniques to overcome the technical limitations of the current colonoscopic examination is important."[36]

Backward View

A problem with tandem colonoscopy is that both times the colon investigation uses a straightforward colonoscopic view. CTC studies have shown that lesions can be missed in locations behind folds or in flexures not visible with the standard colonoscopic forward-viewing optics. This finding may partially explain the recent publications[37–39] reporting colonoscopy's lack of protection against cancer in the right colon. It is possible that a backward view, looking behind folds, may discover more lesions than would be ordinarily seen with forward-viewing instruments. This theory has been investigated, and retroflexion in the right colon is possible in 95% of examinations,[40] with the finding of a 10% increase in discovery of polyps previously hidden behind folds, some greater than 1 cm in diameter. Another study using special tip-bending scopes reported that the standard pediatric variable-stiffness colonoscope could be retroflexed 78% of the time when attempted in the right colon.[41] Peer Medical, Ltd. (Caesarea, Israel), which has recently merged with EndoChoice, Inc. (Atlanta, GA, USA), has developed a 330° retroview colonoscope with 2 sidefacing electronic chips in addition to the standard straight forward-viewing lens. Each has its own lens water-cleaning device and 2 LED lights. The images are displayed on 3 screens in a discontinuous fashion (not panoramic). This device is currently undergoing clinical testing.

The Third Eye Retroscope

An auxiliary disposable endoscope has been developed by Avantis Medical Systems (Sunnyvale, CA, USA) that has the capability of viewing the area behind the forward-facing colonoscope, providing an image of the proximal aspects of folds and of the valleys in between haustral folds (**Fig. 2**). This device is the Third Eye Retroscope (TER), a probe-based mini endoscope capable of being used with a pediatric colonoscope. The device is 2.0 mm in diameter with a 3.1-mm viewing portion containing the video camera chip. The jointed device turns 180° as it emerges from the biopsy/accessory channel of the parent colonoscope. The device has its own LED light source to illuminate the dark areas not previously visible behind (distal to) the tip of the colonoscope, and has a dedicated power supply (**Fig. 3**). As the camera portion of the mini endoscope emerges from the biopsy channel of the scope, its 2 spring-like joints each bend at 90° to place the video lens facing the face plate of the colonoscope, with the ideal position approximately 2 cm from lens to lens. The light source is located between the 2 limbs of the TER. To prevent the automatic shutter adjustment on the main colonoscope that would automatically decrease light intensity from intraluminal brightness (the light from the TER), a polarizing filter hood is affixed to the colonoscope before the case begins, which circumvents the automatic light adjustment. The images are shown on a monitor in split-screen fashion, with the traditional colonoscopic

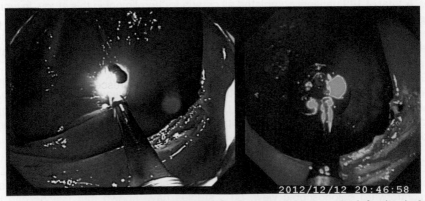

Fig. 2. The split screen image shows the normal colonoscopic view on the left. The shaft of the Third Eye Retroscope (TER) has been passed through the biopsy/accessory channel and its lens and light source are pointed toward the colonoscope face plate. The image on the right is the view from the TER exiting the biopsy channel as it looks back at the colonoscope. Note the illumination behind the tip of the colonoscope as both examine the proximal and distal defects from a recent polypectomy site. In addition, the TER shows another polypectomy site located distal to the colonoscope tip (at 10 o'clock).

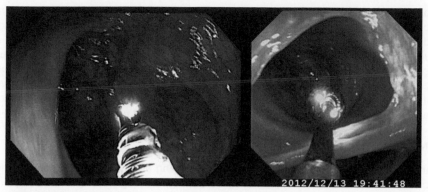

2012/12/13 19:41:48

Fig. 3. On the right frame (TER view), the colonoscope has been withdrawn just past the hepatic flexure and the TER visualizes the transverse colon in which the colonoscope is seen; the TER also shows the ascending colon in the lower part of the picture.

image on the left and the TER view on the right (Video 1). Debris on the lens is washed away by the integrated water jet of the 180 series colonoscope.

Four studies have shown the efficacy of a retroview of the colon.[42–45] The first was a pilot study[42] in 24 patients, among whom 4 additional polyps were found using the TER that would not have been seen with the standard colonoscopic view.

A multicenter prospective study in 8 centers[43] investigating a total of 249 patients showed a 13.2% increase in polyp detection using the TER.

The learning curve for TER use was investigated through having gastroenterologists with no previous TER experience test the rate of polyp discovery with the device. This study[44] showed that the technique is easy to master, as evidenced by the fact that the number of polyps detected on the first 5 of 20 cases examined was the same as in the last 5 patients. The increase in adenoma detection went from 15.4% to 25% in these 20 cases. These findings show a definite but rapid ability to learn the technique of using the TER.

A randomized controlled study called the Third Eye Retroscope Randomized Clinical Evaluation (TERRACE)[45] involved a tandem trial to compare TER colonoscopy with standard colonoscopy. Segments of the colon were examined with the colonoscope and then with the TER to evaluate the degree to which the polyp detection rate was increased using the TER. A 23.2% additional adenoma detection rate was seen, even after correction for the "second-pass effect" that invariably occurs in tandem studies. This study showed that not only smaller polyps but also larger polyps can be missed with standard colonoscopy.

These investigators reexamined their data[46] and found that the patients who were investigated for screening purposes had a low increased adenoma detection rate (<5%) with the TER compared with the standard colonoscopic view. However, if the indication was surveillance postpolypectomy or a diagnostic workup for symptomatology, the TER found additional adenoma/polyps in approximately 36% and 55% of investigations, respectively. These groups are considered to be at above-average risk for colon cancer, and the finding of increased lesions is of great significance.

Capsule Colonoscopy

A capsule study of the large bowel is another method for screening. The capsule has evolved from the small bowel capsule to one that is suitable for colonoscopic investigation. The preparation for the capsule involves filling the colon with fluid so the capsule may easily pass through the large bowel, taking pictures both forward and backward as it traverses the large intestine. Achieving the 2 goals of a clean colon and one filled with fluid requires multiple cathartics and a considerable amount of liquid ingestion. Because of the long transit time to reach the cecum, the capsule becomes dormant for several hours as it passes through the small bowel before becoming active again to take images of the large bowel. The accuracy is lower than colonoscopy for polyps, although it does seem to be a technique of emerging interest.

SUMMARY

Many different techniques for colon cancer screening are available. The fecal immunochemical test is best for fecal-based screening, although the DNA investigation may be more specific when further developed. CTC is as good as colonoscopy for detecting colon cancer and is almost as good as colonoscopy for detecting advanced adenomas, but it is poor for detecting small polyps (<5 mm in diameter), and its ability to recognize flat lesions such as sessile serrated polyps is limited. The flexible sigmoidoscopic examination markedly decreases the incidence of cancer in the visualized segments, but colonoscopy is currently the best procedure for evaluating the large bowel. However, colonoscopy has been shown to miss polyps and adenomas and has been criticized in its inability to protect against right colon cancer. Techniques for retroflexion or backward view of the colon have been investigated, with all showing increased polyp detection. Further developments in colonoscope technology should bring new instruments to discover hidden lesions throughout the colon.

SUPPLEMENTARY DATA

Supplementary data related to this article can be found online at http://dx.doi.org/10.1016/j.giec.2013.03.013.

REFERENCES

1. Berger BM, Ahlquist DA. Stool DNA screening for colorectal neoplasia: biological and technical basis for high detection rates. Pathology 2012;44:80–8.
2. Simons PC, Van Steenbergen LN, De Witte MT, et al. Miss rate of colorectal cancer at CT colonography in average-risk symptomatic patients. Eur Radiol 2013; 23(4):908–13.
3. Sakamoto T, Mitsuzaki K, Utsunomiya D, et al. Detection of flat colorectal polyps at screening CT colonography in comparison with conventional polypoid lesions. Acta Radiol 2012;53:714–9.
4. Sosna J, Sella T, Sy O, et al. Critical analysis of the performance of double-contrast barium enema for detecting colorectal polyps > or = 6 mm in the era of CT colonography. AJR Am J Roentgenol 2008;190:374–85.
5. Thomas S, Atchley J, Higginson A. Audit of the introduction of CT colonography for detection of colorectal carcinoma in a non-academic environment and its implications for the national bowel cancer screening programme. Clin Radiol 2009;64:142–7.
6. Stevenson G. Colon imaging in radiology departments in 2008: goodbye to the routine double contrast barium enema. Can Assoc Radiol J 2008;59:174–82.
7. Atkin WS, Edwards R, Kralj-Hans I, et al, UK Flexible Sigmoidoscopy Trial Investigators. Once-only flexible sigmoidoscopy screening in prevention of colorectal cancer: a multicentre randomised controlled trial. Lancet 2010;375:1624–33.

8. Hoff G, Grotmol T, Skovlund E, et al, Norwegian Colorectal Cancer Prevention Study Group. Risk of colorectal cancer seven years after flexible sigmoidoscopy screening: randomised controlled trial. BMJ 2009;338:b1846.

9. Chaparro M, Gisbert JP, Del Campo L, et al. Accuracy of computed tomographic colonography for the detection of polyps and colorectal tumors: a systematic review and meta-analysis. Digestion 2009;80:1–17.

10. Pickhardt PJ, Nugent PA, Mysliwiec PA, et al. Location of adenomas missed by optical colonoscopy. Ann Intern Med 2004;141:352–9.

11. Hixson LJ, Fennerty MB, Sampliner RE, et al. Prospective blinded trial of the colonoscopic miss-rate of large colorectal polyps. Gastrointest Endosc 1991;37: 125–7.

12. Rex DK, Cutler CS, Lemmel GT, et al. Colonoscopic miss rates of adenomas determined by back-to-back colonoscopies. Gastroenterology 1997;112:24–8.

13. Heresbach D, Barrioz T, Ponchon T. Miss rate for colorectal neoplastic polyps: a prospective multicenter study of back-to-back video colonoscopies. Endoscopy 2008;40:284–90.

14. Bensen S, Mott LA, Dain B, et al. The colonoscopic miss rate and true one-year recurrence of colorectal neoplastic polyps. Polyp Prevention Study Group. Am J Gastroenterol 1999;94:194–9.

15. Chaparro Sánchez M, del Campo Val L, Maté Jiménez J, et al. Computed tomography colonography compared with conventional colonoscopy for the detection of colorectal polyps. Gastroenterol Hepatol 2007;30:375–80.

16. Roberts-Thomson IC, Tucker GR, Hewett PJ, et al. Single-center study comparing computed tomography colonography with conventional colonoscopy. World J Gastroenterol 2008;14:469–73.

17. Cornett D, Barancin C, Roeder B, et al. Findings on optical colonoscopy after positive CT colonography exam. Am J Gastroenterol 2008;103:2068–74.

18. Cotton PB, Durkalski VL, Pineau BC, et al. Computed tomographic colonography (virtual colonoscopy): a multicenter comparison with standard colonoscopy for detection of colorectal neoplasia. JAMA 2004;291:1713–9.

19. Regge D, Laudi C, Galatola G, et al. Diagnostic accuracy of computed tomographic colonography for the detection of advanced neoplasia in individuals at increased risk of colorectal cancer. JAMA 2009;301:2453–61.

20. Postic G, Lewin D, Bickerstaff C, et al. Colonoscopic miss rates determined by direct comparison of colonoscopy with colon resection specimens. Am J Gastroenterol 2002;97:3182–5.

21. Whitlock EP, Lin JS, Liles E, et al. Screening for colorectal cancer: a targeted, updated systematic review for the U.S. Preventive Services Task Force. Ann Intern Med 2008;149:638–58.

22. U.S. Preventive Services Task Force. Screening and surveillance for the early detection of colorectal cancer and adenomatous polyps, 2008: a joint guideline from the American Cancer Society, the US Multi-Society Task Force on Colorectal Cancer, and the American College of Radiology. Ann Intern Med 2008;149:627–37.

23. Rex DK, Johnson DA, Anderson JC, et al. American College of Gastroenterology guidelines for colorectal cancer screening 2009 [corrected]. Am J Gastroenterol 2009;104:739–50.

24. Levin B, Lieberman DA, McFarland B, et al. Screening and surveillance for the early detection of colorectal cancer and adenomatous polyps, 2008: a joint guideline from the American Cancer Society, the US Multi-Society Task Force on Colorectal Cancer, and the American College of Radiology. Gastroenterology 2008;134:1570–95.

25. Huh KC, Rex DK. Missed neoplasms and optimal colonoscopic withdrawal technique. In: Waye JD, Rex DK, Williams CB, editors. Colonoscopy principles and practice. 2nd edition. London: Blackwell Publishing; 2009. p. 560–71.
26. Rex DK, Petrini JL, Baron TH, et al. Quality indicators for colonoscopy. Am J Gastroenterol 2006;101:873–85.
27. Barclay RL, Vicari JJ, Doughty AS, et al. Colonoscopic withdrawal times and adenoma detection during screening colonoscopy. N Engl J Med 2006;355: 2533–41.
28. Simmons DT, Harewood GC, Baron TH, et al. Impact of endoscopist withdrawal speed on polyp yield: implications for optimal colonoscopy withdrawal time. Aliment Pharmacol Ther 2006;24:965–71.
29. Waye JD. What constitutes a total colonoscopy? Am J Gastroenterol 1999;94: 1429–30.
30. Rex DK, Chen SC, Overhiser AJ. Colonoscopy technique in consecutive patients referred for prior incomplete colonoscopy. Clin Gastroenterol Hepatol 2007;5: 879–83.
31. Fatima H, Rex DK, Rothstein R, et al. Cecal insertion and withdrawal times with wide-angle versus standard colonoscopes: a randomized controlled trial. Clin Gastroenterol Hepatol 2008;6:109–14.
32. Rex DK, Chadalawada V, Helper DJ. Wide angle colonoscopy with a prototype instrument: impact on miss rates and efficiency as determined by back-to-back colonoscopies. Am J Gastroenterol 2003;98:2000–5.
33. Deenadayalu VP, Chadalawada V, Rex DK. 170 degrees wide-angle colonoscope: effect on efficiency and miss rates. Am J Gastroenterol 2004;99:2138–42.
34. Lieberman D. Colonoscopy: as good as gold? Ann Intern Med 2004;141:401–3.
35. Zauber AG, Winawer SJ, O'Brien MJ, et al. Colonoscopic polypectomy and long-term prevention of colorectal-cancer deaths. N Engl J Med 2012;366:687–96.
36. Ahn SB, Han DS, Bae JH, et al. The Miss Rate for Colorectal Adenoma Determined by Quality-Adjusted, Back-to-Back Colonoscopies. Gut Liver 2012;6(1): 64–70.
37. Nakao SK, Fassler S, Sucandy I, et al. Colorectal cancer following negative colonoscopy: is 5-year screening the correct interval to recommend? Surg Endosc 2013;27(3):768–73.
38. Singh H, Nugent Z, Mahmud SM, et al. Predictors of colorectal cancer after negative colonoscopy: a population-based study. Am J Gastroenterol 2010;105: 663–73.
39. Bressler B, Paszat LF, Chen Z, et al. Rates of new or missed colorectal cancers after colonoscopy and their risk factors: a population-based analysis. Gastroenterology 2007;132:96–102.
40. Hewett DG, Rex DK. Miss rate of right-sided colon examination during colonoscopy defined by retroflexion: an observational study. Gastrointest Endosc 2011; 74:246–52.
41. Kessler WR, Rex DK. Impact of bending section length on insertion and retroflexion properties of pediatric and adult colonoscopes. Am J Gastroenterol 2005;100:1290–5.
42. Triadafilopoulos G, Watts HD, Higgins J, et al. A novel retrograde-viewing auxiliary imaging device (Third Eye Retroscope) improves the detection of simulated polyps in anatomic models of the colon. Gastrointest Endosc 2007;65(1):139–44.
43. Waye JD, Heigh RI, Fleischer DE, et al. A retrograde-viewing device improves detection of adenomas in the colon: a prospective efficacy evaluation (with videos). Gastrointest Endosc 2010;71(3):551–6.

44. DeMarco DC, Odstrcil E, Lara LF, et al. Impact of experience with a retrograde-viewing device on adenoma detection rates and withdrawal times during colonoscopy: the Third Eye Retroscope study group. Gastrointest Endosc 2010; 71(3):542–50.

45. Leufkens AM, DeMarco DC, Rastogi A, et al, Third Eye Retroscope Randomized Clinical Evaluation [TERRACE] Study Group. Effect of a retrograde-viewing device on adenoma detection rate during colonoscopy: the TERRACE study. Gastrointest Endosc 2011;73:480–9.

46. Siersema PD, Rastogi A, Leufkens AM, et al. Retrograde-viewing device improves adenoma detection rate in colonoscopies for surveillance and diagnostic workup. World J Gastroenterol 2012;18:3400.

Colonic Polyps
Are We Ready to Resect and Discard?

Cesare Hassan, MD[a],*, Alessandro Repici, MD[a], Angelo Zullo, MD[a],
Vijay Kanakadandi, MD[b], Prateek Sharma, MD[b]

KEYWORDS

- Electronic chromoendoscopy • Colonoscopy • Polypectomy
- Narrow-band imaging
- Preservation and incorporation of valuable endoscopic innovations

KEY POINTS

- The very low prevalence of advanced neoplasia in diminutive lesions supports the safety of resect and discard or discard policies.
- Although dye-chromoendoscopy or electronic chromoendoscopy at high magnification seem accurate for in vivo polyp prediction, they seem unfeasible in Western countries. Low-magnification electronic chromoendoscopy seems simple to be implemented in these countries, and an adequate, albeit variable, accuracy has been shown.
- The ability of low-magnification electronic chromoendoscopy in meeting American Society for Gastrointestinal Endoscopy thresholds is uncertain, depending on disease prevalence, technical accuracy, and the surveillance interval adopted for low-risk adenomas.

INTRODUCTION

Colorectal cancer (CRC) represents a major cause of morbidity and mortality in Western countries.[1–3] Endoscopic screening has been shown to be effective in reducing CRC incidence and/or mortality,[4–6] and population-based screening is widely recommended in the United States and Europe.[7,8] It has been estimated that greater than 60% of the eligible American population underwent CRC screening, with colonoscopy as the dominating test.[3] Despite that colonoscopy screening has been shown to be cost-effective or cost-saving in the long term,[9,10] screening costs, as well as exploitation of medical and technological resources, mainly incurs in the short term, while the benefits tend

No funding was obtained.

[a] Digestive Endoscopy Unit, IRCCS Istituto Clinico Humanitas, Via Manzoni 56, Rozzano, Milan 20089, Italy; [b] Division of Gastroenterology and Hepatology, Veterans Affairs Medical Center, University of Kansas School of Medicine, 4801 East Linwood Boulevard, Kansas City, MO 64128-2295, USA

* Corresponding author. Digestive Endoscopy Unit, IRCCS Istituto Clinico Humanitas, Via Manzoni 56, Rozzano, Milan 20089, Italy.

E-mail address: cesareh@hotmail.com

to appear only after several years. An annual volume of approximately 14 million colonoscopies has been estimated in the United States, representing a substantial economic and financial burden to the society.[11]

A major determinant of the cost of colonoscopy is represented by polypectomy,[12] seemingly related to the high prevalence of polypoid (or nonpolypoid) lesions in the general population. It has been recently estimated in published US series that up to 42% of subjects will present with at least one polyp at screening colonoscopy; this rate is likely to increase with the widespread implementation of high-definition endoscopy and quality assurance programs for screening colonoscopy.[13,14] Polypectomy costs are partially related to the cost of pathologic examination. When considering diminutive polyps ($\leq$5 mm in size), which represent more than 60% of all polyps detected by colonoscopy during average-risk screening,[13] the additional cost of postpolypectomy pathologic examination is mainly justified by the necessity to differentiate between precancerous adenomatous and hyperplastic polyps—which may require different policies of postpolypectomy follow-up because of the low prevalence of advanced neoplasia.[15,16]

WHAT IS RESECT AND DISCARD STRATEGY?

Despite being proposed and used by Japanese endoscopists since the early 1990s,[17] in vivo characterization of polyp histology with standard chromoendoscopy failed to gain popularity in Western countries. This failure to gain popularity has been related to several reasons, including the need of dye-spraying, which may be tedious and time-consuming. The advent of electronic chromoendoscopy (EC), preserving the benefits of chromoendoscopy without the disadvantages of dye-spraying, opened the door for optical prediction of polyp histology in Western countries. In preliminary studies, EC has been shown to be able to differentiate between adenomatous and hyperplastic histology of diminutive or small polyps with an adequate degree of accuracy, also predicting the correct interval of postpolypectomy surveillance.[18–20] For these reasons, it has been proposed that EC may prevent the need for standard histologic assessment of diminutive lesions, with future management decisions being driven only by the in vivo endoscopic prediction, also named resect and discard policy.[18,21] It has also been suggested that diminutive hyperplastic polyps in the distal colon may be left in situ after characterization (ie, a discard [without resection] policy).[18,21] When considering the high prevalence of such lesions in the general population, these strategies/policies may be expected to result in substantial savings when applied to a program of colonoscopy screening.[12,22] However, an inappropriate application of resect and discard or discard policies could also result in incorrect surveillance timings or in the nonremoval of serious lesions, causing undesired outcomes and risk of medical litigations.[12,22] For this reason, the American Society for Gastrointestinal Endoscopy recently published a white paper providing specific thresholds and criteria to be met before the clinical implementation of such practices.[23]

DISTRIBUTION OF HISTOLOGY WITHIN DIMINUTIVE AND SMALL POLYPS AND NATURAL HISTORY

The clinical application of a resect and discard strategy strictly depends on the histologic distribution among diminutive polyps. Irrespectively of the EC accuracy in polyp characterization, the relative distribution between hyperplastic and adenomatous histotypes would intrinsically affect the chances of false-positive or false-negative results within these lesions. A very high prevalence of hyperplastic lesions may be expected to marginalize the risk of a false-negative result by increasing the negative predictive value at a certain level of sensitivity, but it would also increase the possibility of false-positive results by reducing the positive predictive value, irrespective of the level of specificity. Second, an excessively high prevalence of advanced histology (ie, high-grade dysplasia, villous histology, or invasive cancer) would prevent the application of a resect and discard policy, because of the inability of EC in differentiating between nonadvanced and advanced adenomas. The clinical outcome of the discard strategy would also be affected by the natural history of unresected diminutive lesions. Although there is a general agreement on the lack of malignant potential of diminutive hyperplastic lesions in the distal colon, any false-negative result of polyp characterization would result in the nonremoval of a diminutive adenoma. A less aggressive natural history of such lesion would lead to a "safer" discard policy. Third, the association between some types of serrated lesions and a higher risk of CRC would not support a discard policy for proximal lesions,[24] unless in vivo characterization of polyp histology could reliably predict such a diagnosis.

Distribution of (Advanced) Adenomatous and Hyperplastic Histotypes Within Subcentimetric Lesions

Table 1 lists the available screening series providing estimates on the frequency of adenomatous lesions among subcentimetric lesions collected from a cumulative population of 18,549 subjects.[25–28] In detail, among 15,128 diminutive polyps, 51% were adenomatous, the remaining being nonadenomatous (mostly hyperplastic). It is however possible that these estimates are an overestimation when limiting the analysis to the distal colon, because of the well-known high prevalence of tiny hyperplastic lesions in this location. For instance, in a consecutive series of 235 distal polyps, including 220 polyps ≤5 mm lesions, only 38 were actually adenomatous, corresponding to a 16% overall frequency of adenomatous type.[29] Compared with diminutive polyps, the rate of adenomatous component seemed to be substantially higher in small (6–9 mm) polyps, corresponding to 64% among the identified 3197 small (6–9 mm) lesions (see **Table 1**).[25–28]

Regarding the relative prevalence of advanced neoplasia in subcentimetric lesions, in a previous systematic review including 20,562 subjects who underwent screening colonoscopy, fewer than 1% (0.8%) of patients with diminutive-only lesions had an advanced adenoma, whereas less than 5% (4.9%) of patients with small-only lesions had an advanced adenoma.[13] When restricting this analysis to invasive cancer, less than 0.1% of patients with a subcentimeter polyp as the largest lesion were affected, corresponding to a 0.04% (1:2726) and 0.07% (1:1488) risk for invasive cancer in diminutive and small polyps, respectively. These findings have been confirmed

Table 1
Relative prevalence of adenomatous histotype among diminutive and small lesions in large cohorts of subjects undertaking endoscopic or CTC screening

| Series | ≤5 mm | | 6–9 mm | |
	No.	Rate Adenomatous	No.	Rate Adenomatous
Pickhardt et al,[25,a] 2003	966	64%	262	61%
Lieberman et al,[26,b] 2008	3744	50%	1198	68%
Rex et al,[27,a] 2009	8798	49%	1282	59%
Gupta et al,[28,a] 2012	1620	60%	455	71%
Total	15,128	51%	3197	64%

[a] Per polyp analysis.
[b] Per patient analysis.

recently by a retrospective analysis of 3 screening studies, including 2361 polyps, showing a 0.5% and 1.5% prevalence of advanced neoplasia within diminutive and small polyps, respectively.[28] Similarly, a retrospective analysis on 5124 asymptomatic subjects confirmed a very low risk of advanced neoplasia and invasive cancer in 464 patients with 6- to 9-mm polyps as the largest lesion, corresponding to a 3.9% and 0% risk, respectively.[30] Of note, the prevalence of sessile or traditional serrated adenoma was also shown to be very low in subcentimetric lesions, being cumulatively present in 0.3% to 0.5% and 0.8% to 1.3% of diminutive and small lesions, respectively.[26,28]

All these data would indicate that in the screening setting less than half of all diminutive lesions (<5 mm) will be adenomatous, whereas the risk of advanced neoplasia is extremely low. These probabilities are probably much less in the rectosigmoid colon. On the other hand, nearly 2 of 3 small lesions (6–9 mm) will be adenomatous, and the risk of advanced neoplasia ranges between 1.5% and 5%.

Natural History of Unresected Subcentimetric Lesions

In 2 prospective Northern European endoscopic studies, Hoff and colleagues[31] and Hofstad and colleagues[32] followed up 194 diminutive polyps and 253 polyps ≤10 mm detected for 3 and 2 years, respectively. No diminutive polyp reached a >5 mm size and only 0.5% of ≤10 mm polyps eclipsed the 10-mm threshold after a 1-year time interval; no case of high-grade dysplasia or carcinoma was registered.[31,32] Pickhardt and colleagues[33] followed 128 computed tomographic colonoscopy (CTC)-detected 6- to 9-mm polyps by repeating CTC after 2 years, recommending polypectomy for those polyps with interval growth. Overall, 116 small polyps did not show significant growth at a second CTC, whereas 12 (9.3%) polyps showed an interval growth of 1 mm or more. At histology, all growing lesions were adenomatous, but no cancer was detected[33]; this was recently confirmed by a Japanese study, in which only 2.9% of 408 subcentimetric lesions followed up for 43.1 months reached a size of ≥10 mm, without the occurrence of any invasive cancer.[34] Overall, these studies indicate that, at least in the short term, most of the ≤10-mm polyps do not present any relevant growth and do not progress to invasive cancer. This statement may be reassuring, when considering the (extremely) low risk of discarding an (advanced) adenoma in the distal colon (see later discussion). Natural history of sessile serrated lesions has been only marginally addressed. In a large series, it has been shown that only the presence of a proximal or ≥10-mm sessile serrated lesion is associated with an increased risk of metachronous neoplasia.[24]

METHODS FOR POLYPS CHARACTERIZATION: ADVANCED ENDOSCOPIC IMAGING
White Light

Despite that an in vivo prediction of polyp histology may be to some extent feasible at white-light (WL) endoscopy,[35,36] a WL-based resect and discard policy has never been formally implemented, presumably related to several reasons. First, WL accuracy in polyp characterization has been shown to be suboptimal and consistently inferior to that of more advanced endoscopic techniques.[18,35,36] Second, no clear classification criteria for WL in vivo polyp characterization have been proposed, preventing a clear assessment of interobserver/intra-observer variability.[18,35,36] Third, no formal training has been tested in a controlled environment. Fourth, high-definition WL endoscopy has been shown to be inferior to chromoendoscopy techniques in predicting polyp histology.[37] Fifth, although mucosal or vascular characteristics of some lesions may already be depicted at WL, this is usually more feasible for large rather than for diminutive lesions (ie, those amenable to a resect and discard policy). These limitations overall explain why a systematic policy of postpolypectomy pathologic referral has been universally implemented, at least in Western countries.[38]

(Dye-)Chromoendoscopy

The field of advanced endoscopic imaging, aiming to predict histology of (non-) polypoid colorectal lesions based on endoscopic features reliably, began in the early 1990s, when Japanese endoscopists showed the possibility of accurately discriminating between nonneoplastic and neoplastic histotype by depicting various pit patterns of colorectal lesions after staining with nonabsorbable or absorbable dyes.[17,39,40] Pit pattern–based classification at magnifying endoscopy has since been extensively validated, showing a high accuracy for differentiating between nonneoplastic (pit pattern I-II) and neoplastic lesions (pit pattern III-V), and, among those neoplastic, between precancerous and malignant phenotypes.[41] An adequate level of interobserver and intra-observer agreement was also shown, assuring the reproducibility of the technique.[17,39,40,42] For these reasons, chromoendoscopy gained immediate acceptance among Japanese endoscopists, allowing an early implementation of optical-based endoscopic policies in that country.[34,41,43] Despite all these favorable characteristics, however, chromoendoscopy unexpectedly failed to be implemented in Western countries. Albeit unclear, such failure may be explained by several reasons. First, high-magnification colonoscopes were not readily available in Europe and the United States. Second, chromoendoscopy requires a long learning curve with at least 200 to 300 procedures.[17,35] Third, the technique seems inconvenient to several Western endoscopists, because of the time required for dye spraying and zoom interpretation. Fourth, the excessive staining in the area surrounding the targeted lesion may mask a serious lesion. Fifth, chromoendoscopy has been generally perceived as a technique to differentiate between noninvasive and invasive lesions rather than to discriminate between nonneoplastic and neoplastic features.

High-magnification and Low-magnification Electronic Chromoendoscopy

The development of electronic or virtual chromoendoscopy (EC) revitalized the interest for advanced endoscopic imaging in Western countries. The main advantages of EC are the simple and immediate activation and the wide availability on the new generations of endoscopes. To differentiate between neoplastic (adenomatous) and nonneoplastic (hyperplastic) lesions, EC also exploits the neo-angiogenesis of neoplastic lesions rather than only the mucosal pit pattern. Narrow-band imaging (NBI; Olympus Inc, Shinjuku-Ku, Japan) is based on the modification of the spectral features with an optical color separation filter narrowing the bandwidth of spectral transmittance. In this system, the center wavelengths of the dedicated trichromatic optical filters are 540 and 415 nm, with bandwidths of 30 nm, to optimize hemoglobin light absorption.[44] By use of this narrow spectrum, the contrast of the superficial capillary pattern in the superficial layer is markedly increased, and thus clear visualization of vascular structures may be achieved during endoscopy.[44] The electronic button on the control section of the colonoscope allows switching between WL and NBI views. Differently from the optical-based NBI, flexible spectral imaging color enhancement (FICE) and I-Scan achieve a similar effect with a software-based postprocessing of the endoscopic image.[45,46]

EC had been initially applied in the setting of high-optical magnification (HM-EC) to predict polyp histology. HM-EC allowed the identification of the honeycomb microvascular pattern around the single glands, leading to a "capillary" or vascular pattern classification.[47] Such classification had been shown to have an adequate degree of accuracy for differentiating between adenomatous and hyperplastic lesions.[35,36,44,45,48–61] As shown in **Table 2**, sensitivity and specificity of HM-EC ranged

Table 2
Studies reporting accuracy of EC in differentiating between adenomatous and hyperplastic lesions at high-magnification colonoscopy

Author	Country	No. of Patients	No. of Polyps	Adenomatous Prevalence	Endoscopist	EC-pit Pattern	EC-vascular Pattern	EC-sensitivity	EC-specificity
Machida et al,[44] 2004	Japan	34	43	79%	—	Yes	Yes	100%	75%
Chiu et al,[36] 2007	Taiwan	133	180	78%	Experienced	No	Yes	91%	80%
Su et al,[35] 2006	Taiwan	78	110	59%	Experienced	No	Yes	96%	88%
Hirata et al,[62] 2007	Japan	99	148	89%	—	Yes	No	99%	94%
East et al,[48] 2007	UK	20	31	64%	Experienced	Yes	Yes	77%	50%
Tischendorf et al,[49] 2007	Germany	52	100	63%	Experienced	Yes	Yes	90%	89%
East et al,[50] 2008	UK	62	116	43%	Experienced	Yes	Yes	98%	88%
Sano et al,[51] 2009	Japan	92	150	74%	Experienced	No	Yes	96%	92%
van den Broek et al,[52] 2009	The Netherlands	32	50	44%	Experienced and Inexperienced	Yes	No	88%	56%
van den Broek et al,[52] 2009	The Netherlands	32	50	44%	Experienced and Inexperienced	Yes	No	90%	55%
Wada et al,[53] 2009	Japan	495	617	95%	Experienced	No	Yes	91%	97%
Tischendorf et al,[55] 2010	Germany	131	100	58%	Experienced	No	Yes	92%	89%
Tischendorf et al,[54] 2010	Germany	223	209	77%	Experienced	No	Yes	94%	86%
Ignjatovic et al,[57] 2011	UK	—	80	50%	Experienced and Inexperienced	No	Yes	93%	59%
Ignjatovic et al,[57] 2011	UK	—	80	50%	Experienced and Inexperienced	No	Yes	90%	33%
Sato et al,[58] 2011	Japan	183	424	80%	Experienced and Inexperienced	No	Yes	91%	77%
Gross et al,[56] 2011	Germany	214	434	59%	Experienced and Inexperienced	No	Yes	93%	92%
Gross et al,[56] 2011	Germany	214	434	59%	Experienced and Inexperienced	No	Yes	86%	88%
Takemura et al,[61] 2012	Japan	—	371	87%	Experienced	Yes	Yes	98%	99%
Kuiper et al,[60] 2012	The Netherlands	64	154	37%	Experienced	Yes	No	81%	93%
Yoo et al,[59] 2011	Korea	68	107	93%	Experienced	Yes	No	89%	88%

between 77% and 100%, and 50% and 100%, respectively. HM-EC appeared also to be superior to WL and similar to (dye-)chromoendoscopy for in vivo polyp characterization.[35,36] In contrast to dye chromoendoscopy, the learning curve appeared to be short, and a high degree of reproducibility, at least among expert endoscopists, was shown.[50,54,57,58] The possibility of developing a reliable computer-aided system for predicting the histology of colorectal lesions by HM-NBI has also been shown.[56,61] However, HM-EC shared a major limitation with chromoendoscopy (ie, the nonavailability of HM-endoscopes in Western countries). For this reason, EC had been mainly implemented in association with low-optical magnification (LM-EC) endoscopy in Western countries,[63] also exploiting the higher resolution of high-definition endoscopes.[64]

Different from HM-EC, LM-EC has been relatively ineffective in depicting the microvascular patterns or pit patterns of many subcentimetric polyps.[36] To compensate for this deficiency, a different diagnostic approach has been introduced that mostly exploits a *gestalt* appreciation of the polyp surface, hue, and vascularization (**Fig. 1**).[37,63,65] In detail, adenomatous polyps mainly appear as dark or brown lesions, as an effect of the neoplastic neo-angiogenesis, whereas hyperplastic polyps are usually pale or at best showing isolated lacy vessels on the surface.[19,37,63,65] Second, LM-EC permits the use of a simplified pit pattern in adenomatous lesions, whereas hyperplastic polyps usually show a lack of any pit pattern.[19,37,63,65] However, in a head-to-head comparison, LM-EC was shown to be inferior to HM-EC,[36] and HM-EC has been consistently shown to be superior to either standard or high-definition LM-EC.[37,57,64] The accuracy of LM-EC has shown some variability in preliminary studies, with sensitivity and specificity ranging between 61% and 91%, and between 32% and 98%, respectively (**Table 3**).[18–20,29,37,55,57,63–65,67–74] This range may, at least in part, be explained by a high degree of heterogeneity in the methodology adopted across the studies. First, several studies did not restrict the analysis to diminutive or subcentimetric polyps, substantially changing the expected prevalence of disease.[18–20,29,37,55,57,63–65,67–74] Moreover, different EC-based classifications, based on either pit or vascular patterns, were adopted in these studies, preventing a clear comparison across the series (see **Table 3**),[18–20,29,37,55,57,63–65,67–74] and participating endoscopists already experienced in EC generally achieved better accuracies than less-trained endoscopists (see **Table 3**).[18–20,29,37,55,57,63–65,67–74] Finally, LM-EC has been shown to be largely unable to differentiate between hyperplastic and sessile serrated lesions or adenomas.[63]

To address such variability, a new classification system (NBI International Colorectal Endoscopic [NICE]) has been validated recently with an adequate interobserver and

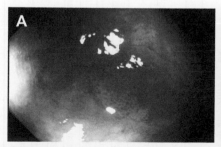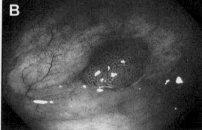

Fig. 1. Appearance of subcentimetric colorectal lesions at narrow-band imaging at low-optical magnification: (*A*) bland, featureless appearance, thin blood vessels coursing across the polyp surface and not surrounding pits (hyperplastic); (*B*) brown color, oval pits, short, thick blood vessels (adenomatous).

Table 3
Studies reporting the accuracy of EC in differentiating between adenomatous and hyperplastic lesions at low-magnification colonoscopy

Author	Country	Setting	No. of Polyps	Adenomatous Prevalence	Endoscopist	EC-pit Pattern	EC-vascular Pattern	EC-sensitivity	EC-specificity
Kuiper et al,[66] 2011	The Netherlands	High	238	49%	Experienced	Yes	No	87%	63%
Chiu et al,[36] 2007	Taiwan	Artificial	180	78%	Experienced	No	Yes	84%	71%
Rastogi et al,[63] 2008	USA	Screening/surveillance	123	59%	Experienced	Yes	No	97%	86%
						No	Yes	86%	97%
Sikka et al,[37] 2008	USA	Artificial	80	61%	Inexperienced	Yes	Yes	95%	90%
Rogart et al,[65] 2008	USA	Unselected	265	49%	Inexperienced	Yes	Yes	80%	81%
Rex,[19] 2009	USA	Unselected	451	51%	Experienced	Yes	Yes	96%	92%
Tischendorf et al,[55] 2010	Germany	Artificial	100	63%	Experienced	No	Yes	92%	89%
Buchner et al,[67] 2010	USA	Unselected	119	68%	Experienced	—	—	77%	71%
Ignjatovic et al,[18] 2009	UK	High	278	71%	Experienced and Inexperienced	No	Yes	94%	89%
Henry et al,[68] 2010	USA	Unselected	126	53%	Experienced	No	Yes	93%	88%
Ignjatovic et al,[69] 2011	UK	Artificial	630	50%	Experienced and Inexperienced	Yes	Yes	87%	84%
Ignjatovic et al,[57,c] 2011	UK	Artificial	80	50%	Experienced. Inexperienced	No	Yes	74%	56%
						No	Yes	61%	32%
Rastogi et al,[70] 2011	USA	Screening/surveillance	—	—	Experienced	Yes	Yes	90%	68%
Gupta et al,[20] 2012	USA	Screening/surveillance	1254	64%	Experienced	Yes	Yes	94%	72%
Hewett et al,[71] 2012	USA	Unselected	236	63%	Experienced	Yes	Yes	98%	69%
Kuiper et al,[72] 2012	The Netherlands	Unselected	108	46%	Experienced	No	No	77%	79%
Hewett et al,[29] 2012	USA	Screening/surveillance	235	16%	Experienced	Yes	Yes	94%	98%
Paggi et al,[73] 2012	Italy	Unselected	511	69%	Experienced	Yes	Yes	95%	66%
Longcroft-Wheaton et al,[64] 2012	UK	Unselected	150	64%	Experienced	Yes	Yes	83%	82%
								93%	81%
Ladabaum et al,[74] 2013	USA	Unselected	2596	65%	Inexperienced	Yes	Yes	91%	40%

intra-observer agreement among experienced and nonexperienced endoscopists (**Table 4**).[71] It has been shown that very short training sessions may be sufficient to reach an adequate EC accuracy, at least in an artificial setting.[75] In the NICE classification, the level of confidence of the endoscopist in in vivo histologic prediction has been introduced, showing a substantial deterioration of LM-EC accuracy when passing from high-level to low-level confidence of diagnosis.[71,74]

RESECT AND DISCARD STRATEGIES/POLICIES

The American Society for Gastrointestinal Endoscopy recently developed a Preservation and Incorporation of Valuable Endoscopic Innovations (PIVI) statement for real-time endoscopic assessment of the histology of diminutive colorectal polyps.[76] In detail, it was determined that:

1. For colorectal polyps ≤5 mm in size to be resected and discarded without pathologic assessment, endoscopic technology (when used with high confidence) used to determine histology of polyps ≤5 mm in size, when combined with histopathologic assessment of polyps >5 mm in size, should provide a ≥90% agreement in assignment of post-polypectomy surveillance intervals when compared with decisions based on pathology assessment of all identified polyps."
2. For a technology to be used to guide the decision to leave suspected rectosigmoid hyperplastic polyps ≤5 mm in size in place (without resection), the technology should provide ≥90% negative predictive value (when used with high confidence) for adenomatous histology."

Resect and Discard (1° PIVI)

Both statements show how the feasibility of in vivo prediction policies is a complex decision-making process that depends on multiple variables, including EC accuracy, level of diagnostic confidence, prevalence of disease, histology of nonassessable polyps, as well as the type of postpolypectomy guidelines adopted.[76] When further analyzing the first statement (ie, resect and discard strategy), the correspondence between the optical prediction and the assignment of postpolypectomy surveillance intervals is not only related to the interaction between EC accuracy and relative

Table 4
The NICE Classification[a] for differentiating between hyperplastic and adenomatous histology

NICE Criterion	Type 1	Type 2
Color	Same or lighter than background	Browner relative to background (verify color arises from vessels)
Vessels	None, or isolated lacy vessels coursing across the lesion	Brown vessels surrounding white structures[b]
Surface pattern	Dark or white spots of uniform size, or homogeneous absence of pattern	Oval, tubular, or branched white structures[b] surrounded by brown vessels
Most likely pathologic abnormality	Hyperplastic	Adenoma

[a] Can be applied using colonoscopes both with or without optical (zoom) magnification.
[b] These structures may represent the pits and the epithelium of the crypt opening.
From Hewett DG, Kaltenbach T, Sano Y, et al. Validation of a simple classification system for endoscopic diagnosis of small colorectal polyps using narrow-band imaging. Gastroenterology 2012;143:599–607.e1; with permission.

prevalence of adenomatous polyps, but also to the recommendations adopted for the surveillance intervals. The recent update from the *US Multi-Society Task Force on Colorectal Cancer* indicates a 10-year interval for distal small (<10 mm) hyperplastic polyps and a 5- to 10-year interval for 1 to 2 tubular adenomas <10 mm, whereas a 3-year interval is recommended for those with advanced histology or $\geq$3 adenomas.[15] When considering the inability of EC in differentiating between adenomas with favorable or advanced histology, the first issue is whether EC-based recommendations may still achieve a 90% agreement based on the available evidence. Because of the very low prevalence of advanced neoplasia within diminutive lesions (0.8%, see discussion above), this may be reasonably excluded. The second issue is whether EC-based differentiation between nonadvanced adenomatous and hyperplastic lesions may provide a >90% agreement in the assignment of the surveillance intervals. This >90% agreement appears to depend mainly on a complex interaction between EC accuracy and on whether a 5-year or a 10-year schedule is chosen for subjects with 1 to 2 tubular adenomas <10 mm. If a 5-year schedule is adopted, the role of EC accuracy is important, because false-negative results would experience an inappropriate surveillance delay at 10 years, whereas those false positives would have a substantial anticipation of the examination at 5 years. When adopting these criteria, some series have reported favorable results (by experienced EC endoscopists) but the majority failed to match the 1° PIVI, especially when EC was performed by less dedicated endoscopists (**Table 5**). On the other hand, if a 10-year schedule is

Table 5
Studies reporting accuracy of EC in matching the desired thresholds for the 2 proposed PIVIs (see text)

Author	Country	No. of Patients	No. of Polyps	Experienced	High/low Confidence	1° PIVI	2° PIVI
Rex,[19] 2009	USA	136	451	Experienced	Yes	Yes	—
Ignjatovic et al,[18] 2009	UK	130	278	Experienced and Inexperienced	Yes	Yes	Yes
Rastogi et al,[70] 2011	USA	—	—	Experienced	No	No	No
Gupta et al,[20] 2012	USA	410	1254	Experienced	No	No/Yes	Yes
Hewett et al,[71] 2012	USA	108	236	Experienced	Yes	—	Yes
Kuiper et al,[72] 2012	The Netherlands	308	108	Inexperienced	Yes	No	—
Hewett et al,[29] 2012	US	31	235	Experienced	Yes	—	Yes
Paggi et al,[73] 2012	Italy	286	511	Experienced	Yes	No	—
Longcroft-Wheaton et al,[64] 2012	UK	51	150	Experienced	No	No/Yes	No
Longcroft-Wheaton et al,[64] 2012	UK	50	143	Experienced	No	Yes	No
Ladabaum et al,[74] 2013	USA	1673	2596	Inexperienced	Yes	No/Yes	Yes

recommended, as also supported by European guidelines,[16,77] the differentiation between ≤2 diminutive polyps between hyperplastic and adenomatous would become irrelevant in the assignment of the surveillance interval, marginalizing any possibility of error. When adopting these criteria, most of the studies succeeded in meeting the 1° PIVI.

Discard (2° PIVI)

The high prevalence of hyperplastic lesions in the rectosigmoid tract undermines the cost-effectiveness of polypectomy. For this reason, a discard (leave-in-place) policy would seem reasonable. This policy has been confirmed by 2 series that specifically applied EC predictions on rectosigmoid lesions (see **Table 5**).[29,74] The failure of meeting the 2° PIVI in other studies would seem to be related mainly to the fact that the analysis was not restricted to rectosigmoid lesions, thereby artificially inflating the relative prevalence of the adenomatous histotype (see **Table 5**). Moreover, the very low risk of neoplastic progression in the few false-negative cases would be marginalized by the favorable natural history (at least at 3–5 years) of unresected adenomas (see discussion above).

SUMMARY

The extremely low prevalence of advanced neoplasia in diminutive lesions, especially in the distal colon, would support the safety of resect and discard or discard policies. This safety is further increased by the low risk of metachronous advanced neoplasia in those with 1 to 2 tubular subcentimetric adenomas.[15] Based on the efficacy, characterization of colorectal lesions with dye-chromoendoscopy or EC at high-optical magnification would presumably assure the highest level of accuracy. On the other hand, high-definition low-magnification EC seems to be reasonably accurate in in vivo histologic prediction, although a high degree of variability has been shown among the available studies. Such an approach may be also expected to be generalizable and reproducible, because of the short-term training period required. When implementing low-magnification EC policies, a major determinant would be represented by the type of surveillance intervals adopted for 1 to 2 low-risk adenomas. If a 10-year interval is adopted, EC-based strategies may be expected to be implemented widely in Western countries, because of an extremely high risk/benefit profile. If, on the other hand, a 5-year interval is adopted, a high level of EC accuracy is required.

REFERENCES

1. Ferlay J, Autier P, Boniol M, et al. Estimates of the cancer incidence and mortality in Europe in 2006. Ann Oncol 2007;18:581–92.
2. Edwards BK, Ward E, Kohler BA, et al. Annual report to the nation on the status of cancer, 1975-2006, featuring colorectal cancer trends and impact of interventions (risk factors, screening, and treatment) to reduce future rates. Cancer 2010;116:544–73.
3. Joseph DA, King JB, Miller JW, et al. Prevalence of colorectal cancer screening among adults–Behavioral Risk Factor Surveillance System, United States, 2010. MMWR Morb Mortal Wkly Rep 2012;61(Suppl):51–6.
4. Winawer SJ, Zauber AG, Ho MN, et al. Prevention of colorectal cancer by colonoscopic polypectomy. The National Polyp Study Workgroup. N Engl J Med 1993;329:1977–81.
5. Atkin W, Kralj-Hans I, Wardle J, et al. Colorectal cancer screening. Randomised trials of flexible sigmoidoscopy. BMJ 2010;341:c4618.

6. Baxter NN, Goldwasser MA, Paszat LF, et al. Association of colonoscopy and death from colorectal cancer. Ann Intern Med 2009;150:1–8.

7. Levin B, Lieberman DA, McFarland B, et al. Screening and surveillance for the early detection of colorectal cancer and adenomatous polyps, 2008: a joint guideline from the American Cancer Society, the US Multi-Society Task Force on Colorectal Cancer, and the American College of Radiology. Gastroenterology 2008;134:1570–95.

8. Rex DK, Johnson DA, Anderson JC, et al. American College of Gastroenterology guidelines for colorectal cancer screening 2009 [corrected]. Am J Gastroenterol 2009;104:739–50.

9. Pignone M, Saha S, Hoerger T, et al. Cost-effectiveness analyses of colorectal cancer screening: a systematic review for the U.S. Preventive Services Task Force. Ann Intern Med 2002;137:96–104.

10. Lansdorp-Vogelaar I, van Ballegooijen M, Zauber AG, et al. Effect of rising chemotherapy costs on the cost savings of colorectal cancer screening. J Natl Cancer Inst 2009;101:1412–22.

11. Seeff LC, Richards TB, Shapiro JA, et al. How many endoscopies are performed for colorectal cancer screening? Results from CDC's survey of endoscopic capacity. Gastroenterology 2004;127:1670–7.

12. Hassan C, Pickhardt PJ, Rex DK. A resect and discard strategy would improve cost-effectiveness of colorectal cancer screening. Clin Gastroenterol Hepatol 2010;8:865–9, 869.e1–3.

13. Hassan C, Pickhardt PJ, Kim DH, et al. Systematic review: distribution of advanced neoplasia according to polyp size at screening colonoscopy. Aliment Pharmacol Ther 2010;31:210–7.

14. Rex DK, Bond JH, Winawer S, et al. Quality in the technical performance of colonoscopy and the continuous quality improvement process for colonoscopy: recommendations of the U.S. Multi-Society Task Force on Colorectal Cancer. Am J Gastroenterol 2002;97:1296–308.

15. Lieberman DA, Rex DK, Winawer S, et al. Guidelines for colonoscopy surveillance after screening and polypectomy: a consensus update by the US Multi-Society Task Force on Colorectal Cancer. Gastroenterology 2012;143:844–57.

16. Atkin WS, Valori R, Kuipers EJ, et al. European guidelines for quality assurance in colorectal cancer screening and diagnosis. First Edition–Colonoscopic surveillance following adenoma removal. Endoscopy 2012;44(Suppl 3):SE151–63.

17. Kudo S, Tamura S, Nakajima T, et al. Diagnosis of colorectal tumorous lesions by magnifying endoscopy. Gastrointest Endosc 1996;44:8–14.

18. Ignjatovic A, East JE, Suzuki N, et al. Optical diagnosis of small colorectal polyps at routine colonoscopy (Detect InSpect ChAracterise Resect and Discard; DISCARD trial): a prospective cohort study. Lancet Oncol 2009;10:1171–8.

19. Rex DK. Narrow-band imaging without optical magnification for histologic analysis of colorectal polyps. Gastroenterology 2009;136:1174–81.

20. Gupta N, Bansal A, Rao D, et al. Accuracy of in vivo optical diagnosis of colon polyp histology by narrow-band imaging in predicting colonoscopy surveillance intervals. Gastrointest Endosc 2012;75:494–502.

21. Rex DK. Reducing costs of colon polyp management. Lancet Oncol 2009;10: 1135–6.

22. Kessler WR, Imperiale TF, Klein RW, et al. A quantitative assessment of the risks and cost savings of forgoing histologic examination of diminutive polyps. Endoscopy 2011;43:683–91.

23. Rex DK, Kahi C, O'Brien M, et al. The American Society for Gastrointestinal Endoscopy PIVI (Preservation and Incorporation of Valuable Endoscopic Innovations) on real-time endoscopic assessment of the histology of diminutive colorectal polyps. Gastrointest Endosc 2011;73:419–22.

24. Schreiner MA, Weiss DG, Lieberman DA. Proximal and large hyperplastic and nondysplastic serrated polyps detected by colonoscopy are associated with neoplasia. Gastroenterology 2010;139:1497–502.

25. Pickhardt PJ, Choi JR, Hwang I, et al. Computed tomographic virtual colonoscopy to screen for colorectal neoplasia in asymptomatic adults. N Engl J Med 2003;349:2191–200.

26. Lieberman D, Moravec M, Holub J, et al. Polyp size and advanced histology in patients undergoing colonoscopy screening: implications for CT colonography. Gastroenterology 2008;135:1100–5.

27. Rex DK, Overhiser AJ, Chen SC, et al. Estimation of impact of American College of Radiology recommendations on CT colonography reporting for resection of high-risk adenoma findings. Am J Gastroenterol 2009;104:149–53.

28. Gupta N, Bansal A, Rao D, et al. Prevalence of advanced histological features in diminutive and small colon polyps. Gastrointest Endosc 2012;75:1022–30.

29. Hewett DG, Huffman ME, Rex DK. Leaving distal colorectal hyperplastic polyps in place can be achieved with high accuracy by using narrow-band imaging: an observational study. Gastrointest Endosc 2012;76:374–80.

30. Pickhardt PJ, Hain KS, Kim DH, et al. Low rates of cancer or high-grade dysplasia in colorectal polyps collected from computed tomography colonography screening. Clin Gastroenterol Hepatol 2010;8:610–5.

31. Hoff G, Foerster A, Vatn MH, et al. Epidemiology of polyps in the rectum and colon. Recovery and evaluation of unresected polyps 2 years after detection. Scand J Gastroenterol 1986;21:853–62.

32. Hofstad B, Vatn MH, Andersen SN, et al. Growth of colorectal polyps: redetection and evaluation of unresected polyps for a period of three years. Gut 1996; 39:449–56.

33. Pickhardt PJ, Kim DK, Cash BD, et al. The natural history of small polyps at CT colonography. Presented at the Annual meeting for the Society of Gastrointestinal Radiologists, Rancho Mirage, CA, Feb 17–22, 2008.

34. Hisabe T, Tsuda S, Matsui T, et al. Natural history of small colorectal protuberant adenomas. Dig Endosc 2010;22(Suppl 1):S43–6.

35. Su MY, Hsu CM, Ho YP, et al. Comparative study of conventional colonoscopy, chromoendoscopy, and narrow-band imaging systems in differential diagnosis of neoplastic and nonneoplastic colonic polyps. Am J Gastroenterol 2006;101: 2711–6.

36. Chiu HM, Chang CY, Chen CC, et al. A prospective comparative study of narrow-band imaging, chromoendoscopy, and conventional colonoscopy in the diagnosis of colorectal neoplasia. Gut 2007;56:373–9.

37. Sikka S, Ringold DA, Jonnalagadda S, et al. Comparison of white light and narrow band high definition images in predicting colon polyp histology, using standard colonoscopes without optical magnification. Endoscopy 2008;40: 818–22.

38. Winawer SJ, Zauber AG, Fletcher RH, et al. Guidelines for colonoscopy surveillance after polypectomy: a consensus update by the US Multi-Society Task Force on Colorectal Cancer and the American Cancer Society. CA Cancer J Clin 2006;56:143–59 [quiz: 184–5].

39. Kato S, Fujii T, Koba I, et al. Assessment of colorectal lesions using magnifying colonoscopy and mucosal dye spraying: can significant lesions be distinguished? Endoscopy 2001;33:306–10.

40. Fu KI, Sano Y, Kato S, et al. Chromoendoscopy using indigo carmine dye spraying with magnifying observation is the most reliable method for differential diagnosis between non-neoplastic and neoplastic colorectal lesions: a prospective study. Endoscopy 2004;36:1089–93.

41. Kudo S, Lambert R, Allen JI, et al. Nonpolypoid neoplastic lesions of the colorectal mucosa. Gastrointest Endosc 2008;68:S3–47.

42. Lambert R, Kudo SE, Vieth M, et al. Pragmatic classification of superficial neoplastic colorectal lesions. Gastrointest Endosc 2009;70:1182–99.

43. Hinoi T, Lucas PC, Kuick R, et al. CDX2 regulates liver intestine-cadherin expression in normal and malignant colon epithelium and intestinal metaplasia. Gastroenterology 2002;123:1565–77.

44. Machida H, Sano Y, Hamamoto Y, et al. Narrow-band imaging in the diagnosis of colorectal mucosal lesions: a pilot study. Endoscopy 2004;36:1094–8.

45. Pohl J, Nguyen-Tat M, Pecho O, et al. Computed virtual chromoendoscopy for classification of small colorectal lesions: a prospective comparative study. Am J Gastroenterol 2008;103:562–9.

46. Lee CK, Lee SH, Hwangbo Y. Narrow-band imaging versus I-Scan for the real-time histological prediction of diminutive colonic polyps: a prospective comparative study by using the simple unified endoscopic classification. Gastrointest Endosc 2011;74:603–9.

47. Konerding MA, Fait E, Gaumann A. 3D microvascular architecture of precancerous lesions and invasive carcinomas of the colon. Br J Cancer 2001; 84:1354–62.

48. East JE, Suzuki N, Saunders BP. Comparison of magnified pit pattern interpretation with narrow band imaging versus chromoendoscopy for diminutive colonic polyps: a pilot study. Gastrointest Endosc 2007;66:310–6.

49. Tischendorf JJ, Wasmuth HE, Koch A, et al. Value of magnifying chromoendoscopy and narrow band imaging (NBI) in classifying colorectal polyps: a prospective controlled study. Endoscopy 2007;39:1092–6.

50. East JE, Suzuki N, Basset P, et al. Narrow band imaging with magnification for the characterization of small and diminutive colonic polyps: pit pattern and vascular pattern intensity. Endoscopy 2008;40:811–7.

51. Sano Y, Ikematsu H, Fu KI, et al. Meshed capillary vessels by use of narrow-band imaging for differential diagnosis of small colorectal polyps. Gastrointest Endosc 2009;69:278–83.

52. van den Broek FJ, van Soest EJ, Naber AH, et al. Combining autofluorescence imaging and narrow-band imaging for the differentiation of adenomas from non-neoplastic colonic polyps among experienced and non-experienced endoscopists. Am J Gastroenterol 2009;104:1498–507.

53. Wada Y, Kudo SE, Kashida H, et al. Diagnosis of colorectal lesions with the magnifying narrow-band imaging system. Gastrointest Endosc 2009;70: 522–31.

54. Tischendorf JJ, Gross S, Winograd R, et al. Computer-aided classification of colorectal polyps based on vascular patterns: a pilot study. Endoscopy 2010; 42:203–7.

55. Tischendorf JJ, Schirin-Sokhan R, Steetz K, et al. Value of magnifying endoscopy in classifying colorectal polyps based on vascular pattern. Endoscopy 2010;42:22–7.

56. Gross S, Trautwein C, Behrens A, et al. Computer-based classification of small colorectal polyps by using narrow-band imaging with optical magnification. Gastrointest Endosc 2011;74:1354–9.
57. Ignjatovic A, East JE, Guenther T, et al. What is the most reliable imaging modality for small colonic polyp characterization? Study of white-light, autofluorescence, and narrow-band imaging. Endoscopy 2011;43:94–9.
58. Sato R, Fujiya M, Watari J, et al. The diagnostic accuracy of high-resolution endoscopy, autofluorescence imaging and narrow-band imaging for differentially diagnosing colon adenoma. Endoscopy 2011;43:862–8.
59. Yoo HY, Lee MS, Ko BM, et al. Correlation of narrow band imaging with magnifying colonoscopy and histology in colorectal tumors. Clin Endosc 2011;44:44–50.
60. Kuiper T, van den Broek FJ, van Eeden S, et al. Feasibility and accuracy of confocal endomicroscopy in comparison with narrow-band imaging and chromoendoscopy for the differentiation of colorectal lesions. Am J Gastroenterol 2012;107:543–50.
61. Takemura Y, Yoshida S, Tanaka S, et al. Computer-aided system for predicting the histology of colorectal tumors by using narrow-band imaging magnifying colonoscopy (with video). Gastrointest Endosc 2012;75:179–85.
62. Hirata M, Tanaka S, Oka S, et al. Magnifying endoscopy with narrow band imaging for diagnosis of colorectal tumors. Gastrointest Endosc 2007;65:988–95.
63. Rastogi A, Bansal A, Wani S, et al. Narrow-band imaging colonoscopy–a pilot feasibility study for the detection of polyps and correlation of surface patterns with polyp histologic diagnosis. Gastrointest Endosc 2008;67:280–6.
64. Longcroft-Wheaton G, Brown J, Cowlishaw D, et al. High-definition vs. standard-definition colonoscopy in the characterization of small colonic polyps: results from a randomized trial. Endoscopy 2012;44:905–10.
65. Rogart JN, Jain D, Siddiqui UD, et al. Narrow-band imaging without high magnification to differentiate polyps during real-time colonoscopy: improvement with experience. Gastrointest Endosc 2008;68:1136–45.
66. Kuiper T, van den Broek FJ, Naber AH, et al. Endoscopic trimodal imaging detects colonic neoplasia as well as standard video endoscopy. Gastroenterology 2011;140:1887–94.
67. Buchner AM, Shahid MW, Heckman MG, et al. Comparison of probe-based confocal laser endomicroscopy with virtual chromoendoscopy for classification of colon polyps. Gastroenterology 2010;138:834–42.
68. Henry ZH, Yeaton P, Shami VM, et al. Meshed capillary vessels found on narrow-band imaging without optical magnification effectively identifies colorectal neoplasia: a North American validation of the Japanese experience. Gastrointest Endosc 2010;72:118–26.
69. Ignjatovic A, Thomas-Gibson S, East JE, et al. Development and validation of a training module on the use of narrow-band imaging in differentiation of small adenomas from hyperplastic colorectal polyps. Gastrointest Endosc 2011;73:128–33.
70. Rastogi A, Early DS, Gupta N, et al. Randomized, controlled trial of standard-definition white-light, high-definition white-light, and narrow-band imaging colonoscopy for the detection of colon polyps and prediction of polyp histology. Gastrointest Endosc 2011;74:593–602.
71. Hewett DG, Kaltenbach T, Sano Y, et al. Validation of a simple classification system for endoscopic diagnosis of small colorectal polyps using narrow-band imaging. Gastroenterology 2012;143:599–607.e1.

72. Kuiper T, Marsman WA, Jansen JM, et al. Accuracy for optical diagnosis of small colorectal polyps in nonacademic settings. Clin Gastroenterol Hepatol 2012;10: 1016–20 [quiz: e79].

73. Paggi S, Rondonotti E, Amato A, et al. Resect and discard strategy in clinical practice: a prospective cohort study. Endoscopy 2012;44:899–904.

74. Ladabaum U, Fioritto A, Mittani A, et al. Real-time optical biopsy of colon polyps with narrow band imaging in community practice does not yet meet key thresholds for clinical decisions. Gastroenterology 2013;144(1):81–91.

75. Raghavendra M, Hewett DG, Rex DK. Differentiating adenomas from hyperplastic colorectal polyps: narrow-band imaging can be learned in 20 minutes. Gastrointest Endosc 2010;72:572–6.

76. Rex DK, Fennerty MB, Sharma P, et al. Bringing new endoscopic imaging technology into everyday practice: what is the role of professional GI societies? Polyp imaging as a template for moving endoscopic innovation forward to answer key clinical questions. Gastrointest Endosc 2010;71:142–6.

77. Denis B, Bottlaender J, Weiss AM, et al. Some diminutive colorectal polyps can be removed and discarded without pathological examination. Endoscopy 2011; 43:81–6.

Surveillance in Inflammatory Bowel Disease
Chromoendoscopy and Digital Mucosal Enhancement

Steven Naymagon, MD*, James F. Marion, MD, AGAF

KEYWORDS

- Dysplasia • Colitis • Inflammatory bowel disease • Colonoscopy
- Chromoendoscopy • Narrow-band imaging • Autofluorescence imaging

KEY POINTS

- Patients with long-standing inflammatory bowel disease have an increased risk of developing colorectal cancer. Performing periodic dysplasia screening and surveillance may diminish this risk.
- Current surveillance practices, the mainstay of which is white-light examination with targeted and random biopsies, are imperfect, and novel approaches are needed.
- Various advanced endoscopic techniques have been studied in an effort to improve the efficacy and efficiency of dysplasia detection.
- To date, chromoendoscopy is the only technique that has consistently yielded positive results in large, well-designed dysplasia-detection trials. Most major society guidelines endorse chromoendoscopy as an adjunctive, accepted, or preferred dysplasia-detection tool.
- Narrow-band imaging, Fuji Intelligent Chromoendoscopy, i-Scan, autofluorescence imaging, and confocal laser endomicroscopy have yielded conflicting outcomes and are not ready for use in clinical practice.
- The widespread use of advanced endoscopic imaging will lead to a paradigm shift in the way gastroenterologists diagnose and treat dysplasia in inflammatory bowel disease.

INTRODUCTION

Inflammatory bowel disease (IBD), including Crohn disease (CD) and ulcerative colitis (UC), results from an inappropriate inflammatory immune response to normal intestinal microbiota in a genetically susceptible host.[1] IBD involving the colon predisposes

Henry D. Janowitz Division of Gastroenterology, Icahn School of Medicine at Mount Sinai, One Gustave Levy Place, New York, NY 10029, USA
* Corresponding author.
E-mail address: steven.naymagon@mountsinai.org

Gastrointest Endoscopy Clin N Am 23 (2013) 679–694
http://dx.doi.org/10.1016/j.giec.2013.03.008
1052-5157/13/$ – see front matter © 2013 Elsevier Inc. All rights reserved.

patients to numerous clinical consequences, including an increased risk of developing colorectal cancer (CRC). The precise risk of cancer, which in the past may have been overestimated because of reliance on outdated evidence, remains unclear, with more recent studies estimating the relative risk of CRC in UC to be between 1 and 2.75.[2] Meta-analyses have shown that duration and extent of disease greatly affect the risk of neoplasia, with nearly one-fifth of patients developing cancer after 30 years.[3] Although most of the literature on neoplasia in IBD is based on data from studies of UC, the risk of cancer appears to be similar in Crohn colitis if at least one-third of the colonic mucosa is involved.[4]

The progression to carcinoma in IBD likely stems from chronic inflammation of the colonic mucosa. There are considerable data supporting the hypothesis that carcinogenesis in IBD typically follows a stepwise pattern from inflammation, to dysplasia, to carcinoma.[5] This pattern provides a rationale for screening and surveillance practices aimed at identifying neoplasia at an early stage. Although there have been no randomized controlled trials demonstrating a mortality benefit, there is indirect evidence justifying dysplasia screening and surveillance in IBD. Retrospective studies have demonstrated that colonoscopic surveillance decreases CRC-related mortality in patients with UC. In addition, having undergone 2 or more colonoscopies offers even more protection.[6,7] Based on such studies, periodic colonoscopic dysplasia surveillance is currently considered the standard of care for all patients with long-standing UC and Crohn colitis.

Although the practice of colonoscopic surveillance is widely accepted, its specific implementation can be controversial. At present the most common surveillance technique involves white-light endoscopic (WLE) examination of the colon with resection or biopsy of any suspicious lesions, as well as random 4-quadrant biopsies taken every 10 cm throughout the length of the colon. The rationale for obtaining nontargeted biopsies is based on the observation that dysplasia in IBD can be difficult, or impossible, to detect using standard endoscopic equipment. To achieve adequate sensitivity for dysplasia detection in flat colonic mucosa, it has been estimated that between 33 and 64 random-biopsy specimens must be obtained at colonoscopy.[8]

However, it is important to point out that most data supporting the random 4-quadrant biopsy methods predate modern endoscopic equipment, and numerous recent studies have called this technique into question for several reasons. First, obtaining the requisite 33 random biopsies still evaluates only a small fraction of the colonic mucosa. Second, practicing gastroenterologists may not strictly follow the random-biopsy protocol. A survey of more than 300 gastroenterologists in the United States found that nearly half of the respondents took less than the recommended number of biopsies,[9] which may stem from the significant time and cost associated with the protocol. Third, the random-biopsy protocol has repeatedly proved to be a very low yield technique. Van den Broek and colleagues[10] reported a dysplasia-detection rate of 0.2% for random biopsies compared with 23% for targeted biopsies. Moreover, only 1 of 475 (0.002%) patients had a change in management based on the results of a nontargeted biopsy. Fourth, in accordance with the findings of van den Broek, investigators are finding that most dysplastic lesions in IBD are in fact detectable using modern endoscopic modalities.[11] Finally, there is evidence that the rates of CRC and dysplasia may be decreasing in UC patients overall.[12] This smaller, more elusive target may further limit our ability to detect existing neoplasia using outdated techniques.

Frustration with current surveillance practices and a sense that the dysplasia target has shrunk have led investigators to seek more innovative ways of approaching this problem. Our growing understanding of the natural history of dysplasia and CRC in

IBD has paralleled the evolving sophistication and resolution of endoscopic tools used to detect it. Naturally the two have become intertwined, and novel endoscopic modalities have been used in the quest to uncover neoplasia. This review aims to outline the available endoscopic technologies for dysplasia detection in IBD, consider the evidence supporting their use, and assess which modalities are ready for use in clinical practice.

DYSPLASIA-DETECTION TECHNIQUES
White-Light and High-Definition White-Light Endoscopy

> Most dysplasia in IBD is visible using modern WLE equipment. HD endoscopes will continue to make WLE an important tool for the detection of dysplasia in IBD.

Two large retrospective studies have demonstrated that most dysplasia in IBD is visible using standard WLE. In their institutional experience, Rutter and colleagues[11] reported that 77.3% of neoplastic lesions were macroscopically visible at colonoscopy. On a per-patient basis, 89.3% of patients had macroscopically detectable neoplasia. Rubin and colleagues[13] achieved similar results at their institution, reporting per-patient sensitivities for dysplasia and cancer of 71.8% and 100%, respectively. Based on these studies, as well as others reporting similar results, it is currently accepted that the majority of neoplastic lesions in UC patients are visible with modern endoscopic equipment. This paradigm again highlights the questionable value of obtaining nontargeted biopsies of endoscopically normal-appearing colonic mucosa.

The advent of modern high-definition (HD), or high-resolution, colonoscopy has further improved the quality of white-light examinations. HD refers to the pixel density of a system. Standard-definition endoscopes produce an image signal of 100,000 to 400,000 pixels, whereas high-resolution or HD endoscopes produce signal images with resolutions that range from 850,000 pixels to more than 1 million pixels. Resolution is distinct from magnification, which involves simply enlarging an image without affecting pixel density.[14]

HD colonoscopy has been shown to improve adenoma detection rates in average-risk patients by improving the ability to detect subtle mucosal changes.[15] Subramanian and colleagues[16] compared the yield of dysplastic lesions detected by standard WLE with that of HD endoscopy in a retrospective cohort of patients with UC or Crohn colitis. An adjusted prevalence ratio of detecting a dysplastic lesion on targeted biopsy of 2.99 (95% confidence interval [CI] 1.16–7.79) for HD colonoscopy was found. WLE is likely to continue to play a vital role in dysplasia detection in IBD with the continued development of HD colonoscopy technologies (**Fig. 1**).

Narrow-Band Imaging

> NBI is a widely available and convenient endoscopic imaging modality. However, several studies have failed to demonstrate its efficacy for the detection of dysplasia in IBD patients.

Narrow-band imaging (NBI) is a technology that uses specialized light filters to modulate the intensity of various constituents of the white-light spectrum. Most NBI systems have narrow-band filters with the absorption property of hemoglobin that allow them to highlight vascular architecture and structures of the mucosal surface.[17] NBI is widely available on newer model endoscopes, making it an attractive option as an adjunct

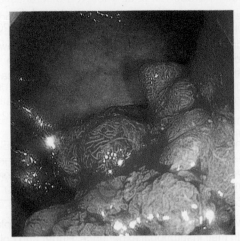

Fig. 1. Colonic adenocarcinoma visualized using high-definition white-light endoscopy. The enhanced resolution allows visualization of the Kudo pit pattern of the lesion, suggesting that it is a neoplasm.

to current dysplasia-detection tools in IBD. Unfortunately, most well-designed randomized studies have failed to show a difference in dysplasia detection using NBI in comparison with WLE.

Dekker and colleagues[18] performed a prospective, randomized, crossover study in which 42 patients with long-standing UC underwent colonoscopies with both NBI and WLE (**Fig. 2**). Neoplasia was detected in 4 patients by both techniques, in another 4 patients by NBI only, and in another 3 patients by WLE only. These results showed no statistical difference between the two modalities. Of note, significantly more non-neoplastic, or false-positive, biopsies were taken using NBI. A similarly designed study compared a newer-generation NBI system with HD WLE in patients with UC. Again, there was no difference between the two modalities in the number of dysplastic lesions detected.[19] A more recent parallel-group trial of patients with UC randomized to receive colonoscopy with NBI or WLE was discontinued early because a

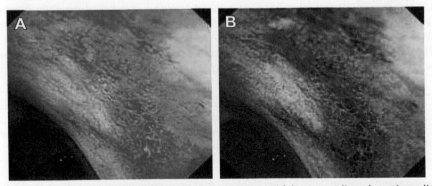

Fig. 2. A flat lesion with low-grade neoplasia in a patient with long-standing ulcerative colitis, viewed by white-light endoscopy (A), and narrow-band imaging, showing dark discoloration of the lesion (B). (*From* Dekker E, van den Broek FJ, Reitsma JB, et al. Narrow-band imaging compared with conventional colonoscopy for the detection of dysplasia in patients with longstanding ulcerative colitis. Endoscopy 2007;39(3):218; with permission from Thieme.)

prespecified midpoint analysis showed no difference in the primary outcome of dysplasia detection between the two groups.[20]

The dysplasia-detection capability of NBI has also been compared with that of chromoendoscopy. In a prospective, randomized, crossover study, Pellisé and colleagues[21] enrolled 60 patients with UC to undergo colonoscopy with both chromoendoscopy and NBI in random order. The study showed a similar dysplasia-detection rate for NBI and chromoendoscopy. However, NBI also resulted in a higher rate of missed lesions, with an odds ratio for missed neoplasia of 4.21. Although this did not reach statistical significance, it was a key finding. Based on the high miss rate (ie, high specificity but low sensitivity) and because the study was somewhat underpowered, the investigators concluded that NBI cannot be recommended for use in dysplasia surveillance in IBD patients at present.

There are likely several reasons for the shortcomings of NBI in the realm of dysplasia detection in the IBD population. According to Pellisé and colleagues,[21] the lack of sensitivity may be attributed to the fact that NBI principally evaluates vascular patterns rather than alterations in crypt architecture detected by chromoendoscopy. The disruption of the vascular pattern is a well-recognized consequence of chronic colitis, and may hamper the efficacy of this technology in this setting. The importance of vascular-pattern analysis in dysplasia detection is not entirely clear, and analysis of crypt architecture and pit patterns has been more readily accepted in identifying neoplastic lesions.[22] A simpler explanation is that NBI provides a darker image than WLE, which may actually hinder visualization of mucosal lesions.[19]

Chromoendoscopy

Chromoendoscopy involves the application of a topical dye to highlight mucosal architecture. Several large, well-designed studies, as well as a meta-analysis, have demonstrated that chromoendoscopy is superior to WLE for the detection of dysplasia in IBD patients.

Chromoendoscopy is the topical application of dyes to the colonic mucosa to enhance detection and delineation of surface abnormalities. The two dye agents most commonly used in trials, as well as in clinical practice, are methylene blue and indigo carmine. Methylene blue is adsorbed and absorbed by normal colonocytes but not by inflamed or neoplastic colonic mucosa, thus highlighting the pit patterns of mucosal lesions. Indigo carmine is not absorbed by the mucosa but simply pools within colonic crypts, allowing for the demarcation of inflamed or neoplastic lesions.[23] These agents are applied to the entire colonic mucosa using a spray catheter or the water jet channel on a standard colonoscope, and allow for inspection within minutes of application.

Chromoendoscopy has been comprehensively studied as a "red-flag" technology for dysplasia detection in IBD. In a prospective cohort of patients with pancolitis, Matsumoto and colleagues[24] showed that chromoendoscopy using indigo carmine significantly enhances the detection and characterization of flat lesions harboring dysplasia. Kiesslich and colleagues[22] performed a randomized controlled trial comparing conventional colonoscopy with chromoendoscopy using methylene blue in 165 patients with long-standing UC. Chromoendoscopy led to a 3-fold increase in the detection of intraepithelial neoplasia in comparison with conventional colonoscopy (32 vs 10; $P = .003$), and allowed for the differentiation between nonneoplastic and neoplastic lesions with sensitivity and specificity of 93%. The same group of investigators performed a follow-up study in which UC patients were randomized to conventional colonoscopy or chromoendoscopy with endomicroscopy. Chromoendo-scopy led to the detection of 4.75-fold more neoplasias (P = .005) than conventional colonoscopy. Endomicroscopy further enhanced the ability to accurately characterize lesions as neoplastic (accuracy 97.8%).[25] Hurlstone and colleagues[26] compared magnification chromoendoscopy in 350 patients with UC with a group of matched historical controls who had undergone conventional examinations. Significantly more neoplastic lesions were detected in the chromoendoscopy group than in the controls (69 vs 24, $P<.0001$). In a tandem study, Rutter and colleagues[27] performed "back-to-back" white-light and indigo carmine colonoscopic examinations in a cohort of 100 patients with UC, and found 7 dysplastic lesions with chromoendoscopy that were missed during the WLE examination. A similarly designed tandem colonoscopy study by Marion and colleagues[28] demonstrated that chromoendoscopy using methy-lene blue was able to detect more dysplastic lesions than either standard WLE targeting or random biopsies. Targeted biopsies with dye spray yielded 17 dysplastic lesions, compared with 3 lesions from random biopsies and 9 lesions with targeted WLE biopsies (**Fig. 3**).

All the major studies summarized here have been positive in favor of chromoendo-scopy, with a per-patient increase in dysplasia detection of approximately 2- to 3-fold and a per-lesion increase of 4- to 5-fold. The results of the pivotal chromoendoscopy trials were pooled in a recent meta-analysis by Subramanian and colleagues.[29] The 6 studies included in the analysis involved a total of 1277 patients. The overall difference in dysplasia detection between chromoendoscopy and WLE was 7% (95% CI 3.2–11.3) on a per-patient analysis, with a number needed to treat of 14.3. Of note, the increase in diagnosis of flat dysplastic lesions using chromoendoscopy over WLE was 27% (95% CI 11.2–41.9). The investigators concluded that chromoendoscopy is preferable to WLE for the detection of dysplasia in patients with colonic IBD who are undergoing surveillance.

Chromoendoscopy has proved to be an extremely effective dysplasia-detection modality, although several practical limitations remain. Some investigators have found chromoendoscopy to be somewhat less accurate in the setting of severe inflamma-tion, which is often encountered in IBD patients. In a trial by Kiesslich and colleagues,[22] chromoendoscopy was extremely sensitive and specific at identifying

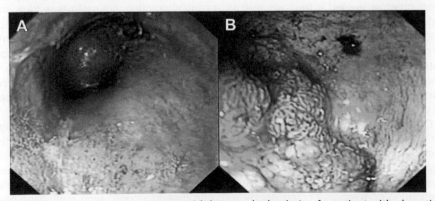

Fig. 3. Colonoscopy of colonic mucosa with low-grade dysplasia of a patient with ulcerative colitis, (A) before methylene blue dye spray and (B) after dye spray. (*From* Marion JF, Waye JD, Present DH, et al. Chromoendoscopy-targeted biopsies are superior to standard colonoscopic surveillance for detecting dysplasia in inflammatory bowel disease patients: a prospective endoscopic trial. Am J Gastroenterol 2008;103(9):2347; with permission from Nature Publishing Group.)

neoplastic lesions in areas of mild inflammation, but could not accurately distinguish inflammation from neoplasia in areas of severely inflamed mucosa. However, this issue exists with other endoscopic modalities as well, making it a global rather than a modality-specific limitation. There was no disadvantage to using dye spray in detecting lesions in inflamed mucosa in other controlled trials comparing it with WLE.[28] It remains unclear whether there are differences in efficacy between methylene blue and indigo carmine, as no studies have compared these two agents. With respect to safety, some investigators have suggested that methylene blue may cause DNA damage in colonocytes.[30] This notion has not been substantiated in clinical trials, and remains a hypothetical risk with unclear clinical relevance.[31] In addition, chromoendoscopy prolongs the length of surveillance procedures by an average of 11 minutes. This difference may be diminished if the random-biopsy protocol is abandoned.[29] Achieving competence in chromoendoscopy, although relatively straightforward, does require training in dye application, pit-pattern analysis, and lesion identification. Chromoendoscopy is currently not part of routine gastroenterology fellowship curricula in most institutions. A concerted effort should be made to integrate this effective technique into the training curricula of the next generation of endoscopists. The clinical impact and long-term clinical outcomes of so efficiently revealing and removing dysplasia, particularly with respect to cancer-related morbidity or mortality, remains unknown. To date, no clinical trials have reported the long-term outcomes of patients who have been enrolled in surveillance programs using chromoendoscopy.

FICE and i-Scan

> FICE and i-Scan are "virtual chromoendoscopy" techniques. FICE has failed to improve the detection of adenoma in average-risk subjects in several studies, whereas i-Scan has shown some positive results. Neither modality has been rigorously studied in the IBD population.

The success and drawbacks of chromoendoscopy have led device manufacturers and investigators to develop and test technologies that might emulate its efficacy while avoiding the associated pitfalls. The goal is to achieve similar resolution and mucosal enhancement without the need to apply a topical dye. Two such "virtual chromoendoscopy" systems are currently available: Fuji Intelligent Chromoendoscopy (FICE; Fujinon, Tokyo, Japan) and i-Scan (Pentax, Tokyo, Japan). These systems differ from NBI in that they do not use light filters but rather a post-processing computer algorithm that modifies a white-light image after it is captured. There is no need to apply a dye, and the system is activated simply with the press of a button.[32] Although there have been no clinical trials assessing the utility of FICE or i-Scan for dysplasia detection in IBD, these modalities have been studied as adjuncts to adenoma detection in screening and surveillance colonoscopy in average-risk populations.

Pohl and colleagues[33] randomized 871 consecutive average-risk subjects to undergo colonoscopy using FICE or standard colonoscopy with targeted indigo carmine chromoendoscopy (**Fig. 4**). The investigators found no significant difference in the adenoma detection rate between the two groups, but did note that FICE was as effective as chromoendoscopy in classifying lesions as benign or neoplastic (sensitivity 92.7% vs 90.4%, $P = .44$). In a similar large prospective study, Aminalai and colleagues[34] randomized 1318 patients to colonoscopy with either FICE or WLE, and found no significant difference in the adenoma-detection rate. Finally, a prospective trial of 359 average-risk subjects randomized to tandem colonoscopy with FICE and HD WLE once again demonstrated no difference in adenoma-detection rate or

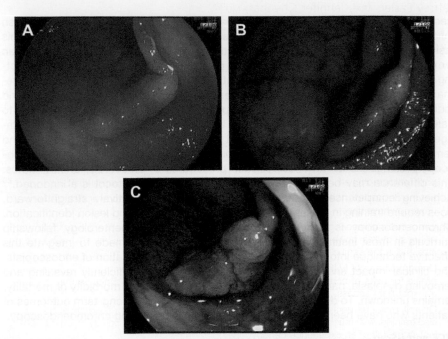

Fig. 4. A flat adenoma visualized with conventional imaging (*A*), Fuji Intelligent Chromoendoscopy (*B*), and after indigo carmine dye spray (*C*). (*From* Pohl J, Lotterer E, Balzer C, et al. Computed virtual chromoendoscopy versus standard colonoscopy with targeted indigocarmine chromoscopy: a randomised multicentre trial. Gut 2009;58(1):75; with permission from BMJ Publishing Group Ltd.)

adenoma-miss rate between the two modalities.[35] The investigators speculated that the failure of FICE to improve detection rates may be attributed to insufficient brightness, greater dependence on ideal bowel preparation than with WLE, and requirement for significant technical skills on the part of the endoscopist. Overall, these investigators were unable to recommend the use of FICE in routine clinical practice.

The evidence supporting i-Scan has been somewhat more positive. In a large prospective trial, Hoffman and colleagues[36] randomly assigned 220 average-risk patients to undergo either a WLE examination or a colonoscopy with i-Scan. The investigators found a 3-fold increase in the number of neoplastic lesions detected by the i-Scan including adenomas, carcinomas, and flat polyps. These investigators also compared i-Scan with chromoendoscopy in a prospective tandem study involving 69 patients undergoing CRC screening.[37] In this study, i-Scan yielded the same number of adenomas as chromoendoscopy. The number of flat lesions detected with i-Scan was significantly more than with WLE and equivalent to chromoendoscopy. Although this technology is still developing and further studies are needed, these results show potential in the realm of dysplasia detection in IBD patients. Namely, if i-Scan can effectively enhance our capability to detect flat dysplasia, which is the rule rather than the exception in IBD, it may become an important tool in the future. Larger, prospective, randomized trials are needed to determine how i-Scan performs in the IBD population in comparison with modern HD colonoscopes (**Fig. 5**).

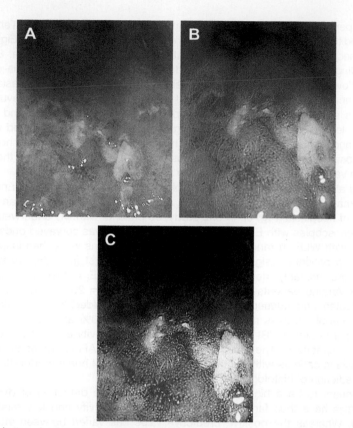

Fig. 5. A lesion harboring low-grade dysplasia in a patient with ulcerative colitis visualized with high-definition white-light endoscopy (*A*), i-Scan mode 1 (*B*), and i-Scan mode 2 (*C*).

Autofluorescence Imaging

AFI is a highly sensitive dysplasia-detection technique that relies on differential emission spectra of normal and neoplastic tissues. Despite promising results in clinical trials, the technical challenges associated with AFI are likely to prevent its widespread use in current practice.

Autofluorescence imaging (AFI) is a technique that uses the differential emission spectra of tissues to construct chromoendoscopy-like images. Because of the presence of endogenous fluorophores in colonocytes, exposure of the mucosa to short-wavelength light leads to the emission (autofluorescence) of longer-wavelength light. The emission spectra of normal and neoplastic cells differ according to the proportion of mitochondria and lysosomes they contain. AFI can therefore act as a red-flag technology by distinguishing between normal, inflamed, hyperplastic, and adenomatous mucosa.[38] Several studies have investigated the role of AFI in dysplasia surveillance in IBD.

Fusco and colleagues[39] studied the long-term effects of fluorescence-guided colonoscopy on the development of dysplasia in 41 UC patients. Thirty-one patients had a negative fluorescence-guided colonoscopy, and were subsequently followed for a mean of 7.8 years with conventional WLE colonoscopies at 2-year intervals. During the study period neoplasia was uncovered in only 2 of these patients (6%). Ten patients were found to have neoplasia on index fluorescence-guided examination. Eight underwent immediate colectomy, with confirmation of intraepithelial neoplasia. Based on these findings, the investigators concluded that AFI is a sensitive dysplasia-detection modality (low miss rate) and has a high positive predictive value for neoplasia.

Messmann and colleagues,[40] using oral and locally applied 5-aminolevulinic acid (5-ALA) as a photosensitizer, examined patients with UC using AFI and revealed dysplastic lesions in 12 of 37 patients. High specificity was also achieved with both systemic and local application of 5-ALA. The negative predictive value of nonfluorescent mucosa for exclusion of dysplasia was high (89%–100%). However, the positive predictive value in this study was very low (13%–21%).

AFI has also been investigated in combination with other modalities. Endoscopic trimodal imaging (ETMI) incorporates WLE, AFI, and NBI for the detection and characterization of neoplasia (**Fig. 6**). In one study, 50 patients with UC underwent surveillance colonoscopies with ETMI. Each colonic segment was surveyed once with AFI and once with WLE, in random order. All detected lesions were then inspected by NBI. Among patients assigned to inspection with AFI first (n = 25), 10 neoplastic lesions were primarily detected and subsequent WLE detected no additional neoplasia. Among patients examined with WLE first (n = 25), 3 neoplastic lesions were detected and subsequent inspection with AFI added 3 neoplastic lesions. Thus, the neoplasia miss rates for AFI and WLE were 0% and 50%, respectively (P = .036). The use of NBI to classify lesions had sensitivity and specificity of 75% and 81%, respectively. The investigators concluded that AFI improves the detection of neoplasia in patients with UC, and that analysis by NBI has a moderate accuracy for the prediction of histology.[41]

AFI appears to be a highly sensitive modality for the detection of dysplasia in IBD. Studies have thus far demonstrated a high sensitivity and low miss rate for dysplasia. Whereas the positive predictive value has varied between studies, the negative predictive value appears to be reliably high. However, owing to numerous practical and technical limitations AFI remains restricted to specialized referral centers. To bring AFI to mainstream practices numerous hurdles will have to be

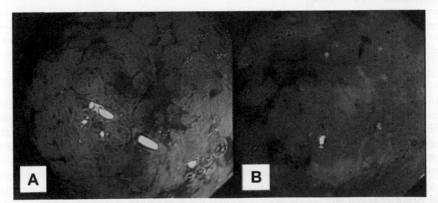

Fig. 6. Images using white-light endoscopy (*A*) and autofluorescence imaging (AFI) (*B*) of a mass, revealing low-grade intraepithelial neoplasia. (*From* van den Broek FJ, Fockens P, van Eeden S, et al. Endoscopic tri-modal imaging for surveillance in ulcerative colitis: randomised comparison of high-resolution endoscopy and autofluorescence imaging for neoplasia detection; and evaluation of narrow-band imaging for classification of lesions. Gut 2008;57(8):1084; with permission from BMJ Publishing Group Ltd.)

overcome, such as investing in the necessary equipment, educating gastroenterologists in the administration of photosensitizers (topical and/or intravenous), and training endoscopists in the interpretation of images produced by AFI.

Confocal Laser Endomicroscopy

Confocal laser endomicroscopy (CLE) is a technique that allows in vivo microscopic examination of the colonic mucosa, thus providing endoscopists with "real-time histology" and possibly obviating biopsy and formal histologic diagnosis. Although this modality is discussed in detail elsewhere in this issue, it does warrant mention here. In the realm of dysplasia surveillance, CLE has been most extensively studied in conjunction with various dysplasia-detection technologies. For instance, in the seminal study by Kiesslich and colleagues[25] discussed earlier, CLE was used as an adjunct to chromoendoscopy to aid in the characterization of detected lesions.

CLE has also been studied as a red-flag modality to aid in the detection of lesions in IBD. Günther and colleagues[42] compared 3 endoscopic surveillance strategies in patients with IBD. One group underwent a WLE examination, a second group underwent a chromoendoscopy examination, and a third group underwent a CLE examination. The investigators uncovered high-grade dysplasia in 2 patients (4% detection rate) when using chromoendoscopy and in 4 patients when using CLE (8% detection rate, $P<.05$). No neoplasia was detected using WLE. These results suggested that CLE may be an effective dysplasia-detection technique. It was noted, however, that the CLE examinations took twice as much time as the chromoendoscopy examinations to complete.

Despite numerous promising findings, CLE is currently not a practical tool for the routine care of IBD patients. CLE requires extensive expertise in both endoscopy and histopathology, a considerable capital investment in the equipment, and a significant amount of time spent per procedure. Taking these considerations into account, it seems that the role of CLE is currently limited to the characterization of lesions detected by red-flag modalities, such as chromoendoscopy, in clinical trials at expert referral centers that have the expertise necessary to acquire and interpret in vivo histologic images.

MAJOR SOCIETY GUIDELINES

The only methods for dysplasia surveillance in IBD that are recommended by the major gastroenterology societies are WLE with random biopsies and chromoendoscopy (**Table 1**). The American College of Gastroenterology (ACG) takes the most conservative stance. In their 2010 statement the ACG recommends "surveillance colonoscopy with multiple biopsies" in patients with long-standing UC.[43] Chromoendoscopy is mentioned as a technique that may enhance the detection of flat lesions, but is not explicitly endorsed by the guidelines. The American Gastroenterologic Association

Table 1
Summary of major gastroenterologic society guidelines on dysplasia surveillance in patients with IBD

	ACG 2010	AGA 2010	BSG 2010
WLE	+	+	±
Random biopsy	+	+	±
Chromoendoscopy	±	+	+

Abbreviations: ACG, American College of Gastroenterology; AGA, American Gastroenterologic Association; BSG, British Society of Gastroenterology; WLE, white-light endoscopy.

(AGA) recommendations in 2010 regarded both the random-biopsy technique and chromoendoscopy as valid surveillance techniques. However, at present the AGA still regards white-light colonoscopy, using standard or HD scopes, with random biopsies as the primary dysplasia-detection technique. Chromoendoscopy with targeted biopsies is considered an acceptable alternative to WLE for endoscopists who have experience with this technique.[44] European guidelines differ from those in North America in that chromoendoscopy is more accepted. The British Society of Gastroenterology (BSG) guidelines recommend pancolonic chromoendoscopy with targeted biopsy of abnormal areas as the primary method of surveillance. If chromoendoscopy is not available, the random-biopsy strategy is considered an acceptable alternative.[45] The other modalities discussed in this review are currently considered investigational.

MODALITIES THAT SHOULD BE USED IN 2013

The currently available dysplasia-detection modalities in IBD are summarized in **Table 2**. The random, 4-quadrant biopsy technique has been shown to have low accuracy for dysplasia detection in numerous prospective, high-quality studies. This technique has also been proved to be impractical because of the significant time and cost necessary to perform the requisite 33 biopsies. However, for historical reasons random biopsies are still incorporated into most society guidelines. Given our current knowledge and endoscopic capabilities, the continued use of nontargeted biopsies as the principal dysplasia-detection technique should be abandoned.

HD WLE continues to play an important role in dysplasia detection in IBD. Most dysplasia in IBD is visible using standard WLE, and the widespread incorporation of HD WLE is likely to improve accuracy even further. Positive results have been reported in prospective studies in average-risk patients as well as in a retrospective cohort of IBD patients. Therefore, targeted HD-WLE remains a practical and valuable dysplasia-detection tool in 2013.

Chromoendoscopy has consistently yielded positive results in numerous well-designed studies in IBD patients. It has been incorporated into most major society guidelines. British guidelines consider chromoendoscopy the first-line dysplasia surveillance modality. The application of dye is relatively straightforward and does not require a significant investment in new equipment or training, making it an extremely practical technique. As more gastroenterologists become familiar with

Table 2
Summary of endoscopic dysplasia-detection modalities in patients with IBD, and recommendations for use

	Demonstrated Accuracy in IBD	Supporting Evidence in IBD	Incorporated into Guidelines	Practicality of Use in Practice	Should be Used in 2013?
Random biopsy	−	−	+	±	±
HD WLE	+	±	+	+	+
Chromoendoscopy	+	+	+	+	+
NBI	−	−	−	±	−
FICE	n/a	n/a	−	±	−
i-Scan	n/a	n/a	−	±	−
AFI	+	+	−	−	−

Abbreviations: AFI, autofluorescence imaging; FICE, Fuji Intelligent Chromoendoscopy; HD WLE, high-definition white-light endoscopy; n/a, not available; NBI, narrow-band imaging.

chromoendoscopy, it should become the primary dysplasia surveillance technique in all IBD patients.

The virtual-chromoendoscopy techniques, including NBI, FICE, and i-Scan, cannot be recommended for use at this time. NBI has been investigated in IBD populations, and the results have been disappointing for both dysplasia detection and lesion characterization. FICE has been studied in non-IBD cohorts and has failed to improve dysplasia detection. i-Scan has had more promising results in adenoma-detection trials in average-risk patients. However, neither FICE nor i-Scan have been rigorously studied in IBD patients. Therefore, despite the "push-of-a-button" convenience of these modalities, there is currently no evidence to support their use.

Although the evidence supporting the efficacy of AFI and CLE in IBD patients has been strongly positive, these techniques have not made the leap from bench to bedside. The significant investments in training and equipment necessary to perform these procedures are prohibitive at present. Therefore, AFI and CLE will remain the tools of clinical investigators and expert referral centers.

SUMMARY

The goal of performing dysplasia surveillance is to prevent cancer and save lives. Despite surveillance practices having been accepted as standard of care for decades, CRC continues to lead to significant morbidity and mortality in IBD patients, suggesting that the current practices are imperfect. The advent of novel endoscopic techniques will allow gastroenterologists to spend more time effectively and efficiently inspecting the colonic mucosa to uncover dysplastic foci, rather than spending the time taking random biopsies of normal-appearing mucosa. Ultimately the goal will be to visualize, delineate, and completely remove any dysplastic lesion, thus sparing patients unnecessary surgeries and, perhaps, even saving lives. Rapid and significant advances have taken place since the days of relying solely on random biopsies to uncover dysplasia. Discerning, detecting, and derailing the natural history of dysplasia in the patient with colitis remains fertile ground for further studies. In the process we can further validate and improve on the tools available to the IBD-endoscopist, and better serve our patients.

REFERENCES

1. Abraham C, Cho JH. Inflammatory bowel disease. N Engl J Med 2009;361(21): 2066-78.
2. Loftus EV. Epidemiology and risk factors for colorectal dysplasia and cancer in ulcerative colitis. Gastroenterol Clin North Am 2006;35(3):517-31.
3. Eaden JA, Abrams KR, Mayberry JF. The risk of colorectal cancer in ulcerative colitis: a meta-analysis. Gut 2001;48(4):526-35.
4. Canavan C, Abrams KR, Mayberry J. Meta-analysis: colorectal and small bowel cancer risk in patients with Crohn's disease. Aliment Pharmacol Ther 2006;23(8): 1097-104.
5. Ullman TA, Itzkowitz SH. Intestinal inflammation and cancer. Gastroenterology 2011;140(6):1807-16.
6. Karlén P, Kornfeld D, Broström O, et al. Is colonoscopic surveillance reducing colorectal cancer mortality in ulcerative colitis? A population based case control study. Gut 1998;42(5):711-4.
7. Lutgens MW, Oldenburg B, Siersema PD, et al. Colonoscopic surveillance improves survival after colorectal cancer diagnosis in inflammatory bowel disease. Br J Cancer 2009;101(10):1671-5.

8. Rubin CE, Haggitt RC, Burmer GC, et al. DNA aneuploidy in colonic biopsies predicts future development of dysplasia in ulcerative colitis. Gastroenterology 1992; 103(5):1611–20.

9. Rodriguez SA, Collins JM, Knigge KL, et al. Surveillance and management of dysplasia in ulcerative colitis. Gastrointest Endosc 2007;65(3):432–9.

10. van den Broek FJ, Stokkers PC, Reitsma JB, et al. Random biopsies taken during colonoscopic surveillance of patients with longstanding ulcerative colitis: low yield and absence of clinical consequences. Am J Gastroenterol 2011. [Epub ahead of print].

11. Rutter MD, Saunders BP, Wilkinson KH, et al. Most dysplasia in ulcerative colitis is visible at colonoscopy. Gastrointest Endosc 2004;60(3):334–9.

12. Jess T, Simonsen J, Jørgensen KT, et al. Decreasing risk of colorectal cancer in patients with inflammatory bowel disease over 30 years. Gastroenterology 2012; 143(2):375–81.

13. Rubin DT, Rothe JA, Hetzel JT, et al. Are dysplasia and colorectal cancer endoscopically visible in patients with ulcerative colitis? Gastrointest Endosc 2007; 65(7):998–1004.

14. Kwon RS, Adler DG, Chand B, et al. High-resolution and high-magnification endoscopes. Gastrointest Endosc 2009;69(3 Pt 1):399–407.

15. Buchner AM, Shahid MW, Heckman MG, et al. High-definition colonoscopy detects colorectal polyps at a higher rate than standard white-light colonoscopy. Clin Gastroenterol Hepatol 2010;8(4):364–70.

16. Subramanian V, Ramappa V, Telakis E, et al. Comparison of high definition with standard white light endoscopy for detection of dysplastic lesions during surveillance colonoscopy in patients with colonic inflammatory bowel disease. Inflamm Bowel Dis 2012;19(2):350–5.

17. Matsumoto T, Kudo T, Iida M. The significance of NBI observation for inflammatory bowel diseases. In: Cohen J, editor. Comprehensive atlas of high resolution endoscopy and narrowband imaging. Oxford (United Kingdom): Blackwell Publishing; 2008. p. 149–60.

18. Dekker E, van den Broek FJ, Reitsma JB, et al. Narrow-band imaging compared with conventional colonoscopy for the detection of dysplasia in patients with longstanding ulcerative colitis. Endoscopy 2007;39(3):216–21.

19. van den Broek FJ, Fockens P, van Eeden S, et al. Narrow-band imaging versus high-definition endoscopy for the diagnosis of neoplasia in ulcerative colitis. Endoscopy 2011;43(2):108–15.

20. Ignjatovic A, East JE, Subramanian V, et al. Narrow band imaging for detection of dysplasia in colitis: a randomized controlled trial. Am J Gastroenterol 2012; 107(6):885–90.

21. Pellisé M, López-Cerón M, Rodríguez de Miguel C, et al. Narrow-band imaging as an alternative to chromoendoscopy for the detection of dysplasia in longstanding inflammatory bowel disease: a prospective, randomized, crossover study. Gastrointest Endosc 2011;74(4):840–8.

22. Kiesslich R, Fritsch J, Holtmann M, et al. Methylene blue-aided chromoendoscopy for the detection of intraepithelial neoplasia and colon cancer in ulcerative colitis. Gastroenterology 2003;124(4):880–8.

23. Kiesslich R, Neurath MF. Chromoendoscopy in inflammatory bowel disease. Gastroenterol Clin North Am 2012;41(2):291–302.

24. Matsumoto T, Nakamura S, Jo Y, et al. Chromoscopy might improve diagnostic accuracy in cancer surveillance for ulcerative colitis. Am J Gastroenterol 2003; 98(8):1827–33.

25. Kiesslich R, Goetz M, Lammersdorf K, et al. Chromoscopy-guided endomicroscopy increases the diagnostic yield of intraepithelial neoplasia in ulcerative colitis. Gastroenterology 2007;132(3):874–82.

26. Hurlstone DP, Sanders DS, Lobo AJ, et al. Indigo carmine-assisted high-magnification chromoscopic colonoscopy for the detection and characterisation of intraepithelial neoplasia in ulcerative colitis: a prospective evaluation. Endoscopy 2005;37(12):1186–92.

27. Rutter MD, Saunders BP, Schofield G, et al. Pancolonic indigo carmine dye spraying for the detection of dysplasia in ulcerative colitis. Gut 2004;53(2): 256–60.

28. Marion JF, Waye JD, Present DH, et al. Chromoendoscopy-targeted biopsies are superior to standard colonoscopic surveillance for detecting dysplasia in inflammatory bowel disease patients: a prospective endoscopic trial. Am J Gastroenterol 2008;103(9):2342–9.

29. Subramanian V, Mannath J, Ragunath K, et al. Meta-analysis: the diagnostic yield of chromoendoscopy for detecting dysplasia in patients with colonic inflammatory bowel disease. Aliment Pharmacol Ther 2011;33(3):304–12.

30. Davies J, Burke D, Olliver JR, et al. Methylene blue but not indigo carmine causes DNA damage to colonocytes in vitro and in vivo at concentrations used in clinical chromoendoscopy. Gut 2007;56(1):155–6.

31. Hardie LJ, Olliver JR, Wild CP, et al. Chromoendoscopy with methylene blue and the risk of DNA damage. Gastroenterology 2004;126(2):623 [author reply: 623–4].

32. Sauk J, Hoffman A, Anandasabapathy S, et al. High-definition and filter-aided colonoscopy. Gastroenterol Clin North Am 2010;39(4):859–81.

33. Pohl J, Lotterer E, Balzer C, et al. Computed virtual chromoendoscopy versus standard colonoscopy with targeted indigocarmine chromoscopy: a randomised multicentre trial. Gut 2009;58(1):73–8.

34. Aminalai A, Rösch T, Aschenbeck J, et al. Live image processing does not increase adenoma detection rate during colonoscopy: a randomized comparison between FICE and conventional imaging (Berlin Colonoscopy Project 5, BE-COP-5). Am J Gastroenterol 2010;105(11):2383–8.

35. Chung SJ, Kim D, Song JH, et al. Efficacy of computed virtual chromoendoscopy on colorectal cancer screening: a prospective, randomized, back-to-back trial of Fuji Intelligent Color Enhancement versus conventional colonoscopy to compare adenoma miss rates. Gastrointest Endosc 2010;72(1):136–42.

36. Hoffman A, Sar F, Goetz M, et al. High definition colonoscopy combined with i-Scan is superior in the detection of colorectal neoplasias compared with standard video colonoscopy: a prospective randomized controlled trial. Endoscopy 2010;42(10):827–33.

37. Hoffman A, Kagel C, Goetz M, et al. Recognition and characterization of small colonic neoplasia with high-definition colonoscopy using i-Scan is as precise as chromoendoscopy. Dig Liver Dis 2010;42(1):45–50.

38. Goetz M. Colonoscopic surveillance in inflammatory bowel disease: state of the art reduction of biopsies. Dig Dis 2011;29(Suppl 1):36–40.

39. Fusco V, Ebert B, Weber-Eibel J, et al. Cancer prevention in ulcerative colitis: long-term outcome following fluorescence-guided colonoscopy. Inflamm Bowel Dis 2012;18(3):489–95.

40. Messmann H, Endlicher E, Freunek G, et al. Fluorescence endoscopy for the detection of low and high grade dysplasia in ulcerative colitis using systemic or local 5-aminolaevulinic acid sensitisation. Gut 2003;52(7):1003–7.

41. van den Broek FJ, Fockens P, van Eeden S, et al. Endoscopic tri-modal imaging for surveillance in ulcerative colitis: randomised comparison of high-resolution endoscopy and autofluorescence imaging for neoplasia detection; and evaluation of narrow-band imaging for classification of lesions. Gut 2008;57(8):1083–9.

42. Günther U, Kusch D, Heller F, et al. Surveillance colonoscopy in patients with inflammatory bowel disease: comparison of random biopsy vs. targeted biopsy protocols. Int J Colorectal Dis 2011;26(5):667–72.

43. Kornbluth A, Sachar DB. Ulcerative colitis practice guidelines in adults: American College of Gastroenterology, Practice Parameters Committee. Am J Gastroenterol 2010;105(3):501–23.

44. Farraye FA, Odze RD, Eaden J, et al. AGA technical review on the diagnosis and management of colorectal neoplasia in inflammatory bowel disease. Gastroenterology 2010;138(2):746–74.

45. Cairns SR, Scholefield JH, Steele RJ, et al. Guidelines for colorectal cancer screening and surveillance in moderate and high risk groups (update from 2002). Gut 2010;59(5):666–89.

Endomicroscopy and Endocytoscopy in IBD

Helmut Neumann, MD, PhD[a],*, Ralf Kiesslich, MD, PhD[b]

KEYWORDS

- Endomicroscopy • Endocytoscopy • IBD • Ulcerative colitis • Crohn's disease
- Molecular imaging

KEY POINTS

- Two types of endomicroscopy systems exist. One is integrated into a standard, high-resolution endoscope (integrated confocal laser endomicroscopy [iCLE]) and one is probe-based, capable of passage through the working channel of a standard endoscope (probe-based CLE [pCLE]).
- Endocytoscopy allows visualization of the superficial mucosal layer. Endoscope-integrated and probe-based devices are available, allowing magnification of the mucosa up to 1400-fold.
- Endomicroscopy can differentiate histologic changes of Crohn's disease (CD) and ulcerative colitis (UC) in vivo in real time and allows for a targeted and tactical biopsy approach.
- Endocytoscopy can discriminate mucosal inflammatory cells during endoscopy and allows determination of histopathologic activity of UC.
- Molecular imaging with fluorescence-labeled probes against disease-specific receptors will enable individualized management of patients with inflammatory bowel disease (IBD).

INTRODUCTION

The incidence of inflammatory bowel diseases (IBDs) with its main entities, CD and UC, is rising. Population-based studies suggest that the overall IBD incidence is 29.6 per 100,000, affecting approximately 1.4 million Americans.[1–3] Patients with IBD suffer from abdominal pain, diarrhea, and often a depressive mood. Moreover, evidence suggests that patients with both UC and CD are at an increased risk for the development of colorectal cancer (CRC). The overall prevalence of CRC in UC patients was recently analyzed in a large meta-analysis and estimated to be 3.7%.[4] CRC is the cause of death in approximately 15% of IBD patients.[5] In this context, it has been shown that patients with course of disease longer than 10 years, pancolitis,

[a] Interdisciplinary Endoscopy, Department of Medicine I, University of Erlangen-Nuremberg, Ulmenweg 18, Erlangen 91054, Germany; [b] Medical Clinic, St. Marienkrankenhaus, Katharina-Kasper gGmbH, Richard-Wagner-Strasse 14, 60318 Frankfurt am Main, Frankfurt, Germany
* Corresponding author.
E-mail address: helmut.neumann@uk-erlangen.de

Gastrointest Endoscopy Clin N Am 23 (2013) 695–705
http://dx.doi.org/10.1016/j.giec.2013.03.006
1052-5157/13/$ – see front matter © 2013 Elsevier Inc. All rights reserved.

left-sided UC, or more proximal disease are at an increased risk.[6] In addition, high rates of multifocal dysplasia and metachronous neoplasia aggravate endoscopic surveillance strategies in these patients. In an attempt to increase diagnostic outcomes of IBD patients, various endoscopic approaches have been introduced.[7] These include red flag technologies, such as magnification endoscopy; dye-based chromoendoscopy techniques (ie, methylene blue and toluidine blue); and dye-less chromoendoscopy techniques, like narrow band imaging (NBI, Olympus, Tokyo, Japan), Fuji Intelligent Color Enhancement (FICE) (Fujifilm, Tokyo, Japan), and i-scan (Pentax Medical, Tokyo, Japan). In addition, several high-resolution endoscopic imaging techniques have been developed, enabling endoscopists to obtain a virtual histology during ongoing endoscopy. These so-called optical biopsy techniques include confocal laser endomicroscopy (CLE; **Figs. 1–3**) and endocytoscopy (**Fig. 4**).

This review focuses on CLE and endocytoscopy for the management of patients with IBD.

TECHNICAL ASPECTS OF CLE

CLE is based on tissue illumination with a low-power laser after application of fluorescence agents, which can either be applied topically (ie, cresyl violet or acriflavine hydrochloride) or systemically (fluorescein sodium). Fluorescein sodium in a dilution of 10% is the most commonly used fluorescence agent. After intravenous injection, fluorescein highlights the extracellular matrix. Adverse events are rare. One recent multicenter study reported transient hypotension without shock (0.5% of patients), nausea (0.39%), injection site erythema (0.35%), self-limited diffuse rash (0.04%), and mild epigastric pain (0.09%).[8] To visualize the cell nucleus fluorescein sodium can be combined with topical application of acriflavine hydrochloride. This dye agent allows for a detailed analysis of the nucleus-to-cytoplasm ratio for diagnosis and grading of intraepithelial neoplasia. Because acriflavine accumulates in nuclei, concerns have been raised regarding a potential mutagenic risk of the drug. Alternatively, cresyl violet can be applied. By cytoplasmic enrichment of cresyl violet, nuclear morphology could be negatively visualized.[9]

Two CE-approved and Food and Drug Administration–approved endomicroscopy devices are available for the daily use in clinical practice. One is integrated into the

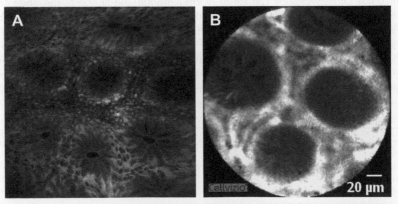

Fig. 1. (A) CLE of noninflamed mucosa using the iCLE. Colonic crypts, surrounded by dark-appearing goblet cells, became evident. (B) Noninflamed mucosa in IBD visualized with the handheld endomicroscopy system (pCLE). Confocal imaging displays colonic crypts and microvessels within the lamina propria.

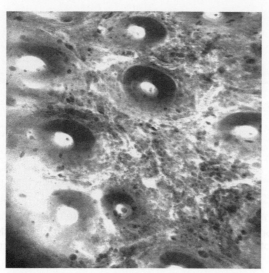

Fig. 2. Confocal imaging using iCLE of inflamed mucosa in IBD. Colonic crypts are variously shaped and irregular. Fluorescein sodium leaked into the lamina propria, thereby highlighting the damage of minute mucosal microvessels.

distal tip of a standard high-resolution video gastroscope or colonoscope (iCLE, Pentax Medical, Tokyo, Japan) and one is probe-based, capable of passage through the working channel of a standard endoscope (pCLE, Cellvizio, Mauna Kea Technologies, Paris, France).[10]

Both systems use an incident 488-nm wavelength laser system. iCLE collects images at a manually adjustable scan rate of 1.6 frames per second with a maximum resolution of 1024 × 1024 pixels (1 megapixel). By pushing a button on the handle of the

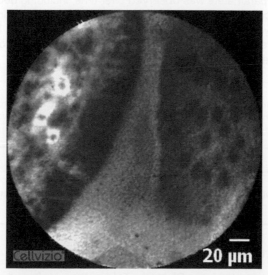

Fig. 3. Using pCLE, mucosal gaps appearing as white incisions of the mucosal surface can be visualized. These gaps are predictive of an acute flare of the disease within the next 12 months.

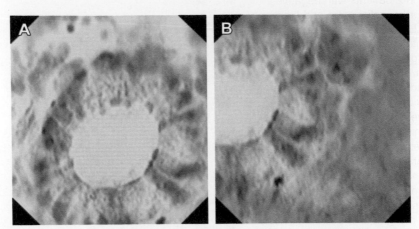

Fig. 4. Endocytoscopy allows assessment of cytologic features, such as the density of cells, the size and shape of nuclei, and the nucleus-to-cytoplasm ratio (*A*). The colonic architecture is clearly visible (*B*).

endoscope, the scanning depth (ranging from 0 μm to 250 μm) and the laser power (ranging from 0 μW to 1000 μW) can be dynamically adjusted. For pCLE, different probes for various indications are available. pCLE devices use a fixed laser power and a fixed imaging plane depth. Confocal images are streamed at a frame rate of 12 frames per second, thereby obtaining real-time videos of the intestinal mucosa. A special computer algorithm (mosaicing) allows reconstruction of single video frames either in real time or postprocessed with an increased field of view of up to 4 mm × 2 mm. **Table 1** provides an overview of main technical aspects of both CLE devices.

One recent study prospectively assessed the learning curve of CLE in patients with IBD.[11] Overall, 26 consecutive patients were included. A significant improvement of CLE performance parameters was observed over time, including decreased confocal imaging time, successful CLE diagnosis, and decline in procedural time. Performance parameters improved significantly after the initial 3 cases. Therefore, it was concluded that CLE may represent an easy-to-learn novel diagnostic method for in vivo analysis of mucosal changes in IBD.

Two different endomicroscopy systems exist. One is integrated into a standard, high-resolution endoscope (iCLE) and one is probe-based, capable of passage through the working channel of a standard endoscope (pCLE).

Both endomicroscopy systems use an incident 488-nm wavelength laser. Nevertheless, resolution, image size and image acquisition are different between both devices.

TECHNICAL ASPECTS OF ENDOCYTOSCOPY

Endocytoscopy (Endocytoscopy, Olympus, Tokyo, Japan) is based on the principle of contact light microscopy permitting visualization of the superficial mucosal layer.[12] Images are displayed on a monitor at 30 frames per second. The endocytoscope is either

Table 1 Technical aspects of iCLE and pCLE		
	iCLE	**pCLE**
Outer diameter (mm)	12.8	1.0; 2.7; 2.6[a]
Length (cm)	120; 180	400; 300[a]
Field of view (μm)	475 × 475	320; 240; 600 μm[2a]
Resolution	0.7	3.5; 1.0[a]
Magnification	×1000	×1000
Imaging plane depth (μm)	0–250 (dynamic)	40–70; 55–65; 70–130 (fixed)[a]

[a] Dependent on various probes. For detailed information, see Neumann and colleageus.[10]

integrated into a handheld device, which can be advanced through the working channel of an endoscope (called pEC), or integrated into a high-resolution endoscope (called iEC). Technical aspects of the system are shown in **Table 2**. Endocytoscopy requires mucolysis with N-acetylcysteine and prestaining of the mucosa with absorptive staining agents, like methylene blue, toluidine blue, or cresyl violet. Usually, the dyes are sprayed onto the mucosa using standard spraying catheters. After an appropriate time of exposure (approximately 60 seconds) to the dye, repeat washing of the mucosa is strictly necessary to remove excess contrast dye before endocytoscopic imaging. Repeat staining is mostly necessary while using absorptive contrast agents. **Table 2** provides an overview of the different endocytoscopy systems. A clear distal cap and mild suction should be used to stabilize the endoscope while obtaining high-magnification imaging of the mucosa. Interpretation of endocytoscopic images is based on architectural details (eg, epithelial structure), cellular features (eg, size and arrangement of cells), and vascular pattern morphology (eg, size and tortuosity). Additionally, endocytoscopy allows the assessment of cytologic features, such as the density of cells, the size and shape of nuclei, and the nucleus-to-cytoplasm ratio. Up to now, endocytoscopy has not been commercially available in Europe or the United States and has mostly been evaluated by Japanese endoscopists for colorectal polyps and early cancer.[13]

Endocytoscopy only allows visualization of the superficial mucosal layer. Endoscope-integrated and probe-based devices are available, allowing magnification of the mucosa up to 1400-fold.

CONFOCAL LASER ENDOMICROSCOPY IN PATIENTS WITH IBD

To date, various studies have proved the benefit of CLE in patients with IBD. Because evidence has shown that patients with IBD are at an increased risk for the development of colitis-associated cancer, guidelines recommend acquiring a large number of biopsy specimens during surveillance colonoscopy.[14] Nevertheless, this buckshot technique is often time consuming and imprecise, so nonpolypoid lesions can be missed.[15] In a large randomized controlled trial, Kiesslich and colleagues[16] evaluated whether chromoendoscopy (methylene blue 0.1%) in combination with CLE was more effective in comparison with the standard surveillance approach of conventional white-light endoscopy. By using chromoendoscopy with endomicroscopy, 4.75-fold more neoplasias could be detected. Moreover, by using targeted and tactical CLE-directed biopsies, 50% fewer biopsy specimens were required. CLE was, therefore,

Table 2
Technical characteristics of endocytoscopy

Type	Probe Based		Endoscope Based		
	XEC-300	**XEC-120**	**XGIF-Q260EC1**	**XCF-Q260EC1**	**GIF-Y0002**
Total length (cm)	380		103	133	103
Functional length (cm)	240		103	133	103
Endoscope working channel (mm)	Requires minimum 3.2-mm working channel		2.8	3.2	2.8
Endoscope magnification	N/A		×85	×110	×380 (×600 digital)
EC magnification	Up to 570-fold	Up to 1390-fold	×580		×380
Field of view (μm)	300 × 300	120 × 120	400 × 400		700 × 600
Horizontal resolution	4.2	1.7	4.0		3.7

Abbreviation: EC, endocytoscopy.

capable of increasing the diagnostic yield of surveillance endoscopy and could also significantly reduce the need for tissue biopsy. These results were confirmed by other groups using either iCLE or pCLE.[17–19] Günther and colleagues[20] included 150 surveillance colonoscopies and compared 3 different endoscopic surveillance strategies for the detection of intraepithelial neoplasia. These included (1) random quadrant biopsies, (2) chromoendoscopy with indigo carmine and subsequent quadrant biopsies, and (3) CLE with random quadrant biopsies and targeted biopsies. In this study, targeted biopsy approaches led to significantly higher detection rates of intraepithelial neoplasia. Accordingly, the investigators concluded that random biopsy protocols should be replaced by targeted biopsy protocols.

Once a lesion in IBD is found, its further differentiation is important for subsequent therapeutic decision making. Although adenoma-like mass lesions are treated endoscopically, dysplasia-associated lesions or masses, which frequently have associated high-grade intraepithelial neoplasia and are associated with CRC in up to 60% of IBD patients, should be managed by aggressive surgical resection.[21–23] In this context, both endomicroscopy systems were proved reliable for the in vivo differentiation of adenoma-like mass and dysplasia-associated lesion or mass lesions, with an overall accuracy of 97%, thus providing the ability to guide therapy in real time.[24,25]

Because pouchitis and dysplasia may affect the reservoir after restorative proctocolectomy, Trovato and coworkers[26] evaluated the efficacy of CLE for in vivo diagnosis of mucosal changes in ileal pouch for UC and familial adenomatous polyposis. Pathologic features were observed in up to 89% of patients and included villous atrophy, inflammation, ulceration, and colonic metaplasia. Dysplasia was not observed. Confocal imaging correlated well with histopathologic analysis and suggests that endomicroscopy may be helpful in the evaluation of morphologic changes in the ileal pouch.

Differentiation between UC and CD is of paramount importance because both disease entities involve different therapeutic management strategies. Because CLE allows on-demand in vivo differentiation of architectural and cellular details during endoscopy, various studies have analyzed if CLE may provide similar features in comparison with histopathology, which was set as the gold standard. In an early study, Watanabe and colleagues[27] examined patients with UC and investigated the features of confocal imaging of inflamed and noninflamed rectal mucosa; 12 patients in the active phase, 5 in the nonactive phase, and 14 control patients were included. CLE was feasible for providing information equivalent to conventional endoscopy. These data were confirmed by a larger study by Li and colleagues,[28] including 73 consecutive patients with UC. Endomicroscopic assessment of crypt architecture and fluorescein leakage showed good correlation with histologic results. More than half of the patients with normal mucosa seen on conventional white-light endoscopy showed acute inflammation on histology, whereas no patients with normal mucosa or with chronic inflammation seen on CLE showed acute inflammation on histology. Therefore, CLE seemed a reliable tool for real-time assessment of inflammatory activity in UC.

Neumann and colleagues[29] evaluated whether CLE is feasible for in vivo diagnosis of CD; 55 consecutive patients with CD and 18 control patients were enrolled, and the colonic mucosa was examined by white-light endoscopy followed by CLE. A significantly higher proportion of patients with active CD had increased colonic crypt tortuosity, enlarged crypt lumen, microerosions, augmented vascularization, and increased cellular infiltrates within the lamina propria. In quiescent CD, a significant increase in crypt and goblet cell number was detected compared with controls. Based on these findings, the Crohn's Disease Endomicroscopic Activity Score was proposed, allowing the assessment of CD activity in vivo.

The interaction of bacteria with the immune system is a key mechanism in the pathogenesis of IBD. In this context, cell shedding has been proposed as a potential mechanism, allowing intraluminal bacteria to penetrate into the intestinal mucosa.[30] In 2007, Kiesslich and colleagues[31] determined if CLE could resolve the presence of human epithelial gaps and whether a proinflammatory cytokine could increase cell shedding. Intestinal mucosa was imaged with CLE after staining with acriflavine, and results were validated by parallel studies of anesthetized mice. CLE could distinguish between epithelial discontinuities (gaps) and goblet cells in human intestine. This preliminary result suggested that the sealing of epithelial gaps had to be considered as a component of the intestinal barrier and has potential implications for intestinal barrier dysfunction in IBD. The data were confirmed by Liu and coworkers,[32,33] who, in addition, found that epithelial gap density was significantly higher in patients with CD than in controls.

Another study aimed at assessing the prognostic value of epithelial gap densities for hospitalization or surgery in the follow-up of patients with IBD[34]: 21 CD patients and 20 UC patients with a median follow-up of 14 months were studied. An increased gap density was accompanied with a significantly higher risk for hospitalization or surgery. Specifically, gap density was found a significant predictor for risk of major events associated with each increase of 1% in gap density. Therefore, increased epithelial gaps in the small intestine may be predictive for future hospitalization or surgery in IBD patients. One recent pilot study also demonstrated that epithelial cell shedding and barrier loss detected by CLE could predict relapse rates of IBD and has, therefore, the potential to be used as a diagnostic tool for the management of IBD. The sensitivity, specificity, and accuracy of the new grading system to predict a flare in IBD were 63%, 91%, and 79%, respectively.[35]

Recently, the potential of CLE was studied to visualize intramucosal enteric bacteria in vivo in patients with IBD.[36] Initial experiments were performed in mouse models and afterward translated into the human intestine in vivo. For the identification of intramucosal bacteria, CLE had a sensitivity and specificity of 89% and 100%, respectively. Moreover, patients with IBD showed significantly more intramucosal bacteria in comparison with control patients. These data disclosed the emerging potential of CLE as a new diagnostic tool to image living bacteria in vivo.

Because most drugs used for the treatment of IBD are systemically bioavailable, thereby covering the potential of severe side effects, a targeted, individualized approach to inflamed areas of the intestine with specific drugs is highly desirable. One recent work evaluated for the first time the potential of nanoparticle and microparticle uptake into the rectal mucosa of human IBD patients.[37] Two hours after rectal application of fluorescent-labeled placebo nanoparticles and microparticles to 33 patients with IBD and healthy controls, confocal imaging was performed to visualize the particles in inflamed mucosal areas. The investigators observed a significantly enhanced accumulation of microparticles in ulcerous lesions, whereas nanoparticles were only visible in traces on mucosal surfaces of all patients. It was concluded that nanoparticles may not be required for local drug delivery to intestinal lesions in humans, thereby minimizing the risk of unintended translocation into the blood system. These results are fascinating and imply an outlook on individualized therapy for patients with IBD.

Endomicroscopy can differentiate histologic changes of CD and UC in vivo in real time and allows for a targeted and tactical biopsy approach.

ENDOCYTOSCOPY IN PATIENTS WITH IBD

Few data are available on the use of endocytoscopy in patients with IBD. Bessho and coworkers[38] evaluated the correlation between endocytoscopy and conventional histopathology for real-time diagnosis of microstructural features in UC. The investigators proposed an endocytoscopy score to determine histopathologic activity of UC; 55 patients with UC were included and evaluated using an endocytoscope with 450-fold magnification. Matts endoscopic and histopathologic grade was determined in every case to evaluate disease severity. The endocytoscopy score, consisting of shape and distance between crypts, and the visibility of superficial microvessels showed a strong correlation with Matts histopathologic grades. In addition, the endocytoscopic score showed high reproducibility with substantial kappa values. A recent study aimed at determining the reliability of endocytoscopy for the discrimination of mucosal inflammatory cells and intestinal inflammatory disease activity in patients with IBD.[39] Overall, 40 IBD patients were included. For vital staining, either methylene blue or toluidine blue was used. Endocytoscopy was reliable to distinguish single inflammatory cells, including neutrophilic, basophilic, and eosinophilic granulocytes and lymphocytes. Sensitivity and specificity ranges among different cell types were between 60% and 89% and 90% and 95%, respectively. Interobserver agreement was substantial whereas intraobserver agreement was almost perfect. Moreover, concordance between endocytoscopy and histopathology for grading of intestinal disease activity was 100%. Taken together, endocytoscopy might have the potential to assess histologic activity in vivo during ongoing endoscopy. Nevertheless, further research in this field is recommended.

Endocytoscopy can discriminate mucosal inflammatory cells during endoscopy and allows determination of histopathologic activity of UC.

SUMMARY

Optical biopsy techniques, including CLE and endocytoscopy, have revolutionized our understanding of how to diagnose and manage patients with IBD. Using these advanced endoscopic imaging techniques, endoscopists are now able to diagnose CD-associated and UC-associated histologic changes in vivo in real time and to predict relapse rates in IBD. In addition, advanced endoscopic imaging allows detecting more preneoplastic and neoplastic changes in comparison with standard endoscopic imaging techniques, thereby improving patient outcome. For the near future, it is expected that molecular imaging with fluorescence-labeled probes against disease-specific receptors will enable individualized management of patients with IBD.

REFERENCES

1. Wilson J, Hair C, Knight R, et al. High incidence of inflammatory bowel disease in Australia: a prospective population-based Australian incidence study. Inflamm Bowel Dis 2010;16:1550–6.
2. Neurath MF, Travis SP. Mucosal healing in inflammatory bowel diseases: a systematic review. Gut 2012;61:1619–35.
3. Abraham C, Cho JH. Inflammatory bowel disease. N Engl J Med 2009;361: 2066–78.
4. Eaden JA, Abrams KR, Mayberry JF. The risk of colorectal cancer in ulcerative colitis: a meta-analysis. Gut 2001;48:526–35.
5. Svrcek M, Cosnes J, Beaugerie L, et al. Colorectal neoplasia in Crohn's colitis: a retrospective comparative study with ulcerative colitis. Histopathology 2007;50: 574–83.
6. Ullman T, Odze R, Farraye FA. Diagnosis and management of dysplasia in patients with ulcerative colitis and Crohn's disease of the colon. Inflamm Bowel Dis 2009;15:630–8.
7. Neumann H, Neurath MF, Mudter J. New endoscopic approaches in IBD. World J Gastroenterol 2011;17:63–8.
8. Wallace MB, Meining A, Canto MI, et al. The safety of intravenous fluorescein for confocal laser endomicroscopy in the gastrointestinal tract. Aliment Pharmacol Ther 2010;31:548–52.
9. Goetz M, Toermer T, Vieth M, et al. Simultaneous confocal laser endomicroscopy and chromoendoscopy with topical cresyl violet. Gastrointest Endosc 2009;70: 959–68.
10. Neumann H, Kiesslich R, Wallace MB, et al. Confocal laser endomicroscopy: technical advances and clinical applications. Gastroenterology 2010;139: 388–92.
11. Neumann H, Vieth M, Atreya R, et al. Prospective evaluation of the learning curve of confocal laser endomicroscopy in patients with IBD. Histol Histopathol 2011; 26:867–72.
12. Neumann H, Fuchs FS, Vieth M, et al. Review article: in vivo imaging by endocytoscopy. Aliment Pharmacol Ther 2011;33:1183–93.
13. Kudo SE, Wakamura K, Ikehara N, et al. Diagnosis of colorectal lesions with a novel endocytoscopic classification—a pilot study. Endoscopy 2011;43: 869–75.
14. Farraye FA, Odze RD, Eaden J, et al. AGA medical position statement on the diagnosis and management of colorectal neoplasia in inflammatory bowel disease. Gastroenterology 2010;138:738–45.
15. Connell WR, Lennard-Jones JE, Williams CB, et al. Factors affecting the outcome of endoscopic surveillance for cancer in ulcerative colitis. Gastroenterology 1994; 107:934–44.

16. Kiesslich R, Goetz M, Lammersdorf K, et al. Chromoscopy-guided endomicro-scopy increases the diagnostic yield of intraepithelial neoplasia in ulcerative co-litis. Gastroenterology 2007;132:874–82.
17. van den Broek FJ, van Es JA, van Eeden S, et al. Pilot study of probe-based confocal laser endomicroscopy during colonoscopic surveillance of patients with longstanding ulcerative colitis. Endoscopy 2011;43:116–22.
18. Hlavaty T, Huorka M, Koller T, et al. Colorectal cancer screening in patients with ulcerative and Crohn's colitis with use of colonoscopy, chromoendoscopy and confocal endomicroscopy. Eur J Gastroenterol Hepatol 2011;23:680–9.
19. Rispo A, Castiglione F, Staibano S, et al. Diagnostic accuracy of confocal laser endomicroscopy in diagnosing dysplasia in patients affected by long-standing ulcerative colitis. World J Gastrointest Endosc 2012;4:414–20.
20. Günther U, Kusch D, Heller F, et al. Surveillance colonoscopy in patients with in-flammatory bowel disease: comparison of random biopsy vs. targeted biopsy protocols. Int J Colorectal Dis 2011;26:667–72.
21. Neumann H, Vieth M, Langner C, et al. Cancer risk in IBD: how to diagnose and how to manage DALM and ALM. World J Gastroenterol 2011;17:3184–91.
22. Blackstone MO, Riddell RH, Rogers BH, et al. Dysplasia-associated lesion or mass (DALM) detected by colonoscopy in long-standing ulcerative colitis: an indication for colectomy. Gastroenterology 1981;80:366–74.
23. von Roon AC, Reese G, Teare J, et al. The risk of cancer in patients with Crohn's disease. Dis Colon Rectum 2007;50:839–55.
24. Hurlstone DP, Thomson M, Brown S, et al. Confocal endomicroscopy in ulcerative colitis: differentiating dysplasia-associated lesional mass and adenoma-like mass. Clin Gastroenterol Hepatol 2007;5:1235–41.
25. De Palma GD, Staibano S, Siciliano S, et al. In-vivo characterization of DALM in ulcerative colitis with high-resolution probe-based confocal laser endomicro-scopy. World J Gastroenterol 2011;7(17):677–80.
26. Trovato C, Sonzogni A, Fiori G, et al. Confocal laser endomicroscopy for the detection of mucosal changes in ileal pouch after restorative proctocolectomy. Dig Liver Dis 2009;41:578–85.
27. Watanabe O, Ando T, Maeda O, et al. Confocal endomicroscopy in patients with ulcerative colitis. J Gastroenterol Hepatol 2008;23:286–90.
28. Li CQ, Xie XJ, Yu T, et al. Classification of inflammation activity in ulcerative colitis by confocal laser endomicroscopy. Am J Gastroenterol 2010;105:1391–6.
29. Neumann H, Vieth M, Atreya R, et al. Assessment of Crohn's disease activity by confocal laser endomicroscopy. Inflamm Bowel Dis 2012;18:2261–9.
30. Günther C, Martini E, Wittkopf N, et al. Caspase-8 regulates TNF-α-induced epithelial necroptosis and terminal ileitis. Nature 2011;477:335–9.
31. Kiesslich R, Goetz M, Angus EM, et al. Identification of epithelial gaps in human small and large intestine by confocal endomicroscopy. Gastroenterology 2007; 133:1769–78.
32. Liu JJ, Madsen KL, Boulanger P, et al. Mind the gaps: confocal endomicroscopy showed increased density of small bowel epithelial gaps in inflammatory bowel disease. J Clin Gastroenterol 2011;45:240–5.
33. Liu JJ, Wong K, Thiesen AL, et al. Increased epithelial gaps in the small intestines of patients with inflammatory bowel disease: density matters. Gastrointest En-dosc 2011;73:1174–80.
34. Turcotte JF, Wong K, Mah SJ, et al. Increased epithelial gaps in the small intestine are predictive of hospitalization and surgery in patients with inflammatory bowel disease. Clin Transl Gastroenterol 2012;3:e19.

35. Kiesslich R, Duckworth CA, Moussata D, et al. Local barrier dysfunction identified by confocal laser endomicroscopy predicts relapse in inflammatory bowel disease. Gut 2012;61:1146–53.
36. Moussata D, Goetz M, Gloeckner A, et al. Confocal laser endomicroscopy is a new imaging modality for recognition of intramucosal bacteria in inflammatory bowel disease in vivo. Gut 2011;60:26–33.
37. Schmidt C, Lautenschlaeger C, Collnot EM, et al. Nano- and microscaled particles for drug targeting to inflamed intestinal mucosa-A first in vivo study in human patients. J Control Release 2013;165:139–45.
38. Bessho R, Kanai T, Hosoe N, et al. Correlation between endocytoscopy and conventional histopathology in microstructural features of ulcerative colitis. J Gastroenterol 2011;46:1197–202.
39. Neumann H, Vieth M, Neurath MF, et al. Endocytoscopy allows accurate in vivo differentiation of mucosal inflammatory cells in IBD: a pilot study. Inflamm Bowel Dis 2012. http://dx.doi.org/10.1002/ibd.23025.

Optical Molecular Imaging in the Gastrointestinal Tract

Jennifer Carns, PhD[a], Pelham Keahey, BS[a], Timothy Quang, BS[a],
Sharmila Anandasabapathy, MD[b],
Rebecca Richards-Kortum, PhD[a],*

KEYWORDS

- Optical molecular imaging • White light endoscopy • Narrow band imaging
- Autofluorescence imaging • Chromoendoscopy • Confocal laser endomicroscopy
- High-resolution microendoscopy • Optical coherence tomography

KEY POINTS

- Widefield and high resolution imaging modalities used in preclinical and clinical evaluation for the detection of colorectal cancer and esophageal cancer are reviewed.
- Recent clinical studies have evaluated the sensitivity and specificity of widefield imaging techniques. The effectiveness of narrow band imaging has varied between studies, while the increased sensitivity demonstrated by autofluorescence imaging has often been accompanied by high false positive rates. With the aid of a contrast agent, chromoendoscopy has proven to be more effective than white light imaging in identifying neoplastic changes.
- High resolution techniques including probe based confocal laser endomicroscopy, high resolution microendoscopy, and optical coherence tomography provide images of cellular architecture for smaller fields of view and have proven useful for targeting biopsies and for the real time assessment of margins following endoscopic mucosal resection.
- In many cases, widefield techniques and high resolution imaging can combine molecular and morphologic imaging to yield increased sensitivity and specificity.
- Preclinical approaches to enhance image contrast using vital dyes and molecular specific targeted contrast agents are being developed for both widefield and high resolution techniques.

 Video of high-resolution microendoscopy for the early detection of esophageal neoplasia accompanies this article at http://www.giendo.theclinics.com/

INTRODUCTION

Gastrointestinal (GI) neoplasia is a leading contributor to global cancer mortality and morbidity.[1] Early detection of cancers of the GI tract significantly improves patient

[a] Department of Bioengineering, Rice University, 6100 Main Street, MS 142, Houston, TX 77005, USA; [b] Department of Gastroenterology, Mount Sinai Medical Center, One Gustave L. Levy Place, Box 1069, New York, NY 10029-6574, USA
* Corresponding author.
E-mail address: rkortum@rice.edu

Gastrointest Endoscopy Clin N Am 23 (2013) 707–723
http://dx.doi.org/10.1016/j.giec.2013.03.010
1052-5157/13/$ – see front matter © 2013 Elsevier Inc. All rights reserved.

outcomes; however, current clinical practice often fails to detect these cancers until they are at an advanced stage, when treatment is more invasive, more expensive, and less successful.[1–3] This review highlights the potential of new optical molecular imaging techniques to improve early detection of GI cancers, with a focus on 2 important sites: colorectal cancer and esophageal cancer.

Colorectal cancer is a leading cause of cancer-related deaths worldwide.[1] In the United States, it is the third most common cancer amongst men and women and accounts for 9% of all cancer deaths. The 5-year survival rate increases from 64% to 90% when detection occurs during the early stages of development.[4] Because the prognosis of late-stage colorectal cancer is so poor, it is important to accurately screen patients. Colorectal cancer can be prevented by the removal of colorectal polyps before they progress to cancer. Although colonoscopy is highly sensitive and has the potential to prevent approximately 65% of colorectal cancers from developing, some polyps can still be missed, prompting the need for increasingly sensitive imaging techniques.[5,6]

The incidence of esophageal adenocarcinoma (EAC) is rapidly increasing worldwide. Approximately 24,000 cases of EAC are diagnosed each year in the United States. The 5-year survival rate for late-stage EAC is only 2.8%, whereas for local-staged tumors it is 49.3%.[4] However, with earlier diagnosis, the 5-year survival rate for stage 0 EAC exceeds 95%.[7] Barrett's esophagus (BE) is a benign treatable condition of the esophagus that arises because of acid reflux. Individuals with BE are at higher risk of developing precancerous lesions, which can progress to EAC. Because of this increased risk, it is recommended that individuals with BE undergo routine endoscopic examination at regular intervals to facilitate detection and treatment of precancers and early cancers. However, using standard, white light endoscopy (WLE), it can be difficult to identify early neoplastic lesions. Thus, routine endoscopic surveillance of BE also includes random 4-quadrant biopsies taken every 1 to 2 cm along the Barrett's segment.[3,4] Studies have shown that random 4-quadrant biopsies can have miss rates up to 48%.[8,9] Furthermore, random 4-quadrant biopsies taken every 2 cm can miss up to half of the cancers found when a protocol of 1 cm is used.[10]

Thus, there is an important need for new approaches that can improve the ability to identify early neoplastic lesions in the GI tract. This need has prompted the development of new optical imaging modalities to improve recognition and enable in vivo characterization of suspicious lesions in the GI tract. These approaches leverage both endogenous optical contrast as well as the use of contrast agents targeted against biomarkers that are associated with early neoplasia. This review summarizes recent advances in optical molecular imaging techniques to recognize early neoplastic disease in the GI tract. New approaches that are in clinical evaluation are first discussed; these approaches are based primarily on endogenous optical contrast or the use of vital dyes to enhance image contrast. Approaches in development and preclinical evaluation are then described, including the development of molecular-specific targeted contrast agents.

CLINICAL STUDIES

Several complementary widefield and high-resolution imaging techniques are being evaluated to assist in the endoscopic detection and characterization of early neoplasia in the GI tract. Widefield imaging modalities are designed to survey large areas of tissue, whereas high-resolution imaging is limited to smaller fields of view but can achieve subcellular resolution. A variety of studies have been conducted to evaluate the performance of widefield imaging and high-resolution imaging techniques in the clinical setting. An overview of these emerging technologies and the results of several recent clinical studies are provided in this section.

Widefield Imaging

With the development of high-definition WLE (HD-WLE), the spatial resolution of standard WLE has been drastically improved.[11] Narrow band imaging (NBI) is a complementary widefield technique that can assist in tissue characterization by enhancing the visibility of vasculature in the tissue via illumination with narrow bands of blue and green light, selected to match spectral regions with increased hemoglobin absorbance.[12] Neoplastic changes are often accompanied by an increase in microvasculature density. Hemoglobin is known to absorb wavelengths between 400 and 550 nm. The visualization of microvasculature can therefore be enhanced by using optical filters to pass only 2 bands of illumination. Generally, green (530–550 nm) and blue (390–445 nm) wavelengths are used. The absorption of blue and green light by hemoglobin causes the vasculature to appear darker than surrounding tissue without the need of a contrast agent.

Several clinical studies have been conducted to assess the effectiveness of NBI for detecting early neoplasia, but they have produced varying results. Some recent studies performed with the Olympus GIFQ240 (Olympus, Center Valley, PA) have shown advantages of NBI compared with HD-WLE.[13,14] In a single-center study involving 75 cites on 21 patients with BE, Singh and colleagues[13] compared diagnoses made with NBI and HD-WLE with histology results and found that the NBI diagnosis agreed with the histology results more often than HD-WLE (88.9% vs 71.9%). Muto and colleagues[14] conducted a multicenter randomized trial comparing the detection rates of NBI and HD-WLE for early superficial esophageal squamous cell carcinoma (ESCC), a condition unrelated to BE. Of the 121 patients with histologically confirmed superficial ESCC, 63 patients with a total of 107 lesions were evaluated primarily with NBI followed by a secondary evaluation with HD-WLE, and the remaining 58 patients with a total of 105 lesions were evaluated primarily with HD-WLE followed by NBI. In the first group, NBI alone detected 104 of the 107 lesions, whereas in the second group, HD-WLE alone detected only 58 of the 105 lesions, yielding sensitivities of 97% and 55%, respectively. However, when the results of the secondary evaluations were considered, HD-WLE did not find any additional lesions in the first group, but the addition of NBI with HD-WLE in the second group increased the sensitivity to 95%.

However, other recent studies performed with the Olympus H180 have indicated that the performance of NBI and HD-WLE are similar.[15,16] Sharma and colleagues[16] investigated the detection rate of intestinal metaplasia (IM) and neoplasia, the detection rate of neoplasia specifically, and the number of overall biopsies performed in 123 patients with BE for evaluations with NBI and HD-WLE. Half of the patients were randomly selected to receive HD-WLE examination, in which biopsies of visible lesions were taken followed by random 4-quadrant biopsies for every 2 cm of the BE segment. The remaining patients received NBI examination, in which biopsies were first taken of visible lesions, followed by targeted biopsies of areas detected by NBI. All patients returned within 3 to 8 weeks to receive the alternative procedure from a different endoscopist. Both modalities identified 104 of 113 patients with IM, showing a detection rate of 92%. Patients who were missed by the first procedure were found to have IM in the subsequent procedure. NBI resulted in a total of 267 biopsies, whereas the standard 2-cm protocol resulted in 321 biopsies with HD-WLE. Histology was used to classify each biopsy as no IM, IM, low-grade dysplasia, high-grade dysplasia (HGD), or EAC. NBI did detect significantly more areas for any form of neoplasia, but when the analysis was limited to areas with HGD or EAC, there was no statistical difference between the 2 modalities. However, NBI did require fewer biopsies per patient (3.6 vs 7.6, respectively). Pasha and colleagues[17] analyzed a series of randomized controlled trials to determine the detection rate and miss rate for colon polyps and adenomas by NBI and HD-WLE. They evaluated 6 studies for the detection of adenomas and the detection of patients with polyps, 4 studies for the detection of patients with adenomas, and 5 studies for the detection of adenomas less than 10 mm, flat adenomas, and the number of flat adenomas per patient, and found no statistical difference in the performance of NBI and HD-WLE. These investigators also found no statistical difference in the polyp miss rate (3 studies) or adenoma miss rate (3 studies) between the 2 modalities.

Another widefield imaging technique, autofluorescence imaging (AFI), uses 1 wavelength of light to stimulate endogenous fluorophores in the tissue, triggering the emission of fluorescent light at longer wavelengths. The emitted light can be imaged on a charge-coupled device using an emission filter to block scattered excitation light. Neoplasia is associated with changes in endogenous fluorescence; neoplastic epithelial cells are associated with increased fluorescence from mitochondrial cofactors reduced nicotinamide adenine dinucleotide phosphate and flavin adenine dinucleotide, and collagen in the stroma near neoplastic lesions shows reduced fluorescence.[18] Like NBI, AFI does not require the application of a contrast agent. Although studies have shown that AFI results in an increase in sensitivity for detection of early neoplasia in BE compared with WLE, it has also shown high false-positive rates.[19–23] False-positive rates as high as 40% have been reported using AFI for detection of early neoplasia in BE.[19] The high false-positive rate of AFI is attributed to inflammation, which is also associated with loss of autofluorescence.[20,21] Studies have indicated that when NBI is used in combination with AFI, the false-positive rate can be reduced, but in these studies NBI has misidentified HGD as normal.[19,22]

A recent study by Curvers and colleagues[23] compared the performance of the endoscopic trimodal imaging (ETMI) system (Olympus GIFQ260FZ, available in Europe and Asia) with standard WLE. The ETMI system can perform HD-WLE, AFI, and NBI. The study compared the detection rate of early neoplasia in BE for each modality in 99 patients with low-grade intraepithelial neoplasia. All of the patients underwent 2 consecutive procedures with the ETMI (consisting of HD-WLE followed by AFI and NBI) and standard WLE in random order, each performed by 2 separate endoscopists with no particular expertise in BE or advanced imaging techniques. The endoscopist performing the second procedure was blinded to the results of the first procedure. Targeted biopsies were first taken from areas identified as suspicious, and the imaging modality that detected each suspicious area was noted. Four-quadrant random biopsies every 2 cm were then taken. In **Fig. 1**A–C, images from a patient with no lesions are shown for HD-WLE, AFI, and WLE, respectively. In **Fig. 1**D and E, an early carcinoma is observed with HD-WLE and WLE, respectively. An additional lesion is visible via AFI, indicated by the yellow arrow in **Fig. 1**G, which was not visible in the HD-WLE image of **Fig. 1**F. The NBI image of **Fig. 1**H shows suspicious abnormal blood vessels in the area of the lesion. This study found no significant difference in the overall (targeted + random) detection of dysplasia by ETMI versus standard WLE. There was no significant difference in the targeted detection of dysplastic lesions (low-grade intraepithelial neoplasia, high-grade intraepithelial neoplasia, or carcinoma), with HD-WLE detecting dysplasia in 23 patients compared with 21 patients with standard WLE. However, the addition of AFI led to the detection of an additional 22 dysplastic lesions in 14 patients, increasing the number of detected patients from 21 to 35. NBI was associated with a decrease in the false-positive rate, but was also associated with a reduction in sensitivity. Of the 24 patients with

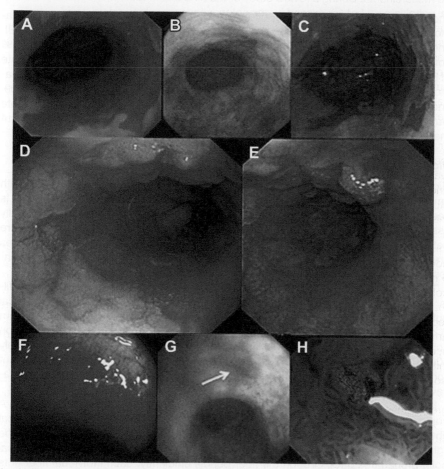

Fig. 1. (*Top row*) Widefield images acquired from endoscopically normal esophagus with (*A*) HD-WLE, (*B*) AFI, and (*C*) standard WLE. (*Middle row*) Widefield images acquired from an early carcinoma with (*D*) HD-WLE and (*E*) WLE; the carcinoma is located at the 12 o'clock position. (*Bottom row*) (*F, G*) An AFI-positive lesion (*arrow*) containing high-grade intraepithelial neoplasia, which was not seen during HD-WLE. (*H*) NBI showed irregular mucosal and vascular patterns and abnormal blood vessels suspicious for dysplasia. (*From* Curvers W, van Vilsteren FG, Baak LC, et al. Endoscopic trimodal imaging versus standard video endoscopy for detection of early Barrett's neoplasia: a multicenter randomized, crossover study in general practice. Gastrointest Endosc 2011;73:201; with permission.)

high-grade intraepithelial neoplasia or carcinoma, random biopsies led to detection in only 6 patients evaluated with ETMI and 7 patients evaluated with standard WLE.

Other widefield imaging techniques have exploited contrast agents to enhance the visibility of neoplastic changes. Chromoendoscopy involves the use of stains, such as Lugol's iodine, to differentiate the areas of stratified squamous epithelium from areas of metaplasia associated with BE.[12] Ishimura and colleagues[24] investigated the use of NBI and chromoendoscopy to assist in the detection of squamous islands for the diagnosis of short-segment BE, which is characterized by segments of metaplasia that are less than 2 to 3 cm in length. The number of identifiable squamous islands was documented first with HD-WLE, followed by NBI, and finally with chromoendoscopy, as shown in **Fig. 2**A–C, respectively. Of the 100 patients evaluated in the study, squamous islands were visible in 48 of the patients using HD-WLE, 71 patients with NBI, and 75 patients with chromoendoscopy. NBI showed a detection rate of 94.7% compared with chromoendoscopy. By contrast, HD-WLE showed a detection rate of 64% when compared with chromoendoscopy. The mean number of detected squamous islands for HD-WLE, NBI, and chromoendoscopy was 0.55 ± 0.06, 1.02 ± 0.09, and 1.76 ± 0.18, respectively. Although chromoendoscopy remains the most accurate way of visibly identifying squamous islands, NBI yielded comparable results without the risk of side effects from the use of Lugol's iodine.

High-Resolution Imaging

High-resolution imaging modalities can achieve subcellular resolution, albeit with small fields of view. This approach, which can provide an image similar to what is seen in histology, is often termed optical biopsy. High-resolution imaging is especially useful for targeting biopsies by providing a live image of the cellular architecture before the biopsy is taken.[25–28] Several different high-resolution imaging modalities are used in vivo; these include confocal laser endomicroscopy (CLE)[24–27] and high-resolution microendoscopy (HRME).[29,30]

The main advantage of CLE over conventional microscopy is the use of a spatial filter to reject out-of-focus light, capturing preferentially from tissue located at the focal point of the imaging system. Because only the light from the focal plane of the system is captured, images can also be acquired at different depths. The typical resolution achievable with CLE is on the order of 1 to 2 μm, with a field of view of approximately 500 to 700 μm². CLE can be used either to image reflected light or to image fluorescent light, typically with exogenous fluorescent contrast agents, such as fluorescein, acraflavine, and proflavine.[24–26,31–33]

In practice, several variations of CLE are used to acquire high-resolution images. A commonly used type of CLE is probe-based CLE (pCLE). pCLE uses a coherent optical fiber bundle composed of more than 10,000 optical fibers as the conduit between the light source and the tissue. Because only the remitted light originating from the focal point propagates back through the fiber bundle efficiently, each individual fiber acts as a spatial filter to reject the out-of-focus light, providing optical sectioning. By scanning the excitation light across the entire bundle, a high-resolution image can be formed. Commercial systems from companies such as Mauna Kea Technologies (Cell-Vizio) and Pentax are available and have been used in several studies.[25–27,32,34] **Fig. 3** shows representative fluorescence images of 4 distinct sites of normal squamous

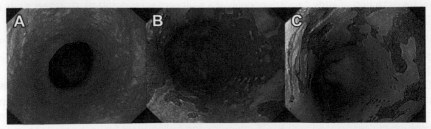

Fig. 2. Endoscopic identification of the squamous islands in short-segment BE with 3 different modalities: WLE (*A*), NBI endoscopy (*B*), and iodine chromoendoscopy (*C*). (*From* Ishimura N, Amano Y, Uno G, et al. Endoscopic characteristics of short-segment Barrett's esophagus, focusing on squamous islands and mucosal folds. J Gastroenterol Hepatol 2012;27:83; with permission.)

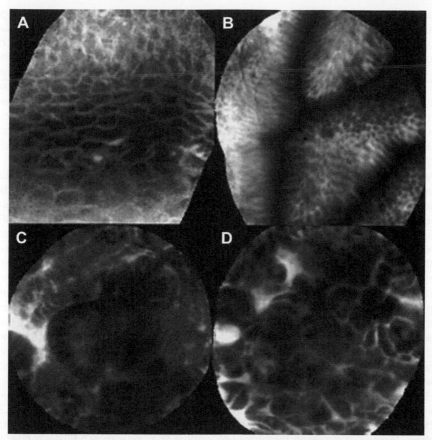

Fig. 3. pCLE imaging of normal squamous epithelium in the esophagus (*A*), BE without dysplasia (*B*), HGD (*C*), and carcinoma (*D*). (*From* Shahid MW, Wallace MB. Endoscopic imaging for the detection of esophageal dysplasia and carcinoma. Gastrointest Endosc Clin N Am 2010;20:17; with permission.)

epithelium in the esophagus, BE, HGD, and squamous cell carcinoma.[33] Fluorescein was the contrast agent used to acquire these images. The variations in tissue architecture between the different sites can be clearly visualized.

Several studies have compared the performance of confocal microendoscopy with HD-WLE examination and NBI in the esophagus and colon. Sharma and colleagues[26] assessed the sensitivity and specificity of pCLE in conjunction with HD-WLE compared with HD-WLE alone in a prospective, randomized, multicenter trial including 101 patients with BE. Images were acquired in fluorescence mode, with fluorescein (2.5 mL, 10%) as the contrast agent. After each site was imaged with pCLE, a biopsy was taken at the same location for histopathologic assessment. The sensitivity and specificity were reported to be 34.2% and 92.7%, respectively, for HD-WLE alone and 68.3% and 87.8% for HD-WLE with pCLE. Of the 120 sites diagnosed with HGD or early carcinoma, HD-WLE alone missed 79 sites, whereas the addition of pCLE reduced the number of missed sites to 38.

Wang and colleagues[32] also used pCLE to image the colon in vivo in a study of 54 patients. Fluorescence images were acquired after the administration of fluorescein.

After imaging, a pinch biopsy was also acquired at each site for histopathology. Image analysis was performed in this study to distinguish between normal mucosa, hyperplasia, tubular adenoma, and villous adenoma. Analysis of each image consisted of calculating the fluorescence contrast ratio, which was defined as the ratio of the mean intensity of the lamina propria to the mean intensity of a crypt in a selected region of interest. Using the fluorescence contrast ratio, the study documented a sensitivity and specificity of 91% and 87%, respectively, when distinguishing between normal and lesional mucosa (including hyperplasia and adenomatous lesions). In addition, high sensitivities and specificities were found when distinguishing hyperplasia from adenoma (97% and 96%) and tubular adenoma from villous adenoma (100% and 92%).

Another use for high-resolution imaging is detecting neoplasia after therapy. Endoscopic mucosal resection (EMR) is generally considered appropriate for flat neoplastic lesions smaller than 1.5 cm that can be easily accessed by the endoscope.[35] High-resolution imaging techniques can be useful in determining the perimeters for EMR, ensuring that all neoplastic areas have been removed. Shahid and colleagues[25] evaluated the diagnostic accuracy of pCLE in detecting residual colorectal neoplasia after EMR in a prospective blind study of 92 patients. The goal was to compare pCLE with chromoendoscopy techniques such as NBI and to assess the diagnostic accuracy of the 2 modalities used together. Fluorescein was used as a contrast agent when performing pCLE. In the study, 92 patients had EMRs performed on a total of 129 sites. The EMR scars were imaged at all 129 sites. Histology determined that 29 sites had residual neoplasia. NBI was able to identify the residual neoplasias with a sensitivity and specificity of 72% and 78%, respectively, whereas pCLE was reported to have sensitivity and specificity of 97% and 77%. When the 2 modalities were combined, a sensitivity and specificity of 100% and 87% was reported.

HRME is another fiber bundle–based confocal technology that offers a portable, low-cost alternative to traditional confocal microendoscopy.[29,30] Similar to pCLE, HRME acquires images by placing the fiber bundle in direct contact with the tissue surface. Instead of scanning through each optical fiber as with pCLE, each fiber in the bundle acts as an individual pixel, which collectively form a high-resolution image that is comparable with other confocal microendoscopy techniques. HRME has been evaluated for use in a few studies for the GI tract.[29,30] In addition, it has been evaluated in a preliminary study in northern China. In this study, the performance of HRME was compared with the performance of chromoendoscopy using Lugol's iodine. Preliminary results have shown that even novice users can be trained to differentiate between normal, dysplastic, and neoplastic tissues with the HRME (Video 1).

PRECLINICAL DEVELOPMENT

In the preclinical setting, many groups are working to develop new contrast agents, including both vital dyes and molecular-targeted agents, to enhance widefield and high-resolution imaging. Also, as imaging techniques have matured, there has been an increased focus on the coregistration of widefield molecular imaging and high-resolution imaging. Some recent developments are highlighted in the following sections.

Widefield Imaging

Although proflavine, a vital dye, has been primarily used clinically as a contrast agent to assist in high-resolution imaging studies, Thekkek and colleagues[21] recently reported on proflavine for use in widefield fluorescence imaging. Proflavine was applied to resected specimens from patients who underwent an EMR, esophagectomy, or colectomy. The contrast agent enhanced visualization of glandular structure in wide-field fluorescence images, including glandular distortion and effacement in Barrett-associated neoplasia, as well as irregularly spaced colonic crypts associated with colonic dysplasia during fluorescence imaging.

Bird-Lieberman and colleagues[36] studied the use of lectins as a molecular-targeted agent to identify progression of BE to carcinoma ex vivo. They examined gene expression profiling data from samples at various stages of progression and determined that upregulation of cell-surface glycan degradation pathways corresponded with progression from BE to EAC. Accordingly, lectins such as wheat germ agglutinin (WGA), helix pomatia agglutinin, and *Aspergillus oryzae* lectin (AOL) all showed reductions in binding to the human esophagus during EAC progression. Histochemical analysis subsequently showed that WGA and AOL had the most significant reduction in binding with progression of BE to EAC. WGA was chosen for further study as a molecular probe because of its common presence in human diets. WGA labeled with fluorescein was applied to resected esophagi ex vivo and imaged using widefield techniques. Both white light imaging and AFI performed without the WGA-fluorescein contrast agent identified no abnormalities. However, after the application of WGA, areas of reduced fluorescence were observed, correlating to areas of reduced WGA binding and dysplasia, as shown in **Fig. 4**. The WGA contrast agent identified areas of dysplasia that would otherwise have been missed with normal WLE and AFI.

In an in vivo *CPC;Apc* mouse model study, Miller and colleagues[37] developed a fiber-optic multispectral scanning endoscope designed to image multiple molecular targets simultaneously for use in early diagnosis of colorectal cancer. These investigators identified 3 peptides (KCCFPAQ, AKPGYLS, LTTHYKL) that showed specific binding to colorectal adenomas and labeled them using fluorescence labels with minimal spectral overlap. Images acquired with the multispectral endoscope could be used to differentiate the emission spectra of 2 of these labels successfully, enabling simultaneous imaging of 2 molecular probes in vivo. Spatially distinguishable binding patterns were apparent during imaging, suggesting different binding targets for the peptides in dysplastic tissue. However, further study into distinguishable dyes for molecular agents and algorithms to account for variations in tissue morphology and orientation are needed.

High-Resolution Imaging: Increasing Accuracy

One of the key limitations of high-resolution imaging is the limited field of view. Consequently, high-resolution techniques sample only a small fraction of the mucosal surface at risk, presenting challenges especially in heterogeneous regions of tissue. Two techniques have been evaluated to overcome this limitation. One option is to couple the use of high-resolution imaging with a widefield imaging system, using the widefield system first to identify areas of suspicion, which can then be characterized by a high-resolution system. Another technique recently developed is video mosaicing, in which consecutive video frames acquired with a high-resolution system are stitched together as the probe is advanced along the tissue. This technique can be especially useful for visualizing the extent of a lesion and giving a broader sense of the overall tissue morphology. Video mosaicing can allow a clinician to acquire high-resolution images from areas approximately 2 to 30× larger than 1 single field of view.[38,39] Although video mosaicing is a promising approach, current publications have only reported its use in postprocessing.

There has also been a focus on developing targeted contrast agents to be used with high-resolution imaging. Goetz and colleagues[31] used fluorescently labeled epidermal

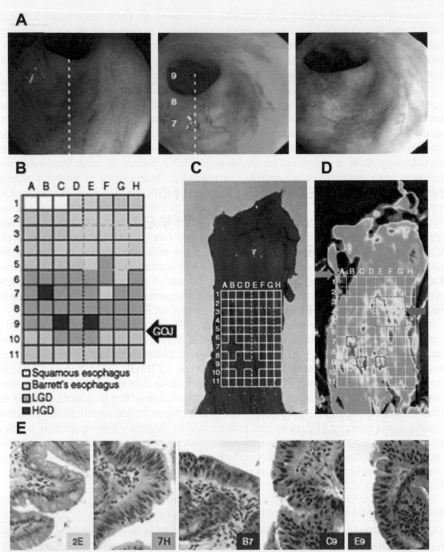

Fig. 4. Whole-organ imaging ex vivo. (*A*) White light (*left*) fluorescence at 490 to 560 nm before the application of WGA (*middle*), fluorescence at 490 to 560 nm after application of WGA and Alexa Fluor 488 (*right*). Areas of low WGA binding appear in purple and high binding in green. The dashed white line is to facilitate orientation between images. (*B*) Grid showing pathologic map of the resected specimen. The black dashed line in (*B*) represents the longitudinal axis shown in (*A*). (*C*) The same specimen opened longitudinally with grid overlay from (*B*). (*D*) Esophagus specimen imaged using an IVIS 200 camera, which quantified fluorescence by color-coded map. The pink arrow marks an area of artifact from the exposed submucosal tissue, and the blue arrow indicates the site of a previous EMR (*outlined with a dashed gray box*). (*E*) Histology from various grid locations. (*From* Bird-Lieberman EL, Neves AA, Lao-Sirieix P, et al. Molecular imaging using fluorescent lectins permits rapid endoscopic identification of dysplasia in Barrett's esophagus. Nat Med 2012;18:319; with permission.)

growth factor receptor (EGFR) antibodies as a contrast agent for detection of colorectal cancer. CLE images were acquired from mice in vivo (n = 68) in addition to ex vivo specimens of human colorectal mucosa. Tumors in the mice were established using human colorectal cancer cell lines with high (SW480) or low (SW620) expression of EGFR. In the rodent model, the confocal probe was scanned across the surface of the tumor to acquire fluorescence images. The tumors were also processed for histology and immunohistochemistry. Images acquired from the mice in vivo were graded on a 0 to 3+ scale by 2 independent investigators according to fluorescence intensity of each image. Mice with a tumor containing the SW480 line were found to have significantly higher mean fluorescence intensity (1.92 ± 0.22) than mice with SW620 tumors (0.59 ± 0.21). The resected, ex vivo human colorectal mucosa specimens were incubated with antibody solution and also imaged. There was a statistically significant difference in the mean fluorescence intensity for neoplasia (2.13 ± 0.30) and normal mucosa (0.25 ± 0.16).

In an in vivo human trial, Hsiung and colleagues[40] showed the use of a specific contrast agent that targets colonic dysplasia with pCLE. The contrast agent used was a fluorescently labeled heptapeptide sequence, which was determined to specifically bind to areas of colonic dysplasia. In this study, polyps were first endoscopically identified. After identification, the peptide was applied and then imaged with pCLE. A neighboring, normal region of mucosa was also imaged. Polyps imaged with pCLE were then biopsied and processed for histology. Characteristic fluorescence images of the colon are displayed in **Fig. 5**. As can be seen, the contrast agent primarily binds

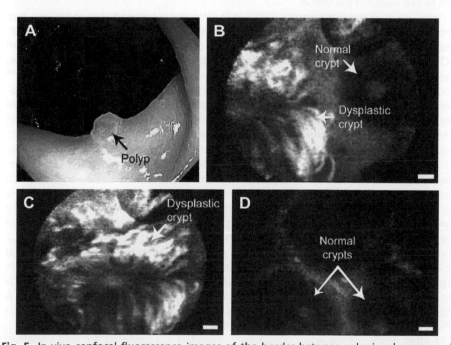

Fig. 5. In vivo confocal fluorescence images of the border between colonic adenoma and normal mucosa, showing peptide binding to dysplastic epithelial cells. The endoscopic view (A), border (B), dysplastic crypt (C), and adjacent mucosa (D) are shown with scale bars of 20 μm. (*From* Hsiung PL, Hardy J, Friedland S, et al. Detection of colonic dysplasia *in vivo* using a targeted heptapeptide and confocal microendoscopy. Nat Med 2008;14:456; with permission.)

to the dysplastic crypts, whereas the normal crypts are unlabeled. A total of 18 polyps were imaged, with 5 representative images selected for each polyp. Analysis of the acquired images consisted of comparison of the mean fluorescence intensity between normal mucosa and the adenoma in three 25-μm × 25-μm regions of interest for each image acquired, yielding a total of 270 different regions of interest. This process resulted in a sensitivity and specificity of 81% and 82%, respectively, when comparing the mean fluorescence intensity between normal tissue and adenomas.

Interferometric Techniques

Various interferometric techniques have been developed to yield morphologic information about the tissue. The light scattered from tissue can be interfered with a reference beam, providing information about the structure of the tissue. Illumination with a source characterized by a low coherence length, a technique known as time domain low coherence interferometry (LCI), can be used to selectively process light scattered from varying depths in the tissue by changing the distance traveled by the reference arm.[41,42] By sweeping the wavelength of the light source, rather than modifying the distance traveled by the reference beam, frequency domain LCI shows further improvements in signal-to-noise ratio and a decrease in data acquisition time.[41,43,44] Furthermore, the angle at which the light is incident on the tissue can be varied using a technique called angle-resolved LCI, yielding information about the angular intensity distribution of the scattered light as a function of depth.[45–47] The detected light can then be processed to yield information about the mean size and relative refractive index of cell nuclei in the tissue.

Optical coherence tomography (OCT) is an imaging interferometric technique that obtains multiple LCI scans, yielding three-dimensional images with micrometer resolution, which provide detailed morphologic information about the tissue. Although OCT has become a clinical resource in ophthalmology, endoscopic OCT has been shown in vivo in the GI tract to provide high-resolution images of the esophagus.[48] Recent work has investigated combining the biochemical information gained from molecular imaging with the high-resolution images obtained from interferometric techniques like OCT. Yuan and colleagues[49] combined fluorescence molecular imaging (FMI) with OCT using a dichroic to simultaneously illuminate the tissue with a different wavelength for each modality. Excised small and large bowels (N = 4) of male C57BL/6J *ApcMin/+* mice were imaged, and fluorescence was obtained using *Ulex europaeus* agglutinin I (UEA-1) conjugated contrast agent, which has been shown to bind to the surfaces of adenomatous polyps as a result of the overexpression of the carbohydrate α-L-fucose on the surface of the polyps. Backscattered and fluorescent light were captured, allowing the scattering coefficient and fluorescence intensity of the tissue to be measured simultaneously. In **Fig. 6**A, an OCT image in which the tissue surface height is color coded reveals 4 hot spots, indicating the presence of 4 raised polyps. Cross-sectional OCT images and histology for the lines in **Fig. 6**A are shown in **Fig. 6**B–I, respectively. The raised polyps are easily distinguished from the surrounding tissue. The tissue scattering coefficient and fluorescence image are shown in **Fig. 6**J, K, and are fused in **Fig. 6**L, showing that the polyps have higher scattering coefficients and fluorescence intensities than the surrounding tissue.

In other work, Iftimia and colleagues[50] reported coregistered ex vivo widefield fluorescence imaging and OCT using colon tissue from *ApcMin* mice. Fluorescence imaging was achieved using poly(epsilon-caprolactone) microparticles labeled with a near-infrared dye and functionalized with an RGD (argenine-glycine-aspartic acid) peptide to recognize the overexpression of αvβ3-integrin receptor. Winkler and colleagues[51] combined OCT and fluorescence microscopy in vivo via endoscope using

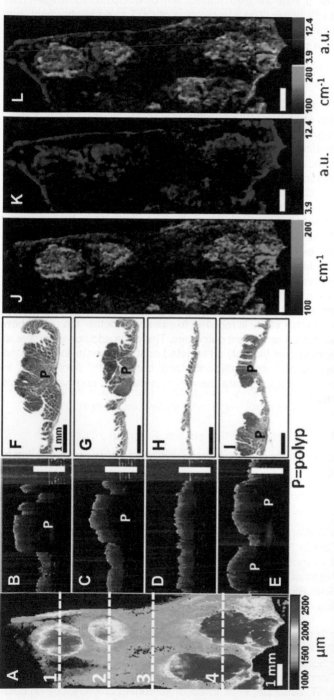

Fig. 6. Coregistered OCT/FMI imaging of intestinal polyps incubated with UEA-1 conjugated liposomes ex vivo. (*A*) OCT en face surface image. Tissue surface height is color coded (ranging from 1 to 2.5 mm). Four polyps (P) are clearly visible as elevated tissue surface height. (*B–I*) Cross-sectional OCT images corresponding to the horizontal lines 1–4 in (*A*). Polyps (P) are visible as protruded masses in (*B*), (*D*), and (*H*). Normal mucosa is shown in (*F*). The scale bars in (*B–H*) are physical distance, and a refractive index of 1.4 for tissue was used for calculating the physical distance. Corresponding histology (*C, E, G, I*) confirms the OCT images. (*J*) Tissue scattering coefficient (μ_s) image ranges from 100/cm to 200/cm. Polyps show higher extinction coefficients. (*K*) Fluorescence image using the UEA-1-conjugated contrast agents. Fluorescence intensities are higher around polyp areas than the surrounding mucosa. (*L*) Fused scattering coefficient and fluorescence image with a scale bar of 1 mm. (*From* Yuan S, Roney CA, Wierwille J, et al. Combining optical coherence tomography with fluorescence molecular imaging: toward simultaneous morphology and molecular imaging. Phys Med Biol 2010;55:191–206; with permission.)

the azoxymethane-treated mouse model of colon cancer. Fluorescence was achieved using the conjugation of a near-infrared fluorescent dye, Cy5.5, to single-chain vascular endothelial growth factor. The combination of OCT and spectroscopy has also been investigated by Robles and colleagues,[52] who showed the combination of both techniques using a source in the visible domain.

SUMMARY

The need to improve the detection and classification of early-stage neoplasia in the esophagus and colon has led to the development of a variety of widefield and high-resolution optical imaging techniques. Although some widefield techniques, such as AFI and NBI, do not require the application of contrast agents, these techniques and others could be enhanced by the use of contrast agents that specifically highlight biochemical changes associated with neoplasia. Widefield fluorescence and high-resolution imaging such as CLE and OCT can combine molecular and morphologic imaging to yield information about the structure and nature of the tissue. Of specific note are the recent advancements in targeted contrast agents, which have been used to highlight areas of dysplasia.

Although optical molecular imaging is promising, several challenges must be overcome before it can be implemented on a large scale. First, larger-scale, multicentral studies are required with appropriate histologic end points to properly assess the diagnostic potential of each modality. In cases in which commercial instruments are not yet available, additional effort is required to ensure standardization of imaging platforms. In the longer term, further study is required to examine whether the use of new modalities has a positive impact on patient outcomes. There are additional barriers to the implementation of approaches that rely on targeted contrast agents, including the identification of biomarkers that are sufficiently and consistently upregulated in neoplasia, the development of appropriate delivery formulations, and navigation of complex regulatory barriers.

SUPPLEMENTARY DATA

Supplementary data related to this article can be found online at http://dx.doi.org/10.1016/j.giec.2013.03.010.

REFERENCES

1. American Cancer Society. Global cancer facts & figures. 2nd edition. Atlanta (GA): American Cancer Society; 2008.
2. Ries L, Melbert D, Krapcho M, et al. SEER cancer statistics review, 1975–2004. Bethesda (MD): National Cancer Institute; 2007.
3. Wang KK, Sampliner RE. Updated guidelines 2008 for the diagnosis, surveillance, and therapy of Barrett's esophagus. Am J Gastroenterol 2008;103:788–97.
4. American Cancer Society. Cancer facts & figures 2012. Atlanta (GA): American Cancer Society; 2012.
5. American Cancer Society. Colorectal cancer facts & figures 2011-2013. Atlanta (GA): American Cancer Society; 2008.
6. Kahi CJ, Imperiale TF, Juliar BE, et al. Effect of screening colonoscopy on colorectal cancer incidence and mortality. Clin Gastroenterol Hepatol 2009;7:770–5.
7. Enzinger PC, Mayer RJ. Esophageal cancer. N Engl J Med 2003;349:2241–52.

8. Vieth M, Ell C, Gossner L, et al. Histological analysis of endoscopic resection specimens from 326 patients with Barrett's esophagus and early neoplasia. Endoscopy 2004;36:776–81.

9. Sharma P, McQuaid K, Dent J, et al. A critical review of the diagnosis and management of Barrett's esophagus: The AGA Chicago Workshop. Gastroenterology 2004;127:310–30.

10. Reid BJ, Petras R, Gramlich TL, et al. The diagnosis of low-grade dysplasia in Barrett's esophagus and its implications for disease progression. Am J Gastroenterol 2000;95:3383–7.

11. Goetz M, Kiesslich R. Advanced imaging of the gastrointestinal tract: research vs. clinical tools? Curr Opin Gastroenterol 2009;25:412–21.

12. Singh R, Mei SC, Sethi S. Advanced endoscopic imaging in Barrett's oesophagus: a review on current practice. World J Gastroenterol 2011;17:4271–6.

13. Singh R, Karageorgiou H, Owen V, et al. Comparison of high-resolution magnification narrow-band imaging and white-light endoscopy in the prediction of histology in Barrett's oesophagus. Scand J Gastroenterol 2009;44:85–92.

14. Muto M, Minashi K, Yano T, et al. Early detection of superficial squamous cell carcinoma in the head and neck region and esophagus by narrow band imaging: a multicenter randomized controlled trial. J Clin Oncol 2010;28: 1566–72.

15. Jayasekera C, Taylor AC, Desmond PV, et al. Added value of narrow band imaging and confocal laser endomicroscopy in detecting Barrett's esophagus neoplasia. Endoscopy 2012;44:1089–95.

16. Sharma P, Hawes RH, Bansal A, et al. Standard endoscopy with random biopsies versus narrow band imaging targeted biopsies in Barrett's oesophagus: a prospective, international, randomized controlled trial. Gut 2011;62:15–21.

17. Pasha SF, Leighton JA, Das A, et al. Comparison of the yield and miss rate of narrow band imaging and white light endoscopy in patients undergoing screening or surveillance colonoscopy: a meta-analysis. Am J Gastroenterol 2012;107:363–70.

18. Monici M. Cell and tissue autofluorescence research and diagnostic applications. Biotechnol Annu Rev 2005;11:227–56.

19. Kara MA, Peters FP, Fockens P, et al. Endoscopic video-autofluorescence imaging followed by narrow band imaging for detecting early neoplasia in Barrett's esophagus. Gastrointest Endosc 2006;64:176–85.

20. Kara MA, Peters FP, Ten Kate FJ, et al. Endoscopic video autofluorescence imaging may improve the detection of early neoplasia in patients with Barrett's esophagus. Gastrointest Endosc 2005;61:679–85.

21. Thekkek N, Anandasabapathy S, Richards-Kortum R. Optical molecular imaging for detection of Barrett's-associated neoplasia. World J Gastroenterol 2011;17: 53–62.

22. Curvers WL, Singh R, Song LM, et al. Endoscopic tri-modal imaging for detection of early neoplasia in Barrett's oesophagus: a multi-centre feasibility study using high-resolution endoscopy, autofluorescence imaging and narrow band imaging incorporated in one endoscopy system. Gut 2008;57:167–72.

23. Curvers W, van Vilsteren FG, Baak LC, et al. Endoscopic trimodal imaging versus standard video endoscopy for detection of early Barrett's neoplasia: a multicenter randomized, crossover study in general practice. Gastrointest Endosc 2011;73:195–203.

24. Ishimura N, Amano Y, Uno G, et al. Endoscopic characteristics of short-segment Barrett's esophagus, focusing on squamous islands and mucosal folds. J Gastroenterol Hepatol 2012;27:82–7.

25. Shahid MW, Buchner AM, Coron E, et al. Diagnostic accuracy of probe-based confocal laser endomicroscopy in detecting residual colorectal neoplasia after EMR: a prospective study. Gastrointest Endosc 2012;75:525–33.

26. Sharma P, Meining AR, Coron E, et al. Real-time increased detection of neoplastic tissue in Barrett's esophagus with probe-based confocal laser endomicroscopy: final results of an international multicenter, prospective, randomized, controlled trial. Gastrointest Endosc 2011;74:465–72.

27. Wallace MB, Sharma P, Lightdale C, et al. Preliminary accuracy and interobserver agreement for the detection of intraepithelial neoplasia in Barrett's esophagus with probe-based confocal laser endomicroscopy. Gastrointest Endosc 2010;72:19–24.

28. Dunbar KB, Okolo P 3rd, Montgomery E, et al. Confocal laser endomicroscopy in Barrett's esophagus and endoscopically inapparent Barrett's neoplasia: a prospective, randomized, double-blind, controlled, crossover trial. Gastrointest Endosc 2009;70:645–54.

29. Muldoon TJ, Anandasabapathy S, Maru D, et al. High-resolution imaging in Barrett's esophagus: a novel, low-cost endoscopic microscope. Gastrointest Endosc 2008;68:737–44.

30. Muldoon TJ, Pierce MC, Nida DL, et al. Subcellular-resolution molecular imaging within living tissue by fiber microendoscopy. Opt Express 2007;15:16413–23.

31. Goetz M, Ziebart A, Foersch S, et al. In vivo molecular imaging of colorectal cancer with confocal endomicroscopy by targeting epidermal growth factor receptor. Gastroenterology 2010;138:435–46.

32. Wang T, Friedland S, Sahbaie P, et al. Functional imaging of colonic mucosa with a fibered confocal microscope for real-time in vivo pathology. Clin Gastroenterol Hepatol 2007;5:1300–5.

33. Shahid MW, Wallace MB. Endoscopic imaging for the detection of esophageal dysplasia and carcinoma. Gastrointest Endosc Clin N Am 2010;20:11–24.

34. Gaddam S, Mathur SC, Singh M, et al. Novel probe-based confocal laser endomicroscopy criteria and interobserver agreement for the detection of dysplasia in Barrett's esophagus. Am J Gastroenterol 2011;106:1961–9.

35. Wang KK, Prasad G, Tian J. Endoscopic mucosal resection and endoscopic submucosal dissection in esophageal and gastric cancers. Curr Opin Gastroenterol 2010;26:453–8.

36. Bird-Lieberman EL, Neves AA, Lao-Sirieix P, et al. Molecular imaging using fluorescent lectins permits rapid endoscopic identification of dysplasia in Barrett's esophagus. Nat Med 2012;18:315–21.

37. Miller SJ, Lee CM, Joshi BP, et al. Targeted detection of murine colonic dysplasia in vivo with flexible multispectral scanning fiber endoscopy. J Biomed Opt 2012;17:021103.

38. Bedard N, Quang T, Schmeler K, et al. Real-time video mosaicing with a high-resolution microendoscope. Biomed Opt Express 2012;3:2428–35.

39. Behrens A, Bommes M, Stehle T, et al. Real-time image composition of bladder mosaics in fluorescence endoscopy. Comput Sci Res Dev 2011;26:51–64.

40. Hsiung PL, Hardy J, Friedland S, et al. Detection of colonic dysplasia in vivo using a targeted heptapeptide and confocal microendoscopy. Nat Med 2008;14:454–8.

41. Drexler W, Fujimoto J. Optical coherence tomography: technology and applications. New York: Springer; 2008.

42. Yang CH, Perelman LT, Wax A, et al. Feasibility of field-based light scattering spectroscopy. J Biomed Opt 2000;5:138.

43. Wax A, Yang C, Izatt JA. Fourier-domain low-coherence interferometry for light-scattering spectroscopy. Opt Lett 2003;28:1230–2.
44. Graf RN, Wax A. Nuclear morphology measurements using Fourier domain low coherence interferometry. Opt Express 2005;13:4693–8.
45. Terry NG, Zhu Y, Rinehart MT, et al. Detection of dysplasia in Barrett's esophagus with *in vivo* depth resolved nuclear morphology measurements. Gastroenterology 2011;140:42–50.
46. Zhu Y, Terry NG, Wax A. Development of angle resolved low coherence interferometry for clinical detection of dysplasia. J Carcinog 2011;10:1–9.
47. Brown WJ, Pyhtila JW, Terry NG, et al. Review and recent development of angle-resolved low-coherence interferometry for detection of precancerous cells in human esophageal epithelium. IEEE J Sel Top Quantum Electron 2008;14:88–97.
48. Zhou C, Tsai TH, Lee HC, et al. Characterization of buried glands before and after radiofrequency ablation by using 3-dimensional optical coherence tomography. Gastrointest Endosc 2012;76:32–40.
49. Yuan S, Roney CA, Wierwille J, et al. Combining optical coherence tomography with fluorescence molecular imaging: towards simultaneous morphology and molecular imaging. Phys Med Biol 2010;55:191–206.
50. Iftimia N, Iyer AK, Hammer DX, et al. Fluorescence-guided optical coherence tomography imaging for colon cancer screening: a preliminary mouse study. Biomed Opt Express 2012;3:178–91.
51. Winkler AM, Rice PF, Weichsel J, et al. *In vivo*, dual-modality OCT/LIF imaging using a novel VEGF receptor-targeted NIR fluorescent probe in the AOM-treated mouse model. Mol Imaging Biol 2011;13:1173–82.
52. Robles FE, Wilson C, Grant G, et al. Molecular imaging true-colour spectroscopic optical coherence tomography. Nat Photonics 2011;5:744–7.

Index

Note: Page numbers of article titles are in **boldface** type.

http://dx.doi.org/10.1016/S1052-5157(13)00059-7
1052-5157/13/$ – see front matter © 2013 Elsevier Inc. All rights reserved.